DESIGN THAT CARES

DESIGN THAT CARES

PLANNING HEALTH FACILITIES FOR PATIENTS AND VISITORS

Third Edition

Janet R. Carpman

Myron A. Grant

with assistance from Elizabeth M. Kirchen

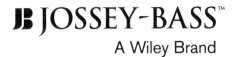

JB JOSSEY-BASS™

A Wiley Brand

Published by Jossey-Bass
A Wiley Brand
One Montgomery Street, Suite 1000, San Francisco, CA 94104–4594—www.josseybass.com

Jossey-Bass books and products are available through most bookstores. To contact Jossey-Bass directly call our Customer Care Department within the U.S. at 800-956-7739, outside the U.S. at 317-572-3986, or fax 317-572-4002.

Wiley publishes in a variety of print and electronic formats and by print-on-demand. Some material included with standard print versions of this book may not be included in e-books or in print-on-demand. If this book refers to media such as a CD or DVD that is not included in the version you purchased, you may download this material at http://booksupport.wiley.com. For more information about Wiley products, visit www.wiley.com.

Library of Congress Cataloging-in-Publication Data

Carpman, Janet Reizenstein, author.
    Design that cares : planning health facilities for patients and visitors / Janet R. Carpman, Myron A. Grant, with assistance from Elizabeth M. Kirchen. – Third edition.
        p. ; cm.
    Includes bibliographical references and index.
    ISBN 978-0-7879-8811-1 (pbk.) — 9781118221631 (pdf) — ISBN 9781118235409 (epub)
    I. Grant, Myron A., author. II. Kirchen, Elizabeth M., author. III. Title.
    [DNLM: 1. Facility Design and Construction.   2. Health Facility Planning.   3. Human Engineering. WX 140]
    RA967
    725'.51–dc23
                                2015036499

Cover design by Wiley
Cover image: © 2016 Carpman Grant Associates, Wayfinding Consultants. Photo credit: Courtesy of Saint Joseph Mercy Ann Arbor.
Photos and illustrations by Myron A. Grant. Photo on page 313 by istockphoto.com.

Printed in the United States of America

THIRD EDITION

PB Printing   10 9 8 7 6 5 4 3 2 1

CONTENTS

To the experienced eye of a careful observing nurse, the daily . . . changes which take place in patients . . . afford a still more important class of data from which to judge of the general adaptation of a hospital for the reception and treatment of the sick. One insensibly allies together restlessness, languor, feverishness, and general malaise with the closeness of wards, defective ventilation, defective structure, bad architectural and administrative arrangements, until it is impossible to resist the conviction that the sick are suffering from something quite other than the disease inscribed on their bed-ticket. . . A vast deal of the suffering, and some at least of the mortality, in these establishments is avoidable.

—Florence Nightingale, 1863[*]

---

[*] *Notes on Hospitals*, Third Edition, London: Longman, Green, Longman, Roberts, and Green, 1863, pp. 6–7. The original of this book is in the Cornell University Library (Medical Library in NYC). There are no known copyright restrictions in the United States on the use of the text. *www.archive.org/details/cu31924012356485*

For our children:

David Carpman, Rachel Carpman, and Adrienne Grant

ACKNOWLEDGMENTS

We are grateful to everyone who contributed to and assisted with the third edition of *Design That Cares: Planning Health Facilities for Patients and Visitors.*

Craig McAllister and David Hughes energetically mined the literature on health facility design and behavior.

Kimberly B. Phalen, PhD, contributed important theoretical and practical information on the benefits of exposure to nature and guidelines for outdoor environments used by patients and visitors.

Peter J. Baker, Anne Bauman, Dick Bauman, Carolyn Burnstein, Bob Collins, Pam Gibb, Diana Raimi, Donald Theyken, and Mary Ellen Weakley helped with photo shoots.

Valerie Fletcher, Christopher Hart, and Ruth Super of the Institute for Human Centered Design, and Kathy Gips of the New England ADA Center, Boston, provided detailed knowledge of design requirements for people with functional limitations and important information about related US legislation and guidelines.

Many colleagues generously forwarded copies of their own research papers. The Center for Health Design went above and beyond to send a whole boxful of useful reports.

Our thanks to the Saint Joseph Mercy Health System, which graciously provided photographic access to two of its Michigan hospital campuses: St. Joseph Mercy Ann Arbor and St. Joseph Mercy Chelsea.

Elizabeth (Betsy) Kirchen skillfully and cheerfully wrestled with the text and references, endlessly delving into a raft of issues and questions to come up with just the right wording. Her passion for the subject matter and attention to detail added immensely to the book's breadth and depth. Betsy also drafted the summaries and pedagogical questions used in each chapter.

We thank draft reviewers David Allison, Kirk Hamilton, Wayne Ruga, PhD, and James Shraiky, who provided thoughtful and constructive comments on the complete draft manuscript.

Our editors at Jossey-Bass, the late Andy Pasternack and Seth Schwartz, ably assisted by Melinda Noack, offered unflagging and sustained support throughout a lengthy writing period.

Finally, we recognize the late Jeptha Dalston, PhD, (then) CEO of the University of Michigan Medical Center, who not only encouraged us to write the first edition of *Design That Cares*, starting in 1984, but also provided financial support and his own brand of Texas-sized good cheer as we went about it. We think he'd be proud that this book continues to influence new generations of health facility decision-makers and students to carefully and caringly consider the needs of patients and visitors in health facility planning and design.

Janet R. Carpman, PhD
Myron A. Grant, MLA
March 2016

In healthcare facilities, where decisions and actions can mean the difference between life and death, where stress levels are high and decision-making time is short, where people experience some of their happiest and saddest moments, and where most individuals feel as if they have lost control over what's happening to and around them, it is critically important to create environments that support patients, families, and staff, and contribute to the quality of care.

With the publication of the first edition of *Design That Cares* some 30 years ago, Jan Carpman, PhD, and Myron Grant, MLA, set out not only to elevate the role of the physical environment and its impact on outcomes for vulnerable patient populations, but also to provide an expansive and accessible tutorial for designers, nondesign professionals, and students who are—or will be—involved in making design decisions. This long-awaited third edition is cause for celebration. It offers a compendium of new research findings, references, design guidelines, and design review questions, as well as overviews and learning objectives. By inference, it shows how our field has grown and continues to grow.

Design That Cares grew out of Carpman and Grant's groundbreaking work at the University of Michigan Medical Center in the 1980s. Their Patient & Visitor Participation Project used empirical research to understand the design-related needs of patients and visitors, with the goal of providing timely, design-relevant findings and recommendations that would help make a multimillion-dollar replacement hospital an exemplar of human-centered design. Carpman and Grant were among the pioneers in what we now know as a worldwide movement for evidence-based health facility design that maximizes patient outcomes and positive customer experience. When my organization, the Center for Health Design, held its first national symposium in 1988, Carpman and Grant were presenters.

Building and renovating health facilities are enormous, complex undertakings. It takes a strong, interdisciplinary team to discuss, imagine, study, debate, and come to consensus on myriad issues over an extended period of time. As members of a hospital planning and design team for six years, Carpman and Grant witnessed scores of medical and health professionals doing their best to understand design issues and options during such a project, but often feeling frustrated and having little influence. With no background in reading architectural plans or in understanding aspects of design—such as scale—nurses, physicians, healthcare administrators, and others often go along with or approve design schemes because of social pressure and time limitations without fully comprehending the behavioral implications. The authors framed *Design That Cares* to include evidence-based findings and guidelines, and especially design review questions, in order to make explicit what decision-makers should ask about proposed design schemes or features, and what design-behavior relationships they should advocate.

At the Center for Health Design, we are strong advocates of design solutions that use an evidence-based design process. A large and growing body of research attests to the fact that physical environments affect patient stress, patient and staff safety, staff effectiveness, and quality of care provided in healthcare settings. Basing planning and design decisions on this research to achieve the best possible outcomes is what evidence-based design is all about. *Design That Cares* contributes to the state of the art by addressing complex issues, including wayfinding, physical comfort, control over social contact, universal design, access to nature, sound and music, and many others. This book is an indispensable resource for making informed design decisions that will affect patients, visitors, and staff over the lifespan of a health facility—often fifty years or more.

I am proud to join the writers of forewords to the first and second editions of *Design That Cares*: Jepha W. Dalston, PhD, former CEO, University of Michigan Medical Center, Ann Arbor and Hermann Hospital, Houston, representing the fields of hospital administration and medical care; and Margaret Gaskie, former senior editor, *Architectural Record*, representing the field of architectural design. My own career in healthcare design is at the nexus of these fields: combining my love of interior design and architecture and my compulsion to help make the (healthcare) world a better place. As they did, I salute Jan Carpman and Myron Grant and *Design That Cares*, third edition, for offering a new generation of present and future health facility design decision-makers jargon-free, compelling, evidence-based guidelines for creating caring environments for patients and families.

Debra Levin, EDAC
President and CEO
The Center for Health Design

The first edition of *Design That Cares* grew out of a quest for information about the design-related needs of patients and visitors. In 1980, when we were hired by the University of Michigan Medical Center to act as what would now be called "customer-experience advocates" during the long, complex, expensive process of designing a huge replacement hospital, there was almost no useful information available about health facility design and its effects on patients. The design needs of family members and visitors were barely on anyone's radar. In the absence of this information and with a commitment to evidence-based decision making, we began conducting our own research. With the existing hospital and its patients as our laboratory, and the fast-moving train of design decision making as our engine, we conducted nearly three dozen distinct studies focusing on patients' and visitors' needs and preferences for health facility design features. Six years later, when the new hospital was complete and we had done our best to use our data to influence scores of design decisions, it was time to publish the information. In the meantime, we had been on the ground floor of a new field. There was finally a nascent body of health facility design literature based on empirical research.

This book was always intended to be different from the vast majority of architecture books and journals. *Design That Cares* is not a compendium of completed projects. Though such publications are useful in order to show designers and design students what has been accomplished across the United States and around the world, they tend not to emphasize the reasons why design decisions were made or how each feature was intended to function. By their visual nature, they emphasize aesthetics over function. Good design, of course, reflects aesthetics, function, and a host of additional considerations and requirements, such as corporate culture, marketing, capital costs, codes and regulations, environmental impacts, operating costs, long-term maintenance, and other requirements.

We wanted *Design That Cares* to consider design from another vantage point: emphasizing function (designing for the needs of patients and visitors) and encouraging creativity on the part of planners and designers. There are endless possibilities for how designs can look while at the same time satisfying functional criteria.

We are delighted that our hunch about the usefulness of this approach has proved to be on target for more than 30 years. As we began writing the third edition, we were gratified to see that the situation we faced in 1980, of having virtually no useful evidence-based information, is long past. There is now an active, productive, prolific community of researchers, designers, and others exploring numerous issues pertaining to patients, visitors, and health facility design. Research has expanded from an exploration of preferences to measures of a variety of physiological effects. The once-radical notion—that health facilities affect patients and visitors and should be designed with their needs in mind—is now an accepted paradigm.

However, paradigms are not enough. We offer this edition of *Design That Cares* to current and future design decision-makers with the hope that its nuanced, evidence-based guidelines will inspire the creation and long-term functioning of health facilities that care for and about their most vulnerable users.

An instructor's supplement is available at www.wiley.com/go/Carpman3e. Comments about this book are invited and can be sent to publichealth@wiley.com.

Janet R. Carpman, PhD
Myron A. Grant, MLA
March 2016

Janet R. Carpman, PhD, and **Myron A. Grant**, MLA, are consultants, designers, and design researchers who believe that environments should respond to the needs and preferences of the people who use them. In the early 1980s, they created and directed the Patient & Visitor Participation Project at the University of Michigan Medical Center, a groundbreaking, six-year-long design research and advocacy effort for a $285 million tertiary care hospital. They went on to establish Carpman Grant Associates, Wayfinding Consultants in 1986, which helps clients create places that are easy to navigate and, as a result, optimize customer experience (www .wayfinding.com). Carpman and Grant have involved thousands of users in hundreds of projects for medical centers, museums, colleges and universities, and other public facilities. In addition to writing three editions of *Design That Cares: Planning Health Facilities for Patients and Visitors*, they are also authors of the award-winning book *Directional Sense: How to Find Your Way Around*, a guide for directionally challenged people. (www .directionalsense.com).

Janet R. Carpman holds degrees from the University of Michigan (PhD, Sociology and Architecture), Harvard University (Master of City Planning) and the University of Rochester (BA, Sociology).

Myron A. Grant holds two degrees from the University of Michigan (Master of Landscape Architecture and Bachelor of Fine Arts).

DESIGN THAT CARES

In the coming decades, healthcare will continue to be an issue of major concern in the United States as it is worldwide. The uncertainties are many. The capacity of the medical professions to treat illness and injury is continually growing, as are the costs associated with such treatment. New legal mandates and constraints upon healthcare delivery are regularly brought into play. The character of society—demographics, experiences, and expectations— is, as always, in transition. Our very understanding of health itself, its sources and conditions, is expanding and evolving.

The healthcare systems of tomorrow will look different from those of the past. Those of us involved in planning and designing healthcare facilities have many issues and questions to consider. No matter how diligent and well informed we are, we cannot know with certainty the nature and rate of future change. Yet some of today's decisions must be based on projections about medicine and society in the year 2030 or 2050. The better we understand the issues involved, the better prepared we will be to meet tomorrow's healthcare demands and contribute to the development of effective, efficient, caring healthcare delivery systems, in the United States and abroad.

Projections and the Direction of Healthcare

Health is an indicator of overall quality of life. The growing popularity of exercise, proper nutrition, and stress-reducing activities shows that many people have a strong interest in health. Individuals in first-world countries,

LEARNING OBJECTIVES
- Understand how ongoing demographic and lifestyle changes in the United States affect demand for and expectations about healthcare.
- Become familiar with some ways in which economic forces and developments in medical practice are transforming the healthcare field and giving rise to an era of healthcare competition.
- Realize how the delivery of high-quality healthcare, in terms of both medical outcomes and human experience, requires attention to supportive health-facility design.
- Grasp the nature and purpose of each phase of the design process, from predesign programming to design, construction, concurrent planning, design review, activation, and post-occupancy evaluation (also known as "Facility Performance Evaluation").

including the United States, are becoming more knowledgeable about their own health and are taking more responsibility for it (Panther, 1984; Spreckelmeyer, 1984).

In addition to less quantifiable developments in social norms and issues, such as customer expectations, ideas about customer experience, gender roles, the role of family and friends in the hospitalization of a loved one, and marketing trends, we can study changes documented by demographers and the US Bureau of the Census. Changes in age distribution, fertility rates, urbanization, work status, and education, too, will all profoundly influence the future of healthcare. What our society looks like, how we live, and how long we live will determine the demands on the healthcare in the next few decades.

Perhaps the most significant demographic trend is the change in age distribution. Because we are living longer and our fertility rate is decreasing, the proportion of older citizens in the US population will continue to grow. In fact, there is a distinction between the "young old" in their sixties and the "old old" in their eighties and above. Whereas in 1930 only 5.4 percent of the US population was over 65 years old, the 2010 figure was 13 percent (Panther, 1984; US Census 2010). In 1930, the median age of the population was 26.4, but by the year 2012 that figure had risen to 37.1 (CIA, 2012; US Government, 1984).

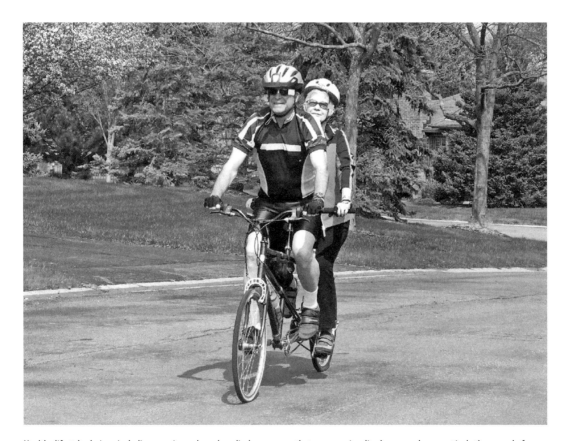

Healthy lifestyle choices, including exercise and good medical care, mean that many seniors live longer and more actively than ever before.

Our longer lifespan is due primarily to an improved standard of living and advances in healthcare. Yet, because of its unique needs, an older population will demand greater services from the healthcare system. Older people tend to have a greater number of chronic health problems, require more visits to the doctor, require a longer period of recuperation after an illness, and need more hospitalization. As a patient grows older, the types of illnesses experienced often shift. And in addition to treating particular illnesses, physicians treating geriatric patients must be concerned with the physiological, sociological, and psychological changes directly related to the aging process (Godfrey-June, 1992).

However, healthcare will have to contend with more changes than just those related to serving an older population. Choices made by couples regarding how many children to have, or whether to have them at all, are profoundly affecting healthcare. In the post–baby-boom years between 1957 and 1973, there was close to a 50 percent decrease in the fertility rate (number of births per 1,000 women of childbearing age) (US Government, 1984). Family planning decisions—to have fewer children, to delay childbirth, or to have no children at all—aided by the availability of effective contraceptives, have already affected the demand for obstetric and pediatric units.

The number of infants born each year does not tell the whole story. Partly because childbirth is now more a matter of choice for many, it is reasonable to speculate that parents-to-be will also want to make more decisions concerning the healthcare their children receive. Both parents, as well as other family members, have already become more involved in the delivery and in infant care. These shifts in birthing participation and the increased popularity of alternative birthing arrangements, such as midwives and birthing rooms, are reshaping obstetric and pediatric healthcare.

Other demographic trends—including greater numbers of women in the workforce, the continued urbanization of America, increases in the number of immigrants and ethnically diverse populations, higher levels of education, and changing occupational profiles—will also put pressure on the healthcare system. With regard to urbanization, not only is the geographic distribution of the population shifting, but residents of urban areas also tend to use physicians' services more often than do their rural counterparts. Changes in the workforce, such as higher levels of education, will also affect the healthcare establishment. As the level of education rises, basic knowledge about medical care also rises. A knowledgeable patient has particular expectations, which may alter the accepted definitions of high-quality care. Changes in these definitions—changes from the patient's and family's points of view—may also result in a public re-examination of the basic policies and practices of healthcare.

Keeping a vigilant eye on lifestyle and demographic trends seems to be a prudent strategy for healthcare decision-makers. Some of the shifts and their effects are easy to track and speculate about, but others are far from certain. Nevertheless, because society is unquestionably in transition and because its changes, the slow as well as the revolutionary, will affect healthcare, it is essential for healthcare leaders to plan for these shifts.

The previously mentioned demographic changes, uncertainties in the general economic climate, and the challenges of healthcare reform make it increasingly important for healthcare

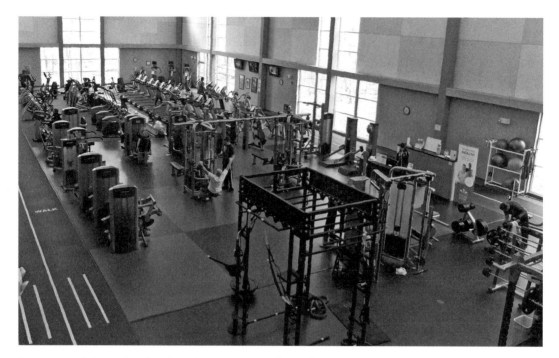

Fitness centers offering a variety of exercise options are an important feature of many health facilities.
Photo credit: Courtesy of Chelsea-Area Wellness Foundation

organizations, whether engaged in renovation or new construction, to "start smart, design smart, and build smart" (Managing Construction Costs, 2012). Since capital improvements and building costs are significant, planning for the long term is essential. Whether planning is for long-term or short-term goals, however, it must not be considered a static process. The long-term strategic plan must have enough elasticity to be altered as the need arises (Michael, 1973). Meeting the needs of consumers requires a dynamic approach to planning.

Healthcare: Changing Within

Rapid developments in science, medical practice, and medical technology, changes in population and age distribution, and the increased role of government regulation are causing a revolution in healthcare. "Old-style" healthcare, dominated by the individual physician's practice and the not-for-profit hospital, is rapidly becoming a thing of the past. Rising healthcare costs, an increasing supply of physicians, an uncertain future for Medicare and Medicaid, limited resources, and other trends have transformed the healthcare field. The age of healthcare competition is upon us (Johnson and Johnson, 1982). Birthing centers, health maintenance organizations, hospices, and big-city hospitals must vie for a piece of the hundreds of billions of dollars ($2.7 trillion in 2011) spent on medical care each year in the United States (NHE Fact Sheet, 2015).

In the competition for patients and their healthcare dollars, the nature of the healthcare facility is changing, too. Some for-profit and not-for-profit hospital chains are springing up, some hospitals are going out of business, and others are being acquired by multi-hospital organizations. Specialty facilities such as substance abuse treatment centers, diagnostic clinics, outpatient surgery centers, sports medicine centers, and freestanding urgent care centers are providing services previously offered only at large hospitals. These changes have thrust healthcare into the world of big business. With intense competition for a market share that will sustain them, healthcare organizations are actively promoting themselves, and the patient is now the marketing target (Block, 1981). For-profit hospitals are introducing such amenities as restaurant-style menus and hotel-like furnishings. Freestanding urgent care clinics are advertising their fast service ("In and out within 30 minutes"), while some hospital emergency rooms post current "wait times" for their ERs online or offer estimates via text message (Detroit Medical Center, 2013; Rice, 2013). To remain solvent and to keep patients coming back, healthcare organizations are nurturing their "high-quality care" images in the media and in the minds of the public.

Design as a Component of High-Quality Healthcare

Designing a healthcare facility is a complex process that must satisfy myriad competing criteria. The design must satisfy the demands of medical technology; that is, spaces must be flexible enough to accommodate complex, newly invented or redesigned equipment. Many facilities must be flexible enough to handle a full range of activities, from a routine physical examination to a life-or-death emergency. The design must satisfy the medical staff, too. It must enhance the efficiency of physicians and nurses who depend on the effectiveness of numerous elements, such as ambient and task lighting, the size and configuration of examination rooms, and the proximity of treatment rooms, ancillary services, and offices. Because sanitary conditions are an essential factor, the needs of maintenance and housekeeping personnel must also be considered. And, in these days of fiscal constraint, economic efficiencies of the design process, including life-cycle costs of the building, must be factored into the design equation. Sustainability and "green" design are also important considerations. Each of these demands on design must be weighed against the others.

In the end, though, after all the floor plans are created and the last coat of paint is on the walls, the healthcare facility will be a place where nurses, physicians, support service staff, patients, and visitors spend part of their lives. People will come to the hospital or doctor's office for a host of reasons. They will travel through the corridors, adjust the patient beds, drink from the water fountains, lie still in MRI machines, visit, wait, use digital devices to send text messages, and go about a variety of daily activities. The design must consider the many ways in which the facility will be experienced—what will be seen, heard, felt, and smelled (Lindell, 1983).

Technical design considerations, however, such as making room for a computerized tomographic (CT) scanner or a crash cart, are of remote concern for many users of a healthcare facility. Of immediate concern is the availability of a comfortable place to wait, the accessibility of restrooms for wheelchair users, or the ability to easily find a particular destination. Designs that favor technological convenience over the needs and preferences of patients and visitors may prove problematic. Good design, therefore, must balance technological needs with human needs.

Designing for the human experience is essential. In choosing a healthcare facility, people consider a variety of factors that together help define the term *high-quality care* (Falick, 1981). Designing with the human experience in mind recognizes that people's images of healthcare facilities are multi-dimensional and that having a facility that is technologically up to date may not be enough to satisfy patients and visitors.

The image patients and visitors have of a facility is affected by their relationships with the healthcare-delivery staff, their belief in the effectiveness of the medical and nursing care being provided, and their impression, good or bad, of the facility itself. The design of a healthcare facility reflects on the quality of care. The challenge of sending a "We Care" message cannot stop with the staff. The message must be designed into the facility itself (Arneill and Frasca-Beaulieu, 2003; Becker and Douglass, 2006; Falick, 1981; Gunn, 1990; Panther, 1984; Spreck-elmeyer, 1984; Tetlow, 1984, 1985).

Attention to customer experience has become as important in the healthcare field as it is in other service industries. Although the food in one restaurant may be virtually the same as in another, the service may be quite different. Likewise, from the moment a patient or visitor arrives at a healthcare facility, the design will convey certain symbolic messages. The nature of these messages is shaped through planning and genuine concern for patients' and visitors' experiences. Humanistic design must be more than just an afterthought. It must move health facility design from its "hospital green" image to a sense of caring for the whole person (Arneill and Frasca-Beaulieu, 2003).

The quality of the physical environment is important far beyond the image it presents, since the therapeutic aspects of design must also be considered. The design of the facility, its wayfinding system, Universal Design features, arrangement of furniture, availability of windows, and accommodation of family members are all part of the patient's journey toward recovery (Canter and Canter, 1979; Petrie, 1980; Remen, 1982).

A substantial and growing body of research continues to show that health-facility design is inextricably linked to patient outcomes (Bilchik, 2002a, 2002b; Bullivant, 2004; Coile, 2002; Egger, 1999; Fowler et al., 1999; Harris et al., 2002; Horsburgh, 1995; Long, 2001; Looker and Stichler, 2003; Martin et al., 1998; Reed, 1995; Simmons, 2003; Solovy, 2006; Stern et al., 2003; Sternberg, 2010; Ulrich, 2003; Ulrich et al., 2008). While much remains to be understood about the mind–body connection, the evidence is strong that what we see, feel, touch, smell, and experience influence the body's ability to heal (Mitchell, 2009). Indeed, it has been suggested that "understanding and reducing stress in the hospital environment is to 21st-century medical care what understanding germ theory and reducing infection were to nineteenth-century care" (Mitchell, 2009).

The therapeutic aspects of design are not meant to be a substitute for medical and nursing care. They can, however, enhance the efforts of healthcare professionals, both by creating a healthier setting for examination, treatment, and recovery as well as stimulating the patient's own immune response. Just as physical design can encourage or discourage the maintenance of sterile conditions and task efficiencies, design can also encourage or discourage certain behaviors and responses. It can enhance or depress the body's ability to heal (Mitchell, 2009; Sternberg, 2010).

Designing for Patients and Visitors

Try to remember the last time you waited to see a physician or dentist. Did you glance through the magazines strewn on the waiting-area table or use your cell phone to check email? Perhaps your heart beat a little more rapidly worrying about what might happen, or you breathed more quickly when you inadvertently overheard a fraught conversation between a patient and a staff member. A routine visit to a physician's or dentist's office can be a profound and memorable experience. Physiological reactions, such as rapid heartbeat or quickened breathing, experienced by many people who visit a healthcare facility may be accompanied by a host of psychological reactions, chief among them stress and anxiety.

Patients and their families and friends (herein also referred to as "visitors") represent particularly vulnerable user groups. They may feel virtually powerless in what they often perceive as an intimidating environment. They visit a healthcare facility under what are often emotionally stressful and physically debilitating conditions. At this time in their lives, they need a supportive, non-stressful environment, and they have little capacity to deal with a complex or confusing one.

It is also important to focus on the design-related needs of patients and visitors because they are healthcare consumers. A large number of healthcare facilities are becoming attuned to their position in a competitive market. It is useful, therefore, to consider those aspects of healthcare delivery, such as the physical environment, that may provide a competitive edge when sensitively designed (Falick, 1981). Patient-centered design can include nearly every aspect of a healthcare facility's environment, from the selection of pleasing lighting, to user-friendly informational carts and kiosks, to an effective wayfinding system (Berry et al., 2000; Carpman, 1992; Jossi, 2005; Levine and Glos, 2000).

If the goal is humanistic design, or "design that cares," then the viewpoints of patients and families must be incorporated into the design process. It is not enough to have input from any single group of users at a healthcare facility. Medical and nursing staff can provide valuable insights about designing the environment to meet their own needs, but even though their primary concern is patient care, their perspective on what is desirable design will not necessarily encompass the views of patients and visitors (Parston, 1983). In redefining patients and visitors as customers and guests, healthcare facilities must focus on their social and psychological needs as well as their physical needs.

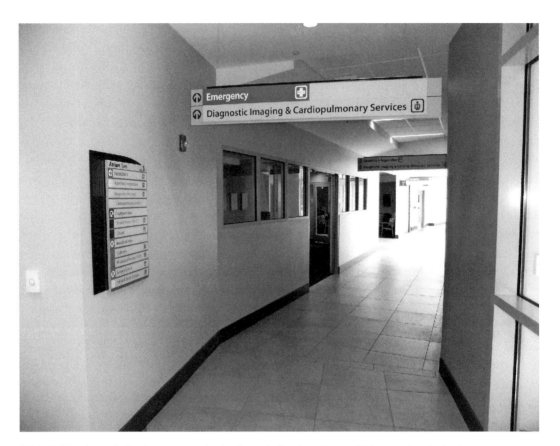

This facility's interior wayfinding signs appear overhead and on walls, directing patients and visitors to various destinations.
Photo credit: Courtesy of St. Joseph Mercy Chelsea

There are other, equally compelling reasons for focusing on patients and visitors. Once they enter the front door, these groups are virtually powerless. Under what are often crisis conditions, patients and visitors are vulnerable to demands on their physical or emotional capacities (Arneill and Frasca-Beaulieu, 2003). Looking forward, patients and visitors must be front and center in the design plans of any healthcare facility.

The design of healthcare facilities has long focused on the functional necessities of the process of delivering healthcare. Unfortunately—and unnecessarily—this approach has often resulted in facility designs that ignore a variety of needs of patients, staff, and visitors. Many researchers have argued that designing healthcare environments that are emotionally and psychologically supportive can foster the process of healing and recovery. A constructed "healing environment" with patients' needs at the forefront has been shown to reduce anxiety and stress, as well as to aid in the healing process (Ulrich, 2000). Positive elements contributing to this include attractive colors, thoughtful acoustics, and well-designed wayfinding elements (Arneill and Frasca-Beaulieu, 2003; Bilchik, 2002a, 2002b; Bullivant, 2004; Coile, 2002; Egger,

1999; Fowler et al., 1999; Harris et al., 2002; Horsburgh, 1995; Long, 2001; Looker and Stichler, 2003; Martin et al., 1998; Reed, 1995; Simmons, 2003; Solovy, 2006; Stern et al., 2003; Ulrich, 2003). And access to positive distractions, such as exposure to nature, can be particularly helpful in creating an environment that lowers stress (Ulrich, 1991).

Stress can become a major obstacle to healing (Ulrich, 1991). Patients feeling stress from unsupportive environments can experience increased blood pressure, muscle tension, and suppressive effects on their immune systems (Frankenhaeuser, 1980; Kennedy, Glaser, and Kiecolt-Glaser, 1990). Stress is also a problem for patients' families and healthcare staff. One study suggests that stress experienced by caregivers of Alzheimer's patients has suppressive effects on the caregivers' own immune functioning (Kiecolt-Glaser and Glaser, 1990). Among staff, stress is associated with low job satisfaction and high rates of burnout (Shumaker and Pequegnat, 1989).

Planners and designers can help reduce this stress by taking into account the interaction between people and their environments. In particular, patients and visitors have needs with respect to wayfinding, physical comfort, regulation of social contact (including matters of privacy and personal territory), and symbolic meaning (Steele, 1973). And in addressing all of these needs, planners must take into account the target population of the facility, as well as the community and cultural heritage of the area (Frasca-Beaulieu, 1999; Shumaker and Reizenstein, 1982).

Wayfinding Ease

The ease with which people find their way around a building affects their level of stress. Large, complex buildings such as hospitals often feel maze-like, particularly for patients and visitors who visit these facilities infrequently. Not being able to find one's way between various destinations can lead to a sense of helplessness and frustration. Signage and graphics can help, but they need to work in conjunction with other features as part of a coordinated wayfinding system (Carpman and Grant, 2002a, 2002b, 2012; Frasca-Beaulieu, 1999).

Physical Comfort

How patients and visitors experience an environment is affected by noise levels, temperature, odors, and lighting, as well as by how capable and successful they are in manipulating their environment or comfortably positioning themselves within it. For example, the degree and types of noise patients will hear if their rooms are located near a lounge or nurses' station will affect their comfort and ability to rest. Likewise, design issues—from the placement of bedside controls to the types of chairs available in waiting areas—affect comfort levels, especially for people with mobility limitations. Additionally, variations in lighting and textures can create a calming environment and are important keys in reducing stress (Frasca-Beaulieu, 1999). Research has shown that patients and visitors pleased with the aesthetics of a healthcare environment are likely to be pleased with the overall experience (Caspari, Eriksson, and Naden, 2006; Hutton and Richardson, 1995).

Control over Social Contact

Patients and visitors need to be able to regulate the amount of interaction they have with others (Giger and Davidhazar, 1990). There may be personal and cultural differences in spatial behavior: proximity to other people and objects, body posture, and movement within a given setting (Giger and Davidhazar, 1990; Smith, 1998). The design must allow for visual privacy, acoustical privacy, social contact, and solitude (Geden and Begeban, 1981). Patients wearing only hospital gowns should not feel as though they are on exhibit (Harris, 1987). Family members dealing with death should have an undisturbed place to grieve. Patients or visitors in need of positive distraction should be able to find effective ways to focus their attention.

Symbolic Meaning

Beyond affecting physical comfort, the environment transmits meaning. What patients and visitors see, hear, and smell tends to blend into a single image. A physical environment that supports the emotional and psychological needs of patients and visitors will be considered positive and caring (Arneill and Frasca-Beaulieu, 2003; Frasca-Beaulieu, 1999). At the same time, environments that make patients and visitors feel unimportant, or even forgotten, send a negative message (Canter and Canter, 1979).

Attending to the needs of patients and visitors will reduce their sense of helplessness and their feeling of being adrift in a strange and complex environment. By attending to these behaviorally-based design issues, the healthcare facility can contribute to a more positive, less stressful experience for patients and visitors. They will have less trouble finding their way between destinations, will feel greater physical comfort, will be able to be social or private depending on their individual needs, and will sense that the facility and its staff care.

The Facility Design Process

Although no two facility design projects progress from abstract idea to concrete form in exactly the same way, every project goes through a series of predictable stages. During each stage, design decision-makers make choices that determine what will be realized in bricks and mortar. It is important to understand the sequence of events and decisions that occur during a project before considering the specific design recommendations made in this book since some design issues come into play only at specific times in the design process. Each stage is complex and time-consuming. For the sake of brevity, we will only outline them here.

Pre-Design Programming

As soon as a design project is shown to be needed and is deemed economically, socially, and politically feasible, the pre-design programming stage can begin. During programming, the project's basic parameters are determined, including its goals and objectives, specific functions, and the types and sizes of spaces it will contain. Building programs vary widely in their comprehensiveness. Some provide only a list of spaces and associated square footages, while others include performance criteria for how the spaces and related systems will be used. The pre-design programming stage usually results in a document that serves as a set of instructions to the design team (Carpman, 1983; Fellows, 1987; Lickhalter, 1987).

Another type of programming—behavioral programming—should be part of the standard planning and design process. This effort thoroughly explores and defines the needs of all users (patients, nurses, family members and visitors, physicians, allied health students, and so on), such as the need for visual and acoustical privacy. These and other behavioral criteria are then translated into design guidelines.

Design

Once the design project's program is set, the design phase can begin. The design phase usually comprises four sub-phases that coincide with the design's evolution from general to specific. These phases are block plans, schematic design, design development, and final construction documents.

Block Plans

Block plans show the building's configuration and its design concept in relation to a particu-lar site. Departments, expressed as gross areas, are shown in relation to other departments, building entrances, vehicular traffic patterns, access points, and internal staff and patient movement patterns. Because block plans do not examine room-by-room detail and are rela-tively easy to prepare, alternative designs can usually be quickly produced. They can be used to evaluate functional adjacencies as well as the flow of people and materials between and among departments. For example, in the case of a large hospital, the emergency department might be located where there is optimum access to a major roadway. In addition, surgery and radiology might be located adjacent to emergency for ease of access to needed facilities and staff.

Schematic Design

Schematic design goes one step further, showing rooms as well as corridors, mechanical spaces, stairs, elevators, and columns. The schematic design phase examines the relationship between all rooms within a department and formalizes the basic net and gross square footages of the building to confirm that the project can be built within budget. It may include an evaluation of the relative merits of different heating, ventilation, air conditioning, plumbing, electrical, fire protection, and other systems.

Design Development

Design development documents refine the schematic design even further. CAD (computer-aided design) drawings are prepared at a larger scale; instead of single-line drawings, dimensions and thicknesses of walls are shown. Room details, including door swings, light fix-ture locations, counters and cupboards, medical equipment, and furniture, appear on design development drawings. Electrical, mechanical, and structural elements are defined.

Construction Documents

Once the design development phase has been completed, the architect and engineers begin construction documents. This detailed set of instructions for the contractor consists of work-ing drawings and specifications—instructions about the quality of the materials and how to build the project. In addition, the construction documents include the agreement between the owner and the contractor, as well as forms that the contractor uses to bid the project. The owner is expected to sign off on all documents at the end of the construction document phase, as well as at the end of each of the other phases. This sign-off means that the owner considers the plans complete.

Concurrent Planning

Interior Design

Interior design typically progresses concurrently with architectural design. Basic interior design services for healthcare facilities often include space planning, which determines the layouts of rooms and achieves both aesthetic and functional goals; color coordination and se-lection of room finishes, furniture, and furnishings; and artwork selection. Interior designers usually work closely with architects and engineers.

Landscape Architecture

Landscape architectural planning also progresses concurrently as part of the total design work. Issues of site planning and exterior design, including vehicular and pedestrian circulation, parking, grading, drainage, exterior seating, selection of vegetation, and location of exterior signs, are typically included as part of the site work.

Wayfinding Planning

While wayfinding planning often occurs late in the project, ideally, it should begin during pro-gramming or early schematic design. Some wayfinding issues need to be considered early on, while decisions are made about site planning, building footprint, and corridor alignments. Wayfinding planning is also needed during later phases, for instance, in order to ensure effective locations for signs at interior decision-points. A wayfinding system incorporates various types of signs, but can and should also include other wayfinding elements. (See chapters 3 and 4.)

Medical Equipment Planning

Medical equipment planning is also part of the design process. It begins at the same time as schematic design, expands into design development, and continues through construction.

During this phase, equipment is selected, its mechanical and electrical requirements are identified, it is purchased, and installed.

Design Review

Design review occurs throughout the design process as the client analyzes design progress by examining floor plans, equipment and specification lists, perspective drawings, digital simulations, three-dimensional models, mockups, and technical specifications. If parts of the design do not meet the performance criteria agreed upon earlier, alternative design approaches are created. (See chapter 11 for a description of how users can participate in Design Review.)

Construction

The construction work for most healthcare-facility projects is awarded through a competitive bid process. During this phase, the owner, usually through the architect or construction manager, responds to questions from potential contractors that may affect the quality or detail of the project. All other things being equal, the contractor with the lowest bid price is usually awarded the contract, and the project then proceeds into construction.

During construction, the owner (again, through the architect or construction manager) inspects the ongoing work in order to ensure compliance with the contract documents. Material substitutions, design modifications, and many other issues must be monitored in order to ensure that the final product is built to fulfill the goals of the program and the operational requirements of its users, as defined by the construction documents.

Activation

Activation is the process of preparing to move into and occupying a new facility. Activation includes strategies for accomplishing the move, planning policies and procedures that will be used in the new facility, orienting staff to the new facility's layout and special features, and training staff to operate in the new surroundings.

Post-Occupancy Evaluation
(also called "Facility Performance Evaluation")

Post-occupancy evaluation (POE), or Facility Performance Evaluation (FPE), which occurs after the environment has been occupied for a period of time, is the systematic assessment of how an environment functions in comparison to the design objectives (Zimring and Reizenstein, 1980, 1981; Zimring et al., 2010). If there are design-related problems, changes are recommended. Post-occupancy evaluation findings can provide valuable information for other buildings, too. Cumulative knowledge gained from this type of evaluation can contribute to the design processes of future projects (Manasc and Adams, 1987).

Summary

○ There is increased demand for a wider variety of healthcare services and higher expectations about those services, as the result of a variety of factors. These include a growing proportion of older people in the US population, an increasing interest in achieving and maintaining good health, shifts in attitudes toward child-bearing and -rearing, and increasing urbanization.

○ Rising healthcare costs, an increasing supply of physicians, an uncertain future for Medicare and Medicaid, limited resources, and other trends such as the growth of specialty facilities have thrust healthcare into the world of big business, where competition is strong to attract and retain patients and their healthcare dollars.

○ Supportive design reduces anxiety and stress, which can be major obstacles to healing and can affect the well-being of patients, families, and staff. Supportive design is an important element in the delivery of high-quality healthcare, both in direct medical terms and as a perceived measure of the quality of care.

○ Certain design decisions—including recommendations made in this book—are appropriate only at particular times in the design process. It is important to understand the sequence of events and decisions that occur during a project. No two design projects progress from abstract idea to concrete form in exactly the same way; however, predictable stages include pre-design programming, design, construction, and activation. Some projects have additional phases which include concurrent planning, design review, and post-occupancy evaluation (Facility Performance Evaluation).

DISCUSSION QUESTIONS

1. What demographic trends are likely to affect healthcare delivery, and in what ways?

2. What developments in healthcare delivery and marketing characterize this age of healthcare competition?

3. What two categories of primary needs must be balanced in the design of a successful healthcare facility?

4. What therapeutic effects—over and above the marketing image of high quality—can a customer-focused, "We Care" environment have upon patients?

5. What are four types of interaction between people and their environments that need to be considered when creating supportive health facility design?

6. What are seven predictable stages of the design process?

References

Arneill, B., and Frasca-Beaulieu, K. Healing environments: Architecture and design conducive to health. In S. Frampton, L. Gilpin, and P. Charmel, editors. *Putting Patients First: Designing and Practicing Patient-Centered Care*, 163–90. San Francisco: Jossey-Bass, 2003.

Becker, F., and Douglass, S. The ecology of the patient visit: Attractiveness, waiting times, and perceived quality of care. *Healthcare Design*, 12–19, November 2006.

Berry, L., Parker, D., Coile Jr., R., Hamilton, D., O'Neill, D., and Sadler, B. The business case for better buildings? *Frontiers* 21(1):3–24, Fall 2004.

Bilchik, G. S. A better place to heal. *Health Forum* 45(4):10–15, July–August 2002a.

_____. New vistas: Evidence-based design projects look into the links between a facility's environment and its care. *Health Facility Management* 15(8):19–24, August 2002b.

Block, L. F., ed. *Marketing for Hospitals in Hard Times.* Chicago: Teach 'em, 1981.

Bullivant, L. U.K.'s "Healthy Hospitals" envisions better health-care design. *Architectural Record* 192(3):32, March 2004.

Canter, D., and Canter, S. Creating therapeutic environments. In D. Canter and S. Canter, editors. *Designing for Therapeutic Environments*, 333–41. New York: John Wiley and Sons, 1979.

Carpman, J. R. Influencing design decisions: An analysis of the impact of the Patient and Visitor Participation Project on the University of Michigan Replacement Hospital Program, 1983. [Available from ProQuest, 789 E. Eisenhower Parkway, Ann Arbor, MI 48108.]

_____. Creating hospitals where people can find their way. Plant Technology and Safety Management Series, Joint Commission on Accreditation of Healthcare Organizations, Number 1, 1991. Reprinted in *Health Facilities '92*, 29th Annual Conference and Technical Exhibition Proceedings, American Society for Hospital Engineering of the American Hospital Association, 1992.

Carpman, J. R., and Grant, M. A. Wayfinding woes: Common obstacles to a successful wayfinding system. *Health Facilities Management*, February 2002a.

_____. Wayfinding: A broad view. In R. Bechtel and A. Churchman, editors. *The New Environmental Psychology Handbook*, 427–42. New York: John Wiley & Sons, 2002b.

_____. *Directional Sense: How to Find Your Way Around.* Boston: Institute for Human Centered Design, 2012.

Caspari, S., Eriksson, K., and Naden, D. The aesthetic dimension in hospitals: An investigation into strategic plans. *International Journal of Nursing Studies*, 43(7):851–59, 2006.

CIA. *The World Factbook.* 2012. /www.cia.gov/.

Coile Jr., R. Competing by design: Healing environments attract patients, reduce costs and help recruit staff. *Physician Executive* 28(4):12–16, July–August 2002.

Detroit Medical Center—DMC. 2013. www.dmc.org/ERwait/.

Egger, E. Designing facilities to be patient-focused. *Health Care Strategic Management* 17(2):1–20, February 1999.

Falick, J. Humanistic design sells your hospital. *Hospitals* 55(4):68–74, February 16, 1981.

Fellows, G. E. Ambulatory surgery design. *AORN* 45(3):708–24, March 1987.

Fowler, E., MacRae, S., Stern, A., Harrison, T., Gerteis, M., Walker, J., Edgman-Levitan, S., and Ruga, W. The built environment as a component of quality care: Understanding and including the patient's perspective. *Journal of Quality Improvement* 25(7):352–62, July 1999.

Frankenhaeuser, M. Psychoneuroendocrine approaches to the study of stressful person-environment transactions. In H. Selye, editor. *Selye's Guide to Stress Research.* Vol. 1, 46–70. New York: Van Nostrand Reinhold, 1980.

Frasca-Beaulieu, K. Interior design for ambulatory care facilities: How to reduce stress and anxiety in patients and families. *Journal of Ambulatory Care* 22(1):67–73, 1999.

Geden, E. A., and Begeban, A. V. Personal space preferences of hospitalized adults. *Research in Nursing and Health* 4:237–41, 1981.

Giger, J. N., and Davidhazar, R. Culture and space. *Advancing Clinical Care,* November–December 1990, 8–11.

Godfrey-June, J. What do the aging want? *Contract Design,* 55–57, March 1992.

Gunn, T. W. Image, architecture, and costs of ambulatory care. *Michigan Hospitals* 26:14–22, 1990.

Harris, P. Dignity in hospital. *British Medical Journal* 294, January 10, 1987.

Harris, P., Ross, C., McBride, G., and Curtis, L. A place to heal: Environmental sources of satisfaction among hospital patients. *Journal of Applied Social Psychology* 32(6):1276–99, 2002.

Horsburgh Jr., C. Healing by design. *New England Journal of Medicine* 333(11):735–40, September 1995.

Hutton, J., and Richardson, L. Healthscapes: The role of the facility and physical environment. *Health Care Management Review* 20(2):48–62, 1995.

Johnson, E., and Johnson, R. *Hospitals in Transition.* Rockville, MD: Aspen Systems Corporation, 1982.

Jossi, F. Patients find a new age of conveniences. *Healthcare Informatics* 22(8):31–33, August 2005.

Kennedy, S., Kiecolt-Glaser, J. K., and Glaser, R. Social support, stress, and the immune system. In B. R. Sarason, I. G. Sarason, and G. R. Pierce, editors. *Social Support: An Interactional View.* Wiley series on personality processes, 253–66. Oxford, England: John Wiley & Sons, 1990.

Kiecolt-Glaser, J., and Glaser, R. Chronic stress and immunity in older adults. Paper presented at the International Congress of Behavioral Medicine, Uppsala, Sweden, June 27–30, 1990.

Levine, H., and Glos, A. Light right. *Health Facilities Management.* 13(5):25–28, May 2000.

Lickhalter, M. How to be a good consumer of programming services. *Journal of Health Administration Education* 6(4, part 1):741–49, 1987.

Lindell, M. The human hospital. *Dimensions in Health Service* 60(5):27–29, May 1983.

Long, R. Healing by design. *Health Facilities Management* 14(11):20–22, November 2001.

Looker, P., and Stichler, J. Healing environments. *Marketing Health Services* 23(2):12–13, Summer 2003.

Managing Construction Costs. *Hospitals and Health Networks.* March 2012. www.hhnmag.com/hhnmag /jsp/articledisplay.jsp?dcrpath=HHNMAG/Article/data/03MAR2012/0312HHN_FEA _VHAgatefold&domain=HHNMAG.

Manasc, V., and Adams, J. Post-occupancy evaluation by hospitals. *Hospital Trustee* 11(5):5–7, September–October 1987.

Martin, D., Diehr, P., Conrad, D., Davis, J., Leickly, R., and Perrin, E. Randomized trial of a patient-centered hospital unit. *Patient Education and Counseling* 34(2):125–33, June 1998.

Michael, D. *On Learning to Plan and Planning to Learn: The Social Psychology of Changing toward Future-Responsive Societal Learning.* San Francisco: Jossey-Bass, 1973.

Mitchell, R. Healthy spaces. *Lancet* 374(9683):18. July 4, 2009. http://download.thelancet.com/pdfs/journals/lancet/PIIS0140673609612216.pdf.

NHE fact sheet: Historical NHE, including sponsor analysis, 2015. www.cms.gov/Research-Statistics-Data-and-Systems/Statistics-Trends-and-Reports/NationalHealthExpendData/NHE-Fact-Sheet.html.

Panther, R. E. Hospital design in the year 2015. In G. S. Lasdon and J. S. Gann, editors. *The Future of Hospital Design: A Discussion among Experts,* 3-11–3-22. Washington, DC: US Department of Health and Human Services, 1984.

Parston, G. Hospital buildings and consumer needs. *Consumer Health Perspectives* 9(5):1–7, September 1983.

Petrie, R. E. Patient well-being is designers' first concern. *Michigan Hospitals* 16(9):12–13, September 1980.

Reed, R. Creating a healing environment by design. *Journal of Ambulatory Care Management* 18(4):16–31, 1995.

Remen, S. Physical surroundings serve as therapeutic catalyst for patients. *Michigan Hospitals* 18(4):20–25, April 1982.

Rice, S. Don't die waiting in the ER. 2013. http://www.cnn.com/2011/HEALTH/01/13/emergency.room.ep/index.html.

Shumaker, S., and Reizenstein, J. E. Environmental factors affecting inpatient stress in acute care hospitals. In G. W. Evans, editor. *Environmental Stress,* 179–223. New York: Cambridge University Press, 1982.

Shumaker, S. A., and Pequegnat, W. Hospital design, health providers, and the delivery of effective health care. In E. H. Zube and G. T. Moore, editors. *Advances in Environment, Behavior, and Design.* Vol. 2, 161–99. New York: Plenum, 1989.

Simmons, J., ed. Designing for quality: Hospitals look to the built environment to provide better patient care and outcomes. *Quality Letter for Healthcare Leaders,* 2–13, April 2003.

Smith, L. Trends in multiculturalism in health care. *Hospital Material Management Quarterly* 20(1):61–70, August 1998.

Solovy, A. Designing a healing environment. *Health Facilities Management* 19(6):30–39, June 2006.

Spreckelmeyer, K. F. Designing for health care in the 21st century. In O. Heyer and S. Graybow, editors. *Proceedings of the International Conference of the Association of Collegiate Schools of Architecture.* Washington, DC, 1984.

Steele, F. Physical Settings and Organization Development. Reading, MA: Addison-Wesley, 1973.

Stern, A. L., MacRae, S., Gerteis, M., Harrison, T., Fowler, E., Edgman-Levitan, S., et al. Understanding the consumer perspective to improve design quality. *Journal of Architectural and Planning Research* 20(1):16–28, Spring 2003.

Sternberg, E. M. *Healing Spaces: The Science of Place and Well-Being.* Cambridge, MA: Belknap Press, 2010.

Tetlow, K. Healing research. *Interiors,* 140–52, October 1984.

_____. New design for physical fitness. *Interiors,* 168–76, October 1985.

Ulrich, R. S. The effect of healthcare architecture and art on medical outcomes. Arts Council England Architecture Week Event, June 25, 2003.

_____. The therapeutic benefits of design. In *Design & Health.* Proceedings of the 2nd Annual International Congress on Design and Health. Karolinska Institute. Stockholm, Sweden. June, 2000:49–59.

_____. Effects of interior design on wellness: Theory and recent scientific research. *Journal of Health Care Interior Design* 3:97–109, 1991.

Ulrich, R. S., Zimring, C., Zhu, X., Dubose, J., Seo, H.-B., Choi, Y.-S., et al. A review of the research literature on evidence-based healthcare design. *Health Environments Research and Design Journal* 1(3), Spring 2008.

US Census 2010. *Age and sex composition: 2010.* www.census.gov/prod/cen2010/briefs/c2010br-03.pdf.

US Government. *Projections of the Population of the United States, by Age, Sex, and Race: 1983 to 2080.* Current Population Reports, Series P-25, No. 952. Washington, DC, 1984.

Zimring, C., Rashid, M., and Kampschroer, K. Facility Performance Evaluation (FPE). *Whole Building Design Guide,* 2014. https://www.wbdg.org/resources/fpe.php.

Zimring, C. M., and Reizenstein, J. E. Post-occupancy evaluation: An overview. *Environment and Behavior* 12(4):429–50, December 1980.

_____. A primer on post-occupancy evaluation. *American Institute of Architects Journal* 70(13):52–58, November 1981.

CHAPTER 2

A LOOK AT CURRENT HEALTHCARE-FACILITY DESIGN RESEARCH

One of the premises of this book is that decisions about designing healthcare facilities should be based on solid information about the needs and preferences of patients and visitors. This chapter explores healthcare-facility design research and describes evidence-based information.

Design Research in Relation to Current Trends in Healthcare

Five current trends in healthcare are of particular relevance for design research: focus on marketing, value of healthcare-facility design, sensitivity to patient experience, recognition of the role and needs of families and visitors, and emphasis on accessibility and Universal Design.

Focusing on Marketing

According to J. L. Quebe, writing in *Health Care Strategic Management*, the retail experience has forever changed the way patients view healthcare facilities:

> The new emphasis on main entries, attractive public areas, and improved signage, all reflect attempts to appeal to a public whose tastes have been largely conditioned by their experience as consumers and by their exposure to the architectural vocabulary of shopping malls and convention hotels. . . Patients who are unable to judge the quality of medical care received now often make choices for services based on their responses to the hospital's image. (Quebe, 1985, p. 4)

LEARNING OBJECTIVES

- Understand the role of design research in identifying the needs and preferences of healthcare consumers—patients, families, and visitors—in a competitive, market-driven healthcare environment.

- Know the value of design research in showing how the physical environment can prevent illness and injury and how healthcare-facility policies can affect patients' healing and recovery times.

- Understand the characteristics of high-quality health-facility design research.

- Become aware of the processes involved in integrating high-quality design research into all stages of the design process.

Competition for patients has fundamentally changed the way health facilities view them; no longer are patients treated as powerless people desperate for medical care, regardless of its conditions. Health facilities must actively market their services. As new medical facilities are built, patients are seen as discerning consumers who make intelligent, well-informed decisions about purchasing healthcare services (Brown and Shoemaker, 2004; Sachner, 1988). As one writer notes:

> Perhaps the most dramatic change in healthcare is the change in consumers. As medical treatment has become accepted as a commodity, the consumer has become more independent, better informed, and choice-conscious. As a result, marketing strategies and facility image are now significant criteria by which the consumer chooses services. (Rostenberg, 1987, p. 15)

Research-based information enables health facilities to tailor design and services to suit the needs and preferences of their customers and ultimately to attract more patients. This type of research, often containing questions about facility design, is exemplified by the "Pebble Project," a collaborative of healthcare organizations, architects, designers, and industry partners whose declared objective is "to identify built environment designs and solutions that improve patient and worker safety, clinical outcomes, environmental performance and operating efficiency" (Bilchik, 2002; Center for Health Design, 2013; Zenisus, 2008).

Indeed, even the exercise of asking hospital consumers what they think can be considered a marketing activity.

BOX 2.1. BENEFITS OF FACILITY DESIGN RESEARCH

1. Research is a tool that lets healthcare organizations know what customers need and prefer.
2. Research can point out how healthcare-facility design features are viewed by customers and staff.
3. Research can show how the physical environment affects patients, visitors, and staff.
4. Research can show how the physical environment can prevent illness and injury.
5. Research can show how healthcare-facility policies affect patients' healing and recovery times.
6. Research can act as a means of communication between patients and healthcare-facility decision-makers by providing data on patient outcomes and satisfaction.
7. Research can identify the needs and preferences of families and visitors.
8. Research is a tool for documenting the way healthcare facilities and design features accommodate the needs of people with disabilities.

Valuing Healthcare-Facility Design

Health-facility design is considered a marketing tool—something that can attract patients to or repel them from a particular facility. Healthcare design also plays a role in recruiting and retaining physicians, nurses, and other staff (Gardner, 1989; Solomon, 1991).

Unlike the quality of medical care, design is something that can readily be understood and judged by the public, for better or worse (Bailey and Leissner, 1995). It has been said that "hospital administrators have found that user-friendly architecture is a good advertising tool" (Doubilet, 1987). Although one hopes the message is an honest one, the strength of design as a marketing tool is almost irresistible: quality architecture will give the image of quality care (Dean, 1986; Johnson, 1987; Lippman, 1991; Solomon, 1991).

Design is also valued as having a strong potential effect on the well-being of patients and visitors. As characterized by *U.S. News & World Report,* healthcare facilities have a long history of seeming like uncaring places:

> Most hospitals are dismally inhospitable. A weakened patient and traumatized family are greeted by harsh lights and cold stainless steel, labyrinths of white corridors, thumping equipment and arid, mysterious smells. The sick rarely have access to medical information, privacy, or a place for quiet talk or grieving. The resulting sense of anxiety and helplessness is the worst imaginable to promote healing. (Horn, 1991, p. 48)

The current approach to healthcare-facility design has many names, including humanistic design, design that cares, evidence-based design, healing environments, and supportive design (Devlin and Arneill, 2003). This type of design is seen as complementary to the healing effects of medications, treatment procedures, surgery, nursing care, policies, and technology and may foster the process of recovery (Ulrich, 1991). Design has been said to be able to enhance the quality of life, even for those who are dying (Leibrock and Birdsong, 1989; Zimring and Bosch, 2008).

Healthcare design should, of course, do no harm. At the least, good healthcare-facility design should support activities essential to achieving desired patient outcomes without imposing additional stressors on the patient beyond those already existing because of illness and treatment (Williams, 1991). However, as some researchers caution:

> All too often, the physical environment represents one of the most neglected and hidden components of both prevention and care. Yet evidence is now being gathered that suggests that poorly designed and planned environments not only create new difficulties both for patients and staff, but also can interfere with treatment effectiveness. What is more, environmental factors have begun to be linked to important outcome measures that are used to assess treatment efficacy. (Winkel and Holahan, 1985, pp. 30–31)

Therefore, hospitals are beginning to be built with patients in mind, starting from the initial stages of the development process and ideally including evidence from patients themselves (Reilling et al., 2004; Stuart, Parker, and Rogers, 2003).

Another role of healthcare-facility design is to help prevent illness and injury. From the design of heating/ventilation/air conditioning (HVAC) systems to the design of stairways and patient bathroom grab bars and the selection of floor coverings, architectural and interior design decisions can directly affect the health and safety of a facility's users.

Sensitivity to Patient Experience

As a result of feedback about current services, patients' expectations, and ideas for improvement, healthcare-facility decision-makers are learning about the perspective of patients (Sahney and Warden, 1991).

In the past, guest relations programs emphasized the importance of treating patients like guests instead of as "faceless ailments to be cured" (Carey, 1985). Such programs deal with amenities such as better food, legible name tags, and more prominent information desks. They also emphasize courtesy on the part of physicians and staff: for example, making eye contact, introducing oneself, explaining procedures as they are done, and addressing patients by name (Carey, 1985).

Information is available on the perspectives of individual patients, for example, in Sue Baier's insightful book, *Bed Number 10* (Baier and Shoemaker, 1989). Factors leading to stress in hospitals can be summarized in a daunting list: unfamiliarity of surroundings, loss of independence, financial concerns, lack of information, threat of severe illness or death, separation from family and friends, problems with pain and medications, and a general feeling of being out of control (Beck, 1982). As researchers have noted, staff may not realize the degree of stress arising from overcrowding, lack of privacy, noise, and intimidating high-technology equipment. Yet all of these factors can "adversely affect the healing process" (Winkel and Holahan, 1985).

Sensitivity to the view from the bed is seen not only as a smart marketing approach, but also as a natural, caring modus operandi. Given that every decision-maker cannot talk to every patient, research provides an opportunity to obtain information from a cross-section of patients about an array of issues.

Units on which patients and families participate in, and take more than the usual responsibility for, their own care (known as *participatory care, cooperative care, progressive patient care,* and other names) are one approach to healthcare delivery and healthcare-facility design. Such approaches emphasize that the healthcare facility does not provide treatment *to* its patients, but rather works in concert *with* them to achieve health. For instance, the Planetree Unit, progenitor of the Planetree Model, of Pacific Presbyterian Medical Center, San Francisco, has some unusual design features for an inpatient unit. There is a completely outfitted kitchen, an attractively decorated lounge, indirect lighting, and patient rooms with floral sheets, pastel cubicle curtains, and bookshelves (Martin et al., 1990).

Careful documentation of the effectiveness of these units offers useful information (Belkin, 1992). In this way, these models of patient care can be clearly compared with the traditional models and their effects on patient recovery and morale can be demonstrated.

Recognizing the Role and Needs of Visitors

Understanding patients' needs usually leads to the recognition that entire families are involved in treatment and recovery. Families and friends have a variety of needs associated with health-care-facility visits or stays, but they may become so focused on the patient's needs that they neglect their own (Carpman, Grant, and Simmons, 1986; Lovejoy, 1987).

Family involvement in patient care has been said to reduce anxiety and fear, foster feelings of usefulness, and provide positive distraction for the patient (D'Alessandro and Dosa, 2001). Families and visitors may play a variety of roles, including caretaker (fulfilling functions the patient is no longer able to accomplish), assistant (acting as a link between the hospital and outside life, continuing previous patterns of living and relating to others), protector (shielding the patient from fears, inadvertent self-inflicted harm, or potential staff mismanagement), companion, witness, and source of emotional support (Lovejoy, 1987).

Visitors need convenient restrooms and places to find food and beverages at all hours. They may need privacy, a change of scene, a place to obtain counseling, and places to relax, reflect, and catch up with work and family responsibilities. Families with children need places where the children can play in a supervised setting (Goldsmith and Miller, 1990). Health facilities also need to be aware and supportive of cultural diversity. Issues such as private and social space, diet and eating habits, and coping mechanisms differ widely among cultures. Moreover, language and cultural barriers can hinder the level of comfort or even the effects of treatment for some patients and their families. Healthcare facilities should ensure that everyone—regardless of language, social, cultural, or ethnic background—feels welcome and is as comfortable as possible (Baker, Hayes, and Fortier, 1998; Clegg, 2003; Davidhizar, Dowd, and Newman-Giger, 1997; Galanti, 2006; Walsh, 2004; Waters, 1999).

Emphasizing Accessibility and Universal Design

Because of changes in attitudes, knowledge, and legislation in the United States, more people with disabilities are able to use public facilities than ever before. As a result of wars, illnesses, injuries, congenital conditions, and life-cycle stages (such as pregnancy and aging), there are large and increasing numbers of people with both temporary and permanent disabilities (also known as functional limitations). (See chapter 9.) Whether it is negotiating a hospital elevator on crutches, feeling unable to stand for long periods of time during pregnancy, or needing to reach a toilet from a wheelchair, most of us will experience some type of disability in our lifetimes, and every disability has design implications.

The Americans with Disabilities Act (ADA) of 1990 is a comprehensive civil rights statute that outlaws discrimination based on physical or mental disability in the areas of employment, access to services provided by public agencies, public accommodations, and telecommunications. The act expressly applies to hospitals and professional offices of healthcare providers (O'Hare and Schmidt, 1991). The ADA requires that covered entities, including hospitals, remove barriers that prevent a person with physical disabilities from having equal access to the facility unless it can be proved that significant cost or other factors make it unreasonable to do so (Kinrade, 2003; Mandelman, 1990).

Universal Design is an inclusion-based design philosophy supporting the idea that aesthetically pleasing environments can be made accessible to and functional for users with a wide range of abilities at little or no extra cost. It emphasizes independence and safety, along with adaptability over time (Behar, 1991).

One way of putting in perspective the cost of making a building accessible and functional for all users is to compare it with the cost of providing staff assistance when patients are limited by the environment and unable to act independently—reaching a phone, operating a bed control, seeing a clock, and so on. The University of Michigan Architecture and Planning Research Laboratory showed, in a full-scale study of hospital patient rooms, that "almost anything that enables the patients to act on their own, without need to call a nurse, saves the hospital money," according to Professor Jonathan King (Fisher, 1985, p. 122).

Conducting High-Quality Healthcare-Facility Design Research

Facility-design research is both an internal component and a natural outgrowth of the five previously-mentioned trends in the healthcare field. Since this research is recognized as valuable and is being employed with greater frequency than ever before, some guidelines may be helpful (Hamilton, 2003; Scalise, 2005).

Design decision-makers—including healthcare administrators, health professionals, facility managers, architects, and interior designers—need to be informed consumers of design research. As informed consumers, design decision-makers will be able to read a journal article or listen to a conference presentation and determine whether it is something worth their attention. Informed consumers of design research will be able to listen to an internal research report and know whether the conclusions are warranted. Informed consumers of design research will know what to ask researchers when they commission their own studies and how to work with researchers to obtain reliable, valid answers to design-related questions.

As design decision-makers consider research papers, articles, e-books or print books, or even anecdotes, some guidelines may be useful. The following research guidelines can become the basis for questions, discussions, and decisions concerning information quality. It is important to note that these are general guidelines only. Each aspect of research requires considerable training, knowledge, and experience. Readers are encouraged to delve more deeply into this topic, if they wish to engage in and/or be informed consumers of design research.

Ensure That Research Is Planned and Carried Out by Trained, Experienced Researchers

This is important because the popular impression seems to be that anyone can put together a questionnaire, especially now that this can be easily done online. Poorly planned and designed questionnaires (or other "measuring instruments") result in low-quality data. There is both science and "art" involved in developing useful questionnaires.

See That the Research Builds On Existing Knowledge

A literature review is the means by which researchers examine the existing theory, method-ologies, studies, findings, debates, conference presentations, and other information related to their topic. Much can be learned and much time saved by not repeating work already com-pleted by others. A literature review summarizes the highlights and shortcomings of related work and includes complete citations.

If the Research Involves Clinical Investigations, Look Into Institutional Review Board Certification

Any research involving human subjects that is supported or conducted by the Department of Health and Human Services (HHS) is governed by the National Research Act of 1974 and the regulations of Title 45 Code of Federal Regulations Part 46 (unless the research is exempt under the terms of the act). Before initiating participation in such research, institutions must commit to compliance through a system of institutional review board (IRB) registration and assurances, under regulation by the Office for Human Research Protections within HHS (US Department of Health and Human Services, 2013).

See That the Research Has a Clearly Stated Purpose Related to Healthcare-Facility Design

For instance, a study of "patient attitudes" is unlikely to produce much, if any, design-relevant information. However, a study comparing inpatient preferences for three different patient room chairs at a particular hospital (with the most-preferred chair to be purchased by the hospital) has a focused, clear, design-relevant purpose.

Provide a Clear Research Design and Related Hypotheses

Although the terms "design research" and "research design" can seem confusing to non-researchers, they are two distinct entities. *Research design* refers to the way the research is for-mulated in order to answer specific questions. It deals with *constructs* and *measures* of those constructs. An example of a construct might be "comfort," and one measure of "comfort" might be "the amount of time a patient can sit in the chair before wanting to get up." Research design also sometimes deals with *experimental groups* and *control groups.*

Hypotheses are possible conclusions researchers establish at the beginning of a project. Even-tually, hypotheses are either supported or unsupported by the findings. For example, one hypoth-esis about chair comfort might be "Chair A will be considered the most comfortable of the three."

Carry Out the Project as Objectively as Possible

Researchers need to avoid bias. For example, studies should not be undertaken to "prove that such-and-such a chair is most comfortable." Researchers should not have a vested interest in a particular outcome.

Single research studies cannot *prove* anything. They can only lend credence to or take credence from a certain hypothesis within the context of many caveats. For instance, one cannot usually generalize findings beyond the population used for the study. Bodies of knowledge grow when *multiple* studies show similar findings for multiple groups in multiple settings over time.

Skillfully Word Questions

The technical term for questionnaires is *measuring instruments,* and the questions that constitute them need to be precise. Even seemingly small changes in question wording can affect responses one way or another.

Problems in question wording can range from a loaded question such as "How long have you been taking antidepressants?" to a multiple-negative question such as "Why don't you think this chair isn't uncomfortable?" to a question with too many fixed responses such as "very, very uncomfortable; very uncomfortable; somewhat comfortable; a little comfortable; a teeny bit comfortable"; and so on.

Use Visual Images, if Possible

One of the difficulties associated with using words alone to ask questions about design issues and features is that respondents form mental images that may or may not conform to the issues and features being queried. If we asked a patient whether she would prefer an inpatient room that looks "homey" or one that looks "institutional," her response will reflect *her* own culture, background, and interpretation of those terms (which may be different from someone else's interpretation) and may not contribute much to our understanding of hospital design and image. On the other hand, when we show digital images, photographs, drawings, or other visual representations of a patient room to a respondent, she can easily tell which ones she *prefers.* Our differences in culture, background, and interpretations of words need not even come into play, and we can learn a great deal about the design features that work together to form a pleasant patient room for her and for other respondents.

Carefully Sample Respondents

Sampling refers to the way in which respondents are selected to participate in a study. Sampling is such a highly developed specialization that many PhD-level researchers work with a sampling consultant to make sure their studies are carried out properly.

There are many types of sampling. Despite its name, *random sampling,* one of the most familiar sampling terms, does not mean that study participants are selected at random. Rather, it means that every member of the population has an equal opportunity to be selected as part of the study. In other words, random sampling requires precision. Some other types of samples include stratified samples, opportunity samples, and stratified random samples.

Make Sure Participants Give Informed Consent

Certain ethical considerations need to guide design research. Study participants need to understand the purpose of the study, whether their identities will be kept confidential, and how much of their time will be required. They must have a choice about whether to participate, and if they decline, they should be treated respectfully.

Use State-of-the-Art Data-Collection Methods

Self-administered questionnaires, focused interviews, behavior mapping, and participant observation are some well-known and time-honored social science data-collection strategies. Physiological data-collection methods include analyses of organ functions (such as heart and brain) and bodily fluids. Administrative data-collection methods might include reviews of patient records for frequency of pain medication requests, aspects of physician progress notes, length of stay, and the like. A design research study should use current methods and follow the associated steps in planning, data-collection, and data analysis.

Use Multiple Data-Collection Methods, if Possible

Because every data-collection method has inherent weaknesses, more than one data-collection method should be used, if possible. In this way, the strengths of one method will compensate for the weaknesses of another. For instance, a researcher might choose to employ fixed-response questions, which are useful in obtaining statistical or *quantitative data,* and open-ended questions, which capture in-depth responses, personal anecdotes, and other details, also known as *qualitative data.*

Use State-of-the-Art Data-Analysis Methods

Just as there are specialists in sampling, there are experts in statistical analysis of quantitative data. A wide variety of statistical tests are available, as are numerous measures for each test. Knowing which statistical methods are appropriate for which types of data, how to carry out the analyses, and how to interpret the various measures of those statistics are all tasks for an expert. There are numerous ways to analyze qualitative data, as well.

State the Limitations of Findings and Their Generalizability

No single design research project is perfect or generalizable to every patient in every hospital in the world. When presenting research findings, responsible researchers state the limits of their studies. For example, they might state that the results should be interpreted within a certain margin of error, or remind readers that only 3 of 200 possible patient chairs were tested. Researchers also need to state how generalizable the findings are (for example, "to all patients in XYZ hospital" or "to female patients between 30 and 50 years old on XYZ hospital's Ob/Gyn unit").

Consider Whether or Not the Research Is Replicable

If a study is ultimately to contribute to the body of accepted knowledge or to the state of the art, other researchers in similar healthcare settings with other respondents should be able to use the same measuring instruments and come up with similar findings. If they cannot, the study is probably not useful beyond the specific institution where the research was conducted.

Make Design Implications Explicit

Often, so much attention is paid to methodological fine points or data analysis details that the point of the design-research study—to learn something about how healthcare-facility design affects behavior, physiology, or preferences—is at best underplayed or at worst forgotten. In order to contribute to the state of the art, the design implications of a study need to be made clear, in conjunction, of course, with all of the associated limitations on generalizability.

Communicate Findings in a Way That Is Clear to Non-researchers

This is one of the most difficult requirements for researchers because they are taught, as are designers and healthcare professionals, to use the jargon of their profession. Unfortunately, that jargon makes research findings almost incomprehensible to people in other professions. Sometimes researchers speak of translating findings into lay terminology. Such translations are necessary for research to contribute to the basic knowledge and understanding of design decision-makers and if it is to influence design decisions.

Research Claims

As awareness of health-facility design and its use in marketing has increased, more people have become eager to jump on its bandwagon. Articles, reports, and even anecdotes that aren't based on carefully collected and analyzed evidence are sometimes presented as "research." On occasion, research is subtly alluded to and sometimes overtly invoked for the purpose of promoting a particular product or perspective, or for lending credence to wholesale claims for "healing environments," "evidence-based design," and other so-called "proven" effects of the environment on behavior.

Recovery and healing are multifaceted, complex processes. Patients' genetic makeups, the precise nature of their illnesses, medical and surgical procedures, medications, health-related behaviors, relationships with family and friends, culture, work responsibilities, the attitudes and practices of staff, the physical environment, and other factors all work together. Ascribing unlimited influence on behavior or patient outcomes to design decisions—an attitude known as "design determinism"—is just as mistaken as saying that the physical environment has no effect on behavior.

Another poorly understood aspect of design research is that environmental features do not function in isolation. For example, lighting exists within a room of a certain size and shape, having certain types of furnishings, certain window sizes and locations, certain colors, and certain floor and ceiling materials. It is difficult to hold all the other variables constant and study a single design feature. Even if we could do that, we still do not know how that feature would function with other furnishings, floor and ceiling materials, and so forth. We need more complex approaches to studying environmental design features in combination.

Integrating Design Research into the Design Process

The primary purpose of healthcare-facility design research, over and above the gathering of information, is to improve design. In this final section we discuss a humanistic design process model that integrates design research. In an admittedly oversimplified model of the traditional design process, decisions are made by clients and high-powered client representatives in conjunction with designers. Goals are met by creating functionally acceptable and aesthetically pleasing spaces and by bringing the project in on time and on budget. A small number of people can be involved, decisions can be based on previously used design concepts, and the client and designer can defer to each other's expertise: the designer's being aesthetics, architectural design, engineering, and code compliance; the client's being function, finances, and corporate culture. The trouble is that this process produces too many poorly designed facilities that do not function effectively or provide caring places for patients, visitors, and staff.

Characteristics of a Humanistic Design Process

Humanistic design supports the needs of patients, visitors, staff, and other health facility users. Adopting a humanistic health-facility design process is more challenging than following a traditional design process since it may take more time, involve more people, and result in more political wrangling within the organization. It will, however, allow organizations to work through the details of how designs will function for users.

A humanistic design process analyzes design alternatives based on a variety of user needs and preferences. Such a design process—and the resulting design—may well save money in the long run by helping prevent the need for renovations. This type of design process will also minimize the need for staff to compensate for ineffective design, such as taking time away from their duties to frequently give directions to patients and visitors attempting to navigate a confusing facility. The value of humanistic design is that it results in some wonderful, caring places for patients, visitors, and staff, places that not only work the day they are opened, but that also accommodate change over time. Humanistic design can and should be both functional and aesthetically pleasing (Carpman, 1991).

Humanistic design shares the following five characteristics: an explicit, shared value system; evidence-based decision-making; participatory design; design review; and post-occupancy evaluation (also known as "Facility Performance Evaluation") (Zimring et al., 2010).

Explicit, Shared Value System

Humanistic design starts with an explicit, shared value system recognizing that a health-facility design project must be practical if it is to be implemented successfully. It must also be politically, economically, and physically feasible. The design must comply with codes, be aesthetically pleasing when completed, and be relatively easy to maintain.

However, where this value system parts company with those of more traditional design projects is in the emphasis it places on the social, emotional, psychological, and physical needs of patients, visitors, and staff. In a humanistic health-facility design project, these needs are placed at the top of the hierarchy of design criteria. For example, within this value system, a patient's need to easily sit down on and rise up from a chair would outweigh a desire to select a particular chair based largely on its appearance. And the nursing staff's need to have a lounge where they can relax for a few minutes, make a private phone call, and put their feet up out of view of physicians, patients, and families would trump an individual's need for an office on the patient floor.

Decisions about the project's goals and objectives and whose needs should take precedence should be discussed and agreed upon before any design-related decisions are made. If a project is to be successful, everyone involved—clients, designers, users, and consultants—should share the same value system.

Evidence-Based Decision-Making

In order to make good design decisions, accurate information is needed about facility users: who they are, what they do within the facility, and which design options they prefer. The two most common mechanisms for identifying users' needs and collecting accurate information are systematic research and consultation with experts. Other techniques for gathering information about users' needs include literature reviews, facility visits, Web searches, interviews and surveys, and simulations. (See chapter 11 for a fuller discussion of these techniques.)

Participatory Design

Humanistic design is achieved through a participatory design process that broadens traditional decision-making responsibilities. (Chapter 11 contains a detailed overview of the benefits and techniques of participation.)

Periodic Design Review

Another component of humanistic health-facility design is periodic, systematic design review. It is not enough to base approval of a set of plans solely on a rudimentary understanding of what is being shown or a claim that the plan will work. A systematic design review of the project must demonstrate that the plan will allow users to function as they need and prefer to do. Design *guidelines* answer the question, "How should this space or design feature function?" Design *review* asks, "Will this space or design feature function as needed?"

Design reviewers should be familiar with relevant design guidelines. They should be skilled at interpreting design graphics, anticipating scenarios that might occur in a given space, and imagining how the space would function under those conditions. Design reviewers should also be skilled at communicating with design decision-makers in a way that is respectful, clear, and useful.

Design review should not end with the first analysis of a design scheme. In most projects, designs go through multiple iterations, from early schematic designs to change orders after construction has begun. Design review is desirable at *every* stage of the process so that changes in the design can be carefully analyzed and the project's progress can be tracked.

Post-Occupancy Evaluation (also known as "Facility Performance Evaluation")

The true test of healthcare-facility design is how it performs over time. Humanistic design does not stop at the dedication ceremony (Shepley and Wilson, 1999). It involves periodic evaluations of how well the design is functioning for all its users. It leads to action when the environment is found to be problematic. Actions might include changes in behavior, policy, scheduling, or design. Periodically attending to the fit between users' needs and environmental design likely means that small problems will not grow into big ones. Such post-occupancy evaluations, also called "Facility Performance Evaluations," give a symbolic message to users that the facility still cares about meeting their needs (Zimring et al., 2010).

Another benefit of this type of evaluation is that other facilities undergoing similar projects can learn from and build upon a project's strengths and avoid its weaknesses. By carefully documenting these evaluations and by making them widely available, we can collectively improve the state of the art in healthcare-facility design.

Objectives for Future Healthcare-Facility Design Research

High-quality health-facility design research has a tremendous amount to offer, and yet its full potential is still unrealized. Meeting the following objectives would dramatically increase the contribution of design research to healthcare-facility design projects.

Awards for Buildings Sensitive to User Needs

Architectural and interior design websites, blogs, magazines, and healthcare design-oriented organizations need to be encouraged to recognize exemplary projects that used healthcare-design research in the design process and that have been occupied long enough to assess their value to all users.

Training for Designers in Research Methods

One way to increase the awareness and sensitivity of professional designers, including future architects, interior designers, landscape architects, graphic designers, and others, is to expose them to design research and its effects while they are in school. When they experience an environment from the perspective of users, their view may be forever altered.

Training for Researchers in Design-Relevant Research

Researchers need to understand and be encouraged to pursue the types of research useful for design decision-making. Researchers also need to present jargon-free findings and use current technology to create effective presentations.

Long-Term Studies of the Effects of Healthcare Facilities on Users

Many studies view particular situations at a single moment in time. Topics for future research include comparisons of the effects of environmental modifications, longitudinal studies of people who have spent prolonged periods in intensive care units, and others (Williams, 1988). Since healthcare facilities are active places involving continual change, research needs to take this dynamic character into account. More evidence is needed regarding the role of design in fostering health and hindering illness (also known as "patient outcomes") (Ulrich, 1991).

Translation of Research Findings into Design Guidelines

Researchers should be encouraged to be explicit about the design implications of their work. Researchers and designers need to work together to create useful sets of design guidelines based on existing research.

More Research Funding

Researchers, designers, administrators, patients, visitors, and other interested parties need to encourage funding of all types and to work with government agencies, healthcare organizations, charitable foundations, and for-profit businesses to encourage them to fund research that can influence health-facility design decision-making.

International Research Agenda

If the field is to progress in a logical, useful way, a prioritized, global agenda must be developed by a committed corps of researchers, designers, administrators, government officials, and others.

Summary

- By ascertaining the needs and preferences of healthcare consumers, design research provides evidence-based information that can enhance a healthcare facility's ability to attract and satisfy patients, families, and visitors; to tailor facilities to their needs; and to attract and retain professional staff.

- Design research can show how to achieve supportive design (also known as "design that cares"). It can reveal how environmental design can complement the healing effects of medications, treatment procedures, surgery, nursing care, policies, and technology, by diminishing the stress that often interferes with treatment effectiveness. Design research can also help decision-makers avoid the danger of illness or injuries resulting from substandard environmental design.

○   High-quality health-facility design research is planned and carried out by trained, experienced researchers. It has a clearly stated purpose, builds on existing knowledge, and is as objective as possible. It has a clear research design and stated hypotheses, samples respondents carefully, skillfully words questions, uses visual images, and makes sure that participants give their informed consent. It uses state-of-the-art data-collection methods—if possible, multiple data-collection methods—and state-of-the-art data analysis methods. It states the limitations of findings and their generalizability, considers whether or not the project is replicable, makes design implications explicit, and communicates findings in a way that is clear to non-researchers.

○   A humanistic design process has the following characteristics:

  –   Explicit, shared value system

  –   Evidence-based decision-making

  –   Participatory design

  –   Periodic design review

  –   Post-occupancy evaluation (also called "Facility Performance Evaluation")

DISCUSSION QUESTIONS

1.   Why is design research important in discovering what healthcare consumers need and prefer?

2.   How can design research contribute to therapeutic outcomes in a healthcare environment?

3.   What contributions does design research make by providing "the view from the bed"?

4.   How is design research valuable in exploring the needs and preferences of patients' families and visitors?

5.   What role can design research play with regard to the legal requirements and social attitudes reflected in the Americans with Disabilities Act (ADA)?

6.   Why is it important that design decision-makers become informed consumers of design research?

7.   What are some characteristics of reliable, professional-quality design research?

8.   What are some characteristics of a design process that seeks to achieve humanistic health facility design?

9.   What contributions can design research make over the course of a humanistic design process?

References

Baier, S., and Shoemaker, M. Z. *Bed Number 10.* Boca Raton, FL: CRC Press, 1989.

Bailey, J., and Leissner, G. Who likes what in health care design? *Health Facilities Management* 8(10): 48–50, October 1995.

Baker, D., Hayes, R., and Fortier, J. Interpreter use and satisfaction with interpersonal aspects of care for Spanish-speaking patients. *Medical Care* 36(10):1461–70, 1998.

Beck, W. C. The patient users. In W. C. Beck and R. H. Meyer, editors. *The Health Care Environment: The User's Viewpoint,* 30–38. Boca Raton, FL: CRC Press, 1982.

Behar, S. Universal design blends function with form. *Group Practice Journal,* 87–88, July–August 1991.

Belkin, L. Hospital study testing the benefits of comfort. *New York Times,* September 26, 1992, p. 16.

Bilchik, G. S. A better place to heal. *Health Forum* 45(4):10–15, 2002.

Brown, K., and Shoemaker, A. Designing facilities around models of care. Washington, DC: The Advisory Board Company, February 2004.

Carey, J. Hospital hospitality. *Newsweek,* 78–79, February 11, 1985.

Carpman, J. R. Socially responsible health facility design: The direction for the new millennium. *Group Practice Journal,* 32–39, July–August 1991.

Carpman, J. R., Grant, M. A., and Simmons, D. A. *Design That Cares: Planning Health Facilities for Patients and Visitors.* Chicago: American Hospital Publishing, 1986.

Center for Health Design. The Pebble Project. 2013. www.healthdesign.org/pebble.

Clegg, A. Older South Asian patient and career perceptions. *Journal of Clinical Nursing* 12:283–290, 2003.

D'Alessandro, D., and Dosa, N. Empowering children and families with information technology. *Archives of Pediatrics and Adolescent Medicine* 155:1131–36, October 2001.

Davidhizar, R., Dowd, S., and Newman-Giger, J. Model for cultural diversity in the radiology department. *Radiologic Technology* 68(3):223, 1997.

Dean, A. O. Emergency unit puts a welcoming face on a hospital. *Architecture,* 65–67, April 1986.

Devlin, A., and Arneill, A. Healthcare environments and patient outcomes. *Environment & Behavior* 35(5):665–94, September 2003.

Doubilet, S. The fittest survive. *Progressive Architecture,* Vol. 68, 5:98–103, 1987.

Fisher, T. Enabling the disabled. *Progressive Architecture,* Vol. 66, 7:119–124, July 1985.

Galanti, G. Applying cultural competence to perianesthesia nursing. *Journal of PeriAnesthesia Nursing* 21(2):97–102, 2006.

Gardner, E. Revamping hospitals' approach to renovation. *Modern Healthcare* 19(15):34–44, April 14, 1989.

Goldsmith, J. C., and Miller, R. Restoring the human scale. *Healthcare Forum* 33(6):22–27, November–December 1990.

Hamilton, D. The four levels of evidence based practice. *Healthcare Design.* 3(4):18–26, November 2003.

Horn, M. Hospitals fit for healing. *U.S. News & World Report,* 48–50, July 22, 1991.

Johnson, K. C. MRI centers: Ten design mistakes to avoid. *Hospitals* 61(7):82–84, April 5, 1987.

Kinrade, S. Acting against discrimination. *Professional Nurse* 18(12):714–15, August 2003.

Leibrock, D., and Birdsong, C. Supportive home environments for people with AIDS. *Journal of Interior Design Education and Research,* 23–28, Spring 1989.

Lippman, H. Is this the ideal hospital? *RN* 54(7):46–49, 1991.

Lovejoy, N. C. Roles played by hospital visitors. *Heart and Lung* 16(5):573–75, September 1987.

Mandelman, J. Disabilities act could spell big changes for providers. *Provider,* 24–25, February 1990.

Martin, D. P., Hunt, J. R., Hughes-Stone, M., and Conrad, D. A. The Planetree model hospital project: An example of the patient as partner. *Hospital & Health Services Administration* 35(4):591–601, Winter 1990.

O'Hare, P. K., and Schmidt, W. T. Required reading: Federal disabilities act increases litigation risks for providers. *Health Progress,* 43–46, April 1991.

Quebe, J. L. The changing landscape of health care. *Health Care Strategic Management,* 4–10, December 1985.

Reilling, J., Knutzen, B., Wallen, T., McCullough, S., Miller, R., and Chernos, S. Enhancing the traditional hospital design process: A focus on patient safety. *Joint Commission Journal on Quality and Safety* 30(3):115–124, 2004.

Rostenberg, B. Alternative health care facilities: Design reflects quality image. *Trustee* 40(4):15–19, April 1987.

Sachner, P. A place of passage. *Architectural Record,* 104–5, November 1988.

Sahney, V. K., and Warden, G. L. The quest for quality and productivity in health services. *Frontiers of Health Services Management* 7(4):7–40, Summer 1991.

Scalise, D. Where the patient and technology meet. *Hospitals & Health Networks.* 79(8):34–38, 2005.

Shepley, M. M., and Wilson, P. Designing for persons with AIDS: A post-occupancy study at the Bailey-Boushay House. *Journal of Architectural and Planning Research* 16(1):17–32, Spring 1999.

Solomon, N. B. Advice from healthcare experts. *Architecture,* 75–81, July 1991.

Stuart, P., Parker, S., and Rogers, M. Giving a Voice to the Community. *Emergency Medicine* 15(4), August 2003.

Ulrich, R. S. Effects of interior design on wellness: Theory and recent scientific research. *Journal of Health Care Interior Design* 3:97–109, 1991.

US Department of Health and Human Services. Guidance on engagement of institutions in human subjects research. 2013. www.hhs.gov/ohrp/policy/engage08.html.

Walsh, S. Formulation of a plan of care for culturally diverse patients. *International Journal of Nursing Terminologies and Classifications* 15(10):17–25, 2004.

Waters, C. Professional nursing support for culturally diverse family members. *Research in Nursing & Health* 22:107–17, 1999.

Williams, M. Design for therapeutic outcomes. Paper presented at the Fourth Symposium of Healthcare Design, November 14–17, 1991, Boston.

Williams, M. A. The physical environment and patient care. *Annual Review of Nursing Research* 6:61–84, 1988.

Winkel, G. H., & Holahan, C. J. (1985). The environmental psychology of the hospital: Is the cure worse than the illness? *Journal of Prevention & Intervention in the Community* 4(1–2), 11–33.

Zenisus, N. The Pebble Project defined. *Healthcare Design* 8(1):30–32, January 2008.

Zimring, C., and Bosch, S. Building the evidence base for evidence-based design. *Environment & Behavior* 40(2):147–50, 2008.

Zimring, C., Rashid, M., and Kampschroer, K. Facility Performance Evaluation (FPE). *Whole Building Design Guide,* 2014. https://www.wbdg.org/resources/fpe.php.

CHAPTER 3

ARRIVAL AND EXTERIOR WAYFINDING

The journey from home to a healthcare facility can be stressful and confusing for first-time or unfamiliar patients and visitors. They need to make decisions at each stage of the journey: traveling to the facility, finding parking, locating the Main Entrance, becoming oriented once inside, and proceeding to first destinations.

There is no one typical experience shared by people traveling to a healthcare facility. Patients and visitors may be traveling from a few blocks away, from across town, from a nearby city, or from even farther away.

This chapter begins by looking at the needs of patients and visitors as they travel to a healthcare facility by car, taxi, or public transit. We examine components of the exterior wayfinding system that assist patients and visitors in making their way to their initial building destinations. Since many patients and visitors drive to health facilities, we also discuss parking facilities. Next, we cover the Main Entrance area, a transition zone where patients and visitors move into the health facility itself. The chapter then describes common first destinations: the Information Desk, the Admitting Department, and a Visitor Information Center.

Traveling to a Healthcare Facility

The design of health facilities should consider the variety of ways patients and visitors will arrive—by car, taxi, van, bus or other public transit—and the need for bus stops, taxi stands, parking areas, and pathways from these to major building entrances. (Some patients will also arrive by ambulance.) Finding the healthcare facility, making one's way to the Main Entrance, and then proceeding to the admitting department or other destination, all relatively

LEARNING OBJECTIVES
- Describe some wayfinding needs of patients and visitors traveling to a healthcare facility.
- Identify components of an effective exterior wayfinding system.
- Become familiar with features of parking facilities designed for patients and visitors.
- Understand some characteristics of a welcoming health facility Main Entrance area.
- Describe some design requirements of typical first destinations within a healthcare facility.

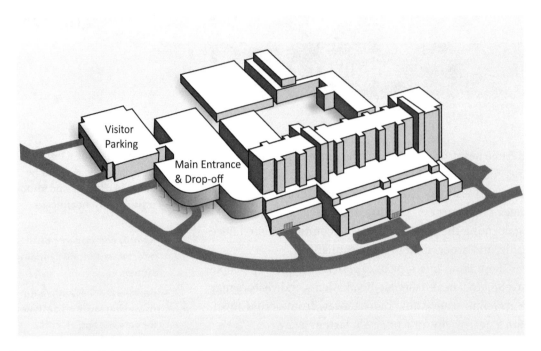

The arrival area at a health facility should be recognizable, provide a weather-protected Drop-off area, and have ample parking nearby. In this conceptual graphic, a canopy helps make the Drop-off and Main Entrance recognizable.

simple tasks under normal circumstances, become anything but routine when complicated by illness, injury, and/or emotional stress. Health facility design can add to stress, be neutral, or sometimes help mitigate it.

Arriving by Car

Many patients and visitors arrive by car, so it is important to provide the environmental and operational support they need. Several issues need to be addressed, including the ease with which drivers can find their way by following exterior signs and environmental cues; the location, availability, and cost of parking; and the parking needs of people with functional limitations.

Arriving by Taxi or Van

When arriving by taxi or van, patients and visitors will not need to worry about finding the way to the facility or locating the Main Entrance, since the drop-off area is usually close to the front door. Phone numbers for local taxi services should be posted near the Main Entrance and be available at information desks.

Arriving by Public Transit

If a public transit system is available, some patients and visitors will use it to travel to health facilities (Reizenstein, Grant, and Vaitkus, 1981). People who live nearby may use the bus system as a regular means of transportation. Visitors from out of town may find it more convenient to use the bus or hotel shuttle for their daily trips from a hotel to the healthcare facility rather than navigating to and from the facility, dealing with traffic, and paying for parking. (Although this discussion focuses on traveling by bus, the guidelines also apply to a rail system.)

Whether or not travelers are familiar with the local bus system, they need information about schedules, pick-up and drop-off points, and fares. Once they arrive at the bus stop closest to the healthcare facility, they also need to be able to find their way to the facility's Main Entrance.

A bus stop located adjacent to the Main Entrance of the healthcare facility will make it easier for users to find their way and will decrease the distance they have to walk. The bus stop should be easily visible from the Main Entrance, so patients and visitors will know how to return to it. Directional signs and maps at bus stops, including information designed for people with functional limitations, will aid wayfinding.

When patients and visitors leave a healthcare facility, they will also need a comfortable, accessible, weather-protected place to wait for their buses. They may have a lengthy wait, during cold or rainy weather. Ideally, the shelter should provide seating, weather protection, and heat, during cold weather. In addition, it should be well lit and safe, especially at night.

Bus schedules, route maps, fare information, information about public transit lines, and related website addresses should be available at the healthcare facility's Information Desk and within the bus shelter.

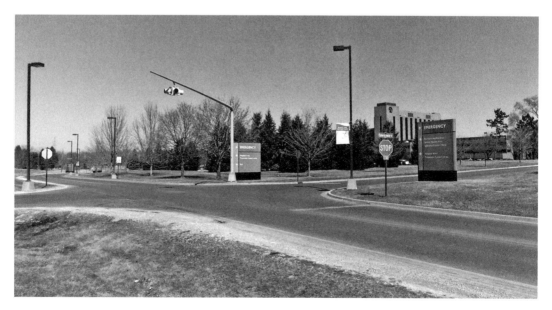

Exterior wayfinding signs provide unfamiliar patients and visitors with directional information at decision-points.
Photo credit: Courtesy of St. Joseph Mercy Ann Arbor

Exterior Wayfinding

Finding their way to a healthcare facility and navigating its roadways and parking areas can be difficult for first-time or otherwise unfamiliar patients and visitors. They need to be able to tell where to enter the healthcare facility site. They must be able to locate the Main Entrance drive and park their cars in a lot or garage. They must then be able to find the correct building within the complex, as well as the correct entrance. Each step of this journey requires "reading" the environment, negotiating decision-points (places where patients and visitors need to decide whether to go right, left, or continue straight ahead) and finding a series of destinations.

Without useful environmental cues and orientation aids (such as signs and maps), unfamiliar patients and visitors may become disoriented, resulting in a series of negative consequences (Carpman, Grant, and Simmons, 1984; Reizenstein et al., 1981). Information for arriving patients and visitors must be conveyed on site through signs, spoken directions, and cues in the environment itself (Rostenberg, 1987). (See Research Box 3.1.)

Some patients and visitors will seek online wayfinding information, use GPS or other digital devices, or receive written instructions or paper maps before a scheduled health facility visit. But not all patients and visitors are able to plan their visits ahead of time, including those coming to the Emergency Room as a result of accident or injury (Rostenberg, 1987).

Exterior Signage

Wayfinding sign messages in and around health facilities need to communicate clearly to unfamiliar patients and visitors. Signs direct users, identify key features of the environment, and inform them about what they should or should not do in order to make their way. Understandable signs help prevent confusion, frustration, and delay. The following example illustrates the problem with signs using wording that is confusing or otherwise incomprehensible to the people reading them:

> On a family swimming expedition as a child, I raced ahead of my parents only to return with the statement that we could not use that beach. "A large sign," I declared, "says 'Presbyterians only—vegetarians not allowed.'" My somewhat startled elders found upon inspection that it actually said "Pedestrians only—vehicles not allowed." (Marks, 1979, p. 94)

When patients and visitors first arrive at an unfamiliar medical complex, the sheer number of buildings may be confusing and hard to differentiate. (See Research Box 3.1.)

Exterior Sign Legibility

Sign messages are not the only factors determining the effectiveness of signs. If a sign cannot be easily seen because of its location or be easily read because of its fonts or letter sizes, its effectiveness will be diminished. When sightlines to an exterior sign are obstructed by trees, or when a sign's background color does not offer sufficient contrast with its text, signs may be of little use.

RESEARCH BOX 3.1 NAMING HOSPITAL BUILDINGS

Recognizing the importance of using understandable terminology for health facility buildings, researchers at the University of Michigan Medical Center conducted two related studies. In the first, patients and visitors were asked to suggest terms for a *parking structure, hospital, ambulatory care facility, medical center,* and *pedestrian bridge,* based on general descriptions of those types of places, e.g., "A building where people park their cars." In the second study, respondents were asked to choose the "best" and "worst" terms from a list (again, based on a general description) (Carpman, Grant, and Simmons, 1984).

Simple, familiar terms were chosen as "best" more often than were more complex or less familiar ones. Consequently, *general hospital* was preferred over *medical pavilion; outpatient clinic* was preferred over *professional office pavilion;* and *University of Michigan Hospitals* was preferred over *University of Michigan Health Sciences Center* and *University of Michigan Health Center.*

Design decision-makers developing an effective and understandable sign system face a complex and sometimes conflicting set of demands. The following are some rules of thumb for planning messages on exterior signs:

· Use destination terms consistently on all signs (for example, don't use the term *outpatient building* on one sign and *clinics* on another) (American Hospital Association, 1979; Marks, 1979).
· Keep sign messages short (no longer than two or three words per message, and fitting on a single line, if possible) so that drivers can read them quickly (Marks, 1979).
· Keep building names and other messages clear enough to be interpreted similarly by all users (American Hospital Association, 1979; Follis and Hammer, 1979; Marks, 1979).
· State messages in positive terms whenever possible (American Hospital Association, 1979; Marks, 1979).
· Use words and phrases that are well within a sixth-grade reading level (American Hospital Association, 1979).

A few suggestions may help ensure sign legibility:

• Mount signs perpendicular to the flow of automobile traffic, so they can be easily seen by drivers (American Hospital Association, 1979; Follis and Hammer, 1979).

• Locate signs within the viewer's 60-degree "cone of vision" (Follis and Hammer, 1979).

• Consider the effect of a sign's color scheme since certain color combinations are more legible than others. The combination black-on-yellow is most legible, followed by (in order) black-on-white, yellow-on-black, white-on-blue, yellow-on-blue, green-on-white, blue-on-yellow, white-on-green, white-on-brown, brown-on-yellow, brown-on-white, yellow-on-brown, red-on-white, yellow-on-red, and red-on-yellow, with white-on-red least legible (American Hospital Association, 1979; Institute for Signage Research, 1979; Passini, 1977; Wechsler, 1979; Weisman, 1985).

- Avoid color combinations that rely on red and green, since color-blind people (approximately 10 percent of the male population) may not be able to distinguish between these two colors (American Hospital Association, 1979; Institute for Signage Research, 1979; Passini, 1977; Wechsler, 1979; Weisman, 1985).

- Consider the legibility of fonts and letter sizes. Letter-size requirements for pedestrian signs are different (smaller) than requirements for vehicular signs.

- Provide outdoor signs that can be seen at night as well as during the day. There are a number of options for lighting exterior signs, including internal illumination, ground-mounted spot lighting, and reflective lettering.

Exterior Sign Messages

As patients and visitors drive to a healthcare facility, they need different levels of information at certain points along the journey. When they are far away, they need more general information and as they approach, they need more specific information. Such hierarchical systems common in large complexes, such as airports, help prevent patients and visitors from being overwhelmed with too much unnecessary information (Huelat, 2007; Selfridge, 1979).

Signs should successively direct drivers to designated highway exits, through the city or town, and to the Main Entrance of the healthcare facility. Along major arrival routes, hospital trailblazer signs should point drivers to the facility. At the site entrance, drivers should be directed to major building destinations. On site, exterior directional signs should provide information, as needed. As patients and visitors reach their building destinations, directional signs should direct them to parking options and building entrances.

Signs Related to Accessibility

Clear signage facilitates independent travel by directing people with mobility limitations to accessible parking areas, accessible routes, and drop-off areas. The international symbol of accessibility should be used consistently and as mandated by ADA guidelines, codes, or other regulations (Harkness and Groom, 1976).

Environmental Cues

Buildings and their surrounding landscapes can act as visual cues that help patients and visitors make wayfinding decisions (Huelat, 2007). When they see what they perceive as a path to their destination, they head toward it. (See Research Box 3.2.) Natural elements such as trees, hedges, and water or rock features can help draw visitors to certain areas (Huelat, 2007). Conversely, when views to destinations are obstructed by shrubs or trees, unfamiliar patients and visitors are unlikely to recognize their destinations and may miss them.

**RESEARCH BOX 3.2 COMPARING ARCHITECTURAL AND
SIGNAGE WAYFINDING CUES**

Designers at the University of Michigan Medical Center faced a potential wayfinding problem
when they tried to determine where to locate the entrances to a new public parking structure
(Carpman et al., 1985). The debate centered on the proposed relationship between the entrances to the parking structure and the circular drop-off drive at the hospital's Main Entrance.
Because the drive and the parking structure needed to be located in close proximity, one proposal was to construct an entrance to the parking structure accessed directly from the circular
drive (see option A on page 44), with an additional entrance from the main road. Proponents
of the scheme believed that this design would give drivers the option of entering the parking
structure after dropping someone off in front of the Main Entrance. It was argued that people
would read and follow signs and would turn into the circle only if they were dropping off a
passenger.

Another proposal was to have both entrances to the parking structure accessed from the main
road, away from the drop-off circle (see option B). Advocates of this scheme felt that having
an entrance located directly off the drop-off circle would attract drivers into the circle, causing
congestion.

Design research was seen as a way of resolving the issue. Rather than asking prospective drivers (in this case, visitors to the hospital) which scenario they would prefer, researchers decided
to ask them what they would actually do and how they would find their way, given a certain
situation.

Using two videotaped drive-throughs of a model of the entry area, the researchers simulated
the drive from the entrance of the medical campus to the drop-off circle. Responses to the
simulation showed that a substantial number of drivers would be drawn into the drop-off circle
when they could see the parking structure entrance. Respondents ignored the sign messages
that directed them to another entrance and instead followed the powerful visual cue. However, when no entrance to the parking structure was visible from the drop-off circle—that is,
when the visual cue was absent—participants were more likely to follow directional signs and
go straight to the parking structure entrance, bypassing the drop-off circle. Findings of the research influenced the initial design of the parking structure, which had no entrances off the
drop-off circle.

Exterior Handheld Maps

A well-designed exterior handheld map can help orient unfamiliar patients and visitors.
Maps can be sent to patients before scheduled appointments, can be available on the facility's

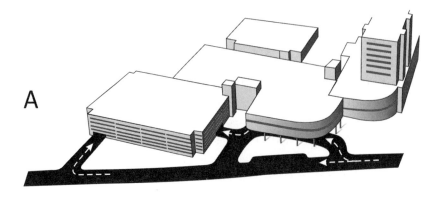

A

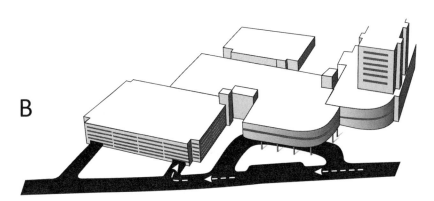

B

Drop-off circle option A shows an entrance to the visitor parking garage from the drop-off circle. Option B shows access to the visitor parking structure from the street, but no access from the drop-off circle.

website, and may be picked up on site. Maps should also be made available by referring physician offices.

Such maps need to be carefully designed to convey information clearly. They should include:

- An area map showing arrival routes from nearby expressways and streets
- A detailed map of the health facility site, showing buildings, parking structures and lots, adjacent streets, and public entrances
- Written directions to the facility

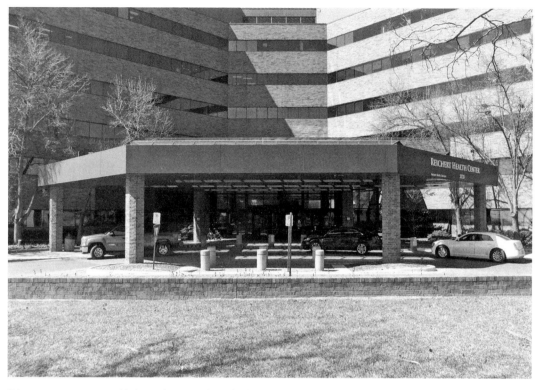

This entrance area is recognizable from a distance and provides shelter as drivers drop off and pick up patients.

Photo credit: Courtesy of St. Joseph Mercy Ann Arbor

Main Entrance Drop-Off Area

Because a health facility's Main Entrance is likely to be the first area experienced by unfamiliar patients and visitors, it should provide a pleasant and friendly first impression (Arneill and Frasca-Beaulieu, 2003; Chance, 1997).

Many healthcare facilities, especially hospitals, provide covered Drop-Off/Pick-Up areas at the Main Entrance. Such areas make the Main Entrance easily recognizable and offer weather protection. Attendants may be posted there to offer assistance.

When designing a Drop-Off/Pick-Up area for a healthcare facility, consider the following:

• Locate the Drop-Off area immediately adjacent to the Main Entrance.

• Provide sheltered access to the building.

• If a Drop-Off area is partially enclosed and likely to have poor air circulation, consider providing an exhaust evacuation system (Cobb, 1990).

• Provide an accessible route between the Drop-Off area and the area inside the Main Entrance. Follow ADA Guidelines, opting for flat surfaces (Cobb, 1990).

- Choose paving materials that are not slippery when wet and that will ensure a smooth ride for patients using wheeled mobility aids, such as wheelchairs.

- Consider stationing an attendant at the Drop-Off area to provide directions and assist patients getting into and out of cars.

- Design the Drop-Off area to allow ample room for cars dropping off and picking up patients, as well as for those driving through.

- In areas that experience snow and ice, consider installing a snow-melting system (Cobb, 1990).

- Provide ample parking near the Main Entrance and mark the route to and from parking with clear signage.

- Locate a taxi stand near the Main Entrance in a place that will not cause congestion in the Drop-Off area.

Parking

Safety, physical comfort, convenience, and accessibility need to be considered when designing health-facility parking lots and garages (Chance, 1997). Decision-makers also need to consider parking rates and whether or not to offer valet parking.

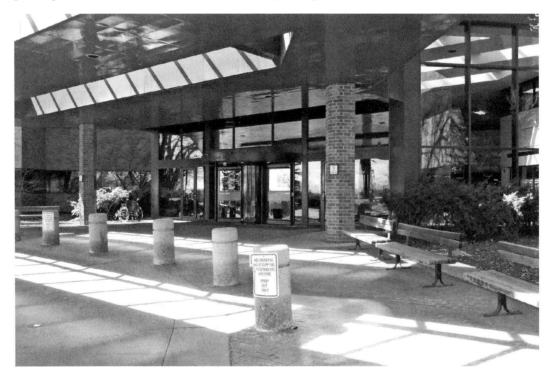

Providing seating at building entrances is important for patients who wait as their drivers park or return from parking. This entrance features bollards, which contribute to safety by separating pedestrian areas from driving lanes.

Photo credit: Courtesy of St. Joseph Mercy Ann Arbor

Valet Parking

Many large medical centers offer valet parking as a service that offsets the difficulties for patients and visitors of searching for parking, walking long distances from parking to the health-facility entrance, and dealing with inclement weather. In addition, valet-parking attendants can greet patients and visitors, assist them with getting into and out of cars, load belongings and medical equipment, and provide wheelchairs, as needed. There is usually an additional charge for valet parking (Thames, 1987).

Parking Lots

Many healthcare facilities provide public parking lots in addition to or in place of parking structures. Drivers typically locate the building entrance they need and then seek a nearby parking lot. The Main Entrance, Day Surgery, Emergency, medical office buildings, and other destinations may have their own parking lots. There may also be large parking lots designated for "Public" or "Patient and Visitor" parking.

Within parking lots, accessible parking spaces should be marked with the universal symbol of accessibility and located close to building entrances. In order to use these spaces, drivers must have special hang tags or license plates.

Aside from finding the correct parking lot and a vacant parking space as they enter the healthcare-facility site, patients and visitors will be most challenged by finding their cars after their visit. Design decision-makers can alleviate the stress associated with "losing" one's car (i.e., forgetting its location) by providing identification signs that help drivers notice and remember where they parked.

Parking lots are typically illuminated by regularly spaced lights located at the top of tall poles. In addition to providing lighting during inclement weather and after dark, these poles provide useful locations for parking lot and row identification signs, which should be placed high enough to see over the tops of cars and vans. In smaller lots with only a few rows, only the lot itself needs a unique label. In larger lots where finding their cars will be challenging for patients and visitors, providing frequent lot/row identification signs will help ensure that they see a sign on the way in, as they exit their cars. If they take note of the lot and row, hopefully they will remember it on the way back.

Health facilities should consider providing emergency communication systems in parking lots, as well as in parking structures.

The following suggestions can help with the design of parking lots:

- In parking lots with more than a few rows, provide row identification signs that are easy to read from a distance.
- At health facilities with multiple parking lots, provide signs that clearly identify the lot and the row, and place signs frequently enough so that drivers will see a sign no matter where they park.
- Provide shuttle buses and lighted shuttle bus shelters in large parking lots.

- Provide emergency call devices at shuttle bus shelters and at other locations in parking lots.

Parking Structures

Many large health facilities build multi-story parking structures in order to provide a large number of sheltered parking spaces in a limited area. However, some patients and visitors are reluctant to use parking structures that they perceive to be confusing or unsafe, even if this is not the case (Anderson, 1994). Logical layouts, effective lighting, and well-thought-out signage can help make parking structures safe, secure, and easy to navigate (New Hospital Garage, 1996).

Healthcare facilities may wish to consider installing commercial safety systems in their parking structures. One author (Speyer, 1987) recommends the following steps:

- Obtain a comprehensive appraisal of threat potential and security needs for the parking structure.
- Develop and document a plan for "adequate or reasonable" security.
- Implement a security system with the aid of a professional security company.
- Make provisions for maintenance and annual testing of the system.
- Keep records of security evaluations and protective measures taken.

Other parking structure concerns involve wayfinding. In addition to the basic layout and vehicular and pedestrian circulation patterns, the following suggestions can make parking structures easier to navigate:

- Provide effective, uniform illumination on parking, driving, and wall surfaces (Kirkpatrick and Cudney, 1992).
- Use lighting to highlight stairs and elevators (Kirkpatrick and Cudney, 1992; New Hospital Garage, 1996).
- Select sign colors that will be legible under various lighting conditions (Kirkpatrick and Cudney, 1992).
- Locate signs at key decision-points (Kirkpatrick and Cudney, 1992).
- Provide pedestrian and vehicular directional signs to help visitors find important destinations such as elevators and stairs (Kirkpatrick and Cudney, 1992).
- Clearly identify parking rows and parking structure levels. Whitewash walls and ceilings to reflect light and create a brighter atmosphere (Anderson, 1994; Kirkpatrick and Cudney, 1992).
- Paint fire-protection elements red for easy identification (Kirkpatrick and Cudney, 1992).

- Provide emergency intercoms or telephones at major entrances, exits, and lobby areas (Kirkpatrick and Cudney, 1992).

If patients or visitors require medical or other emergency attention within the parking area, help needs to be readily available. For instance, the parking structure floor-to-ceiling height must allow ambulance access. Installing and maintaining an emergency communication system, video cameras, and effective lighting within the parking area will provide an extra measure of security. Security guards or attendants should be available to help people in need.

Park-and-Ride Options

In urban areas, finding enough space for parking is an ongoing problem, and patient and visitor parking areas may be located some distance from the main facility. Although perhaps not an optimal solution, a remote parking lot with a frequent shuttle bus may be an acceptable option when visitor parking cannot be provided close by. For example, when visitors to the University of Michigan Medical Center were asked whether they would be willing to park their cars in a parking lot a mile away if it was served by a shuttle bus leaving every 15 minutes, two-thirds said that they would be willing to do so (Reizenstein et al., 1981). Other considerations when healthcare organizations develop a shuttle-bus system include security (especially at night), effective signage, and weather-protected bus shelters with comfortable seating. In addition—and regardless of the location of the parking lot—row/area and directional signs should be legible throughout.

Long-Term Parking Rates

To help recoup the costs of constructing, running, and maintaining parking garages, many healthcare organizations charge for parking. For the patient or companion visiting the facility for a short time, a standard parking fee may seem reasonable, but for patients or visitors spending several hours a day at a facility over a period of weeks or months, the standard parking fee may be seen as a burden (Reizenstein et al., 1981). In setting parking fees, a facility sends a symbolic message. Providing lower long-term fees or free parking for patients and visitors, subsidized by rates charged to other users, might be a useful—and caring—marketing strategy.

Transition between Parking and the Building Entrance Area

Once patients and visitors park in a lot, they need to figure out how to proceed from parking to the needed building entrance, which may or may not be in view. Pedestrian directional signs, identification signs, and exterior You-Are-Here maps will help patients and visitors get where they need to be.

Patients and visitors who park in a structure have a different set of wayfinding challenges. They must find the correct elevator and then determine the correct level on which to exit, in order to proceed to their building. Parking structures located right next to healthcare facilities may be connected on more than one floor. When parking structures serve several buildings, choosing the correct exit (and finding it again on their return) becomes part of the wayfinding puzzle for patients and visitors. In cases like these, it will be helpful to provide vehicular and pedestrian directional signs at decision-points on each level of parking structures. You-Are-Here maps, placed at strategic decision-points, will also help patients and visitors understand where they are and how to get to their destinations without experiencing stress and delays.

The following suggestions can help with planning the transition from parking to building entrance areas:

- In health facilities with several public entrances, provide pedestrian directional signs and You-Are-Here maps at strategic locations at the edges of parking lots.

- In parking structures that connect to buildings on more than one level, provide information about exit floors. Clearly identify exit points.

- In parking structures that serve several buildings, provide pedestrian directional signs and You-Are-Here maps at pedestrian exits.

The Main Entrance Area

In many ways the Main Entrance sets the tone for the healthcare facility (Olsen and Pershing, 1981). It provides a transition zone from the exterior to the interior environment. The Main Entrance is a place to obtain information, become oriented to the layout of the facility, and wait for transportation. When sensitively designed, the Main Entrance area can provide a welcoming and calming environment (Arneill and Frasca-Beaulieu, 2003; Chance, 1997).

Becoming Oriented

As they enter a healthcare facility, patients and visitors want to know where they are and where to go next. Well-designed signs and maps near an Information Desk can help orient them to the facility and introduce its wayfinding system. This will help them recognize directional information as they encounter it throughout the facility.

Although some patients and visitors have little or no trouble finding their way, those who are unfamiliar with the facility may easily become lost (Carpman, Grant, and Simmons, 1984; Reizenstein et al., 1981; Shumaker and Reizenstein, 1982). A wayfinding system consisting of an obvious entrance area, signs, effective lighting, You-Are-Here maps, and other features can help direct visitors and patients from their parking spots or other drop-off points to their destinations (Rostenberg, 1987).

You-Are-Here (YAH) maps aid orientation in and around health facilities. Placing a YAH map at the pedestrian exit of the parking area allows people to gain an overall understanding of the site layout and plan the most direct route to their destinations.

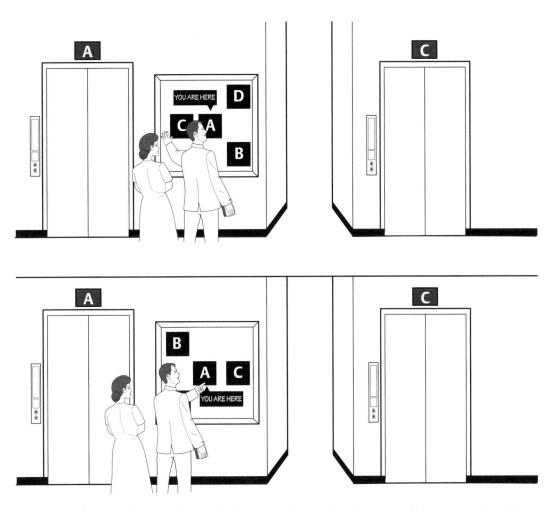

When a You-Are-Here map is misaligned, as in the top drawing, users need to mentally realign the map, which can cause confusion. When a You-Are-Here map is correctly aligned so that forward in space is "up" on the map, it is easier to use.

Source: M. Levine. You-are-here maps: Psychological considerations. *Environment and Behavior* 14(2):221–37, March 1982. Copyright 1982 Sage Publications, Inc. Redrawn, with changes, by permission of Sage Publications, Inc.

In order to effectively orient unfamiliar users, it is essential that YAH map information be presented clearly and the map itself should be oriented so that forward in space is "up" on the map (Levine, 1992). For example, if the visitor is facing east while looking at the map, the map should be oriented so that east is at the top of the map. The map's location should be carefully selected. Being able to identify objects or structures on the map that they can also see around them helps viewers become oriented. Users need at least two points of reference on the map in order for it to be useful. A correctly placed You-Are-Here symbol is one point of reference, and a prominent building or landmark could be the other. Labeling additional objects and buildings will provide more reference points.

Access for People with Functional Limitations

Entering a healthcare facility may be challenging for people with temporary or permanent functional limitations who are trying to make their way from the parking area or drop-off point to the destination entrance (American Hospital Association, 1979; English Tourist Board, 1983; Harkness and Groom, 1976; Kamisar, 1979). In some instances, the journey may require travel from an upper floor of a parking structure, along sidewalks, and across a number of streets. A number of design features can help, including ample parking space width, location of accessible parking close to an exit, an accessible route that does not conflict with automobile traffic, and paving materials that are smooth, rather than bumpy. (See chapter 9.)

Wheelchair users may need to transfer from a car to a wheelchair. This process is easier if the parking space is on a level grade and if the space is wide enough (12 feet or ~3.7 meters) to allow the car door to open to its fullest position. Vans equipped with a side wheelchair lift need 16 feet (~4.9 meters). Although most accessible parking spots should be on a parking structure level with direct access into the health facility, occasionally wheelchair users will have to park elsewhere. It is important that they be able to enter elevator lobbies and elevators. If there is a curb, access ramps should be provided. Elevators should be at least 4 feet

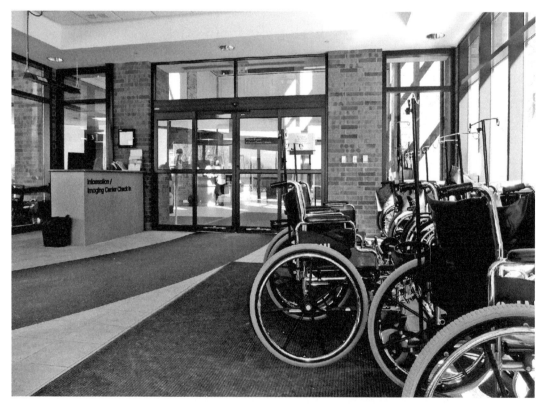

Since some patients need to borrow wheelchairs, it's useful to provide dedicated storage areas at health facility entrances.
Photo credit: Courtesy of St. Joseph Mercy Ann Arbor

3 inches by 5 feet 8 inches (~1.3 meters by ~1.7 meters) to accommodate a wheelchair. Elevator controls should be placed within reach, at a maximum height of 48 inches (1.2 meters) (American Hospital Association, 1979; English Tourist Board, 1983; Harkness and Groom, 1976; Kamisar, 1979). Always follow the most current ADA Guidelines. (See chapter 9.)

Once people with functional limitations reach street level, they may still face barriers. People with vision limitations need to be able to follow the desired route and avoid physical obstacles in their path. They also need to be able to determine an effective route and safely walk along that route. Design features can help, including signage with tactile lettering or Braille; sidewalks free from obstructions such as street furniture and equipment; and sidewalk textural indicators relating to building entrances and transitions to streets. People with hearing limitations need to be able to follow the desired route safely without requiring spoken directions. It is particularly important that signs and maps be available to direct them to their destinations. Warning signals like those used on emergency vehicles should provide visual as well as auditory cues (Carpman, Grant, and Norton, 1984).

Sidewalk design is particularly important for people with mobility limitations:

- Build sidewalks wide enough to allow two wheelchairs to pass easily, at least 5 feet (~1.5 meters) wide (American Hospital Association, 1979; English Tourist Board, 1983; Harkness and Groom, 1976; Kamisar, 1979).

- Eliminate obstructions (such as grates) that may catch wheels or crutches.

- Keep benches or other street furniture away from the circulation path.

- Provide curb cuts at street crossings at a low enough grade to be accessible (American Hospital Association, 1979; English Tourist Board, 1983; Harkness and Groom, 1976; Kamisar, 1979).

- Design grades to be flat enough to allow easy movement. If grades must be greater than 5 percent, provide handrails.

- Avoid the use of brick and other uneven paving materials that might create a bumpy ride for wheelchair users or hazards for people using walkers or pushing strollers.

Sometimes Main Entrance areas can become congested and confusing. Consideration should be given to people, such as seniors or those with functional limitations, who have difficulty moving about, finding their way, or handling their belongings. Staff or volunteers may be needed to give directions, assist patients and visitors with belongings, or provide needed information.

To accommodate some of the needs of patients and visitors in Main Entrance areas, consider the following (English Tourist Board, 1983; Harkness and Groom, 1976):

- Select doors that are easily negotiable by wheelchair users, people using walkers, or people with vision limitations. Turnstiles and revolving doors may prove hazardous to people who move with some difficulty and may be inaccessible for wheelchair users or people with strollers.

- Provide doors that can be easily opened by people with little upper-body strength. The force needed to open a door should not exceed 8 pounds. Consider specifying automatic doors that open with a pressure-sensitive mat, a wall-mounted push plate, or an electronic eye.

- Avoid obstructions at the Main Entrance. For example, mud mats and pressure-sensitive mats should be flush with the floor. This will allow a wheelchair or stroller to easily maneuver over them.

- Provide space out of the flow of traffic for storing wheelchairs.

- Ensure that restrooms are nearby and in view from the Main Entrance.

Waiting in the Main Entrance Area

Patients and visitors waiting to be picked up by a companion, taxi, van, or bus need a comfortable and safe place to wait and a view to the Drop-Off/Pick-Up area. Main Entrance areas need to be large enough to accommodate people arriving, departing, and waiting. These Main Entrance areas need to offer comfortable places to sit, convenient places to put belongings, and access to nearby restrooms. In addition, Main Entrance areas should provide taxi information,

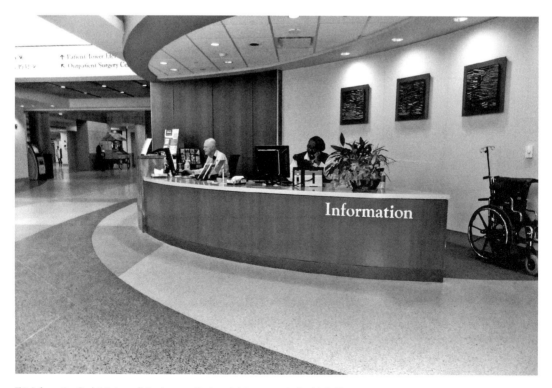

This Information Desk is in immediate view as patients and visitors enter the health facility.

Photo credit: Courtesy of St. Joseph Mercy Ann Arbor

exterior maps, transit schedules, and signs directing users out of the building and back to the bus stop, parking lot, or parking structure.

First Destinations

Patients' and visitors' first contacts with healthcare staff may be at an Information Desk, Admitting or Registration, or a Visitor Information Center.

Information Desk

An Information Desk may serve a variety of functions. It welcomes patients and visitors. It provides a place where they can ask questions about appointments, restrooms, patient room locations, hours of operation, availability of services, public transportation, parking, eating facilities, and the like. Attendants at Information Desks can help orient patients and visitors to the facility by providing maps and directions. Some healthcare facilities, such as those designed following the Planetree model discussed in chapter 2, may have dedicated information-services staff who formally greet patients and visitors, in an effort to create a more welcoming environment (Arneill and Frasca-Beaulieu, 2003).

The effectiveness of Information Desks can be increased by design:

- Provide direct visual access to the Information Desk from the Main Entrance.
- Provide legible signage identifying the Information Desk.
- Provide visual access from the Information Desk to the Main Entrance so staff members can see entering patients and visitors.
- Design the Information Desk to look different from other counters or windows in the Main Entrance area, such as the Cashier, the Security Desk, or the Reception area for the Admitting Department.
- Make the Information Desk accessible and welcoming to all users. Allow enough surrounding circulation space to prevent congestion.
- Provide a portion of the counter that is low enough—30–33 inches (~76–84 centimeters) high—for wheelchair users to talk comfortably with staff or to fill out forms (Harkness and Groom, 1976).
- Provide direction-giving training for Information Desk staff. (See Research Box 3.3.) Consider providing handheld maps patients and visitors can take with them.

Admitting or Registration

Admitting or Registration are often among the first destinations for patients arriving at a healthcare facility. Some admissions procedures require patients and their companions to wait, fill out forms, have interviews with staff, and visit one or more ancillary services before settling into a patient room. During this process, patients and companions need a comfortable place to wait and a private place to hold confidential conversations with hospital staff.

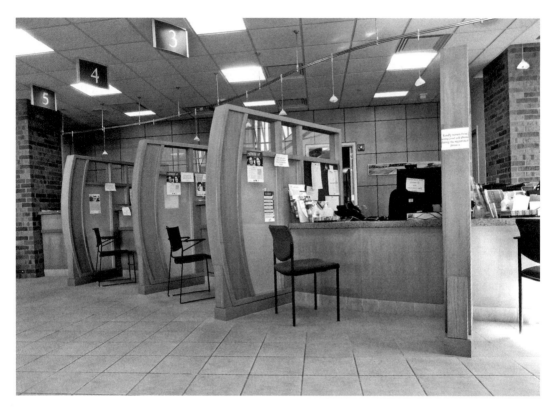

Partial walls at an Admitting or Registration area help protect patients' confidential information by providing some acoustical and visual privacy.

Photo credit: Courtesy of St. Joseph Mercy Ann Arbor

RESEARCH BOX 3.3   USING THE INFORMATION DESK AS A WAYFINDING AID

As part of an entry area analysis during a renovation project, researchers at Bellevue Hospital in New York City examined the relationship between the interaction with Information Desk staff and subsequent wayfinding difficulties (Olsen and Pershing, 1981).

Seventy-four percent of the interviewed patients stopped at the Information Desk before proceeding to their various destinations. Eighty percent of this group thought they had received accurate directions. The important role played by Information Desk staff in orientation is shown by the fact that the vast majority of those who thought they were given accurate directions experienced no major problems finding their destinations. Another 20 percent of interviewed patients and visitors who stopped at the information Desk thought that they had been given incorrect information. As a result, most of these patients and visitors experienced wayfinding difficulties.

Obviously, not all patients and visitors who enter the facility will stop at the Information Desk, but its availability and staffing are crucial for those who are unfamiliar with the facility.

The ability of the facility to meet these needs is linked with environmental design in the following ways (Valenta, 1981) (see Research Box 3.4):

• To help ensure acoustical privacy, provide private offices, tall partitions, acoustic barriers, or spatial separations of task areas.

• Store electronic and written records in ways that ensure patient confidentiality.

• Provide staff and patients with a comfortable conversational distance between one another.

• Keep passageways clear of obstructions, provide chairs that do not tip over easily, and eliminate furniture with protruding or sharp edges.

• Provide accessible pathways to desks, seating areas, and circulation areas.

RESEARCH BOX 3.4 ADMITTING DEPARTMENT DESIGN AND PATIENT NEEDS

The relationship between behavioral needs and design in 26 admitting departments was explored in a detailed study (Valenta, 1981). Four design-related needs were examined: confidentiality (privacy), communication, safety and security, and stress reduction. Although this study examined only the admitting staff's *perceptions of patient needs* and how well they were being met by existing environmental conditions, it provides valuable insights into links between health facility design and behavior.

Confidentiality (privacy)

Admitting staff considered confidentiality to be the patient's most significant need. While being admitted to the hospital, patients must report, both verbally and in writing, a wide range of personal information concerning their health history and financial status as well as current health problems. The researcher found that the overall design of the department and the proximity of spaces within the department affected *perceived* confidentiality and privacy. An open plan, with limited visual and acoustical privacy, was generally disliked by staff. They believed that an open plan compromised both the patient's privacy and their own as well. While partitions and private offices increased the perception of confidentiality, the researcher found that actual acoustical privacy was not appreciably increased in areas with these design features.

Communication

Communication refers to those design features that increase or decrease the ability to have successful conversations. Increasing communication was seen by the staff as the patient's second-most urgent need. Reducing noise levels and other distractions increased communication. Interestingly, symbolic aspects of the design were also considered important. Furniture arrangements (such as the spatial arrangement, proximity of chairs, and the use of a

(continued)

RESEARCH BOX 3.4. (*Continued*)

desk as a potential barrier) were seen as indicators of communication. Other symbolic factors, such as whether patients and staff were supplied chairs of equal quality, were also linked to communication.

Safety and Security

Although admitting staff were naturally concerned about their own security and the security of their belongings, they were more worried about the patient's safety while in the admitting department. In particular, they thought that some chairs could easily be tipped over, that some spaces were too small to allow safe wheelchair access, and that some surfaces had dangerously protruding sharp edges.

Stress Reduction

Being admitted to a hospital is a stress-inducing experience. However, design elements can be used to reduce stress. Admitting staff taking part in this study believed that stress reduction was the patient's least-urgent need, whereas they rated it as their own second-most urgent need (behind communication). Ambient factors seemed to be particularly important in stress reduction: the ability to control noise, thermal comfort (temperature and humidity), and lighting. Staff preferred to have natural light available. They considered easy wayfinding an important stress reducer.

Storage Areas

During winter weather, people bundle up with coats, hats, scarves, and gloves. For outpatients who may be visiting a number of different departments, or visitors who spend hours shuttling between patient rooms, waiting areas, and the cafeteria, keeping track of personal belongings may become a nuisance (Reizenstein et al., 1981). A simple solution to this problem would be to provide coin return lockers or a coat check area where belongings could be checked and securely stored.

Visitor Information

Family members and visitors of hospital patients often experience stress for at least two reasons: worrying about their loved ones and coping with an unfamiliar setting, including rules, procedures, staff, and medical issues. Visitors are often the forgotten users of a hospital. Even though they are present in large numbers, they typically have no official role, no connection with the administration, and no space of their own. Their needs for information and reassurance may not be met (Reizenstein and Grant, 1981).

Visitors may be reluctant to approach the nursing or medical staff for information, fearing that they may not be able to make contact, may not receive understandable answers to questions, or that their patient may be penalized in some way by family members' questions. This fear and isolation leads some visitors to perceive their concerns as insignificant and results in reluctance to find solutions (Reizenstein et al., 1981). One approach to relieving this "invisible visitor syndrome" is to provide a central area where visitors can bring general questions and concerns. In some facilities, Information Desk staff or concierges provide visitors and family members with needed services and information about parking, overnight accommodations, restaurants, shopping, Wi-Fi, and the like (Reizenstein et al., 1981; Zimring, Carpman, and Michelson, 1987). A dedicated Visitor Information Center could provide visitors with more in-depth answers and more opportunity for interaction with helpful staff.

Summary

- The journey from home to a healthcare facility can be stressful and confusing for first-time or unfamiliar patients and visitors. They need to make decisions at each stage of the journey: traveling to the facility, finding parking, locating the Main Entrance, becoming oriented once inside, and proceeding to first destinations.

- Whether traveling by car, taxi, van, or public transit, patients and visitors are often under emotional stress and/or physical duress. They need legible signage with understandable wording. Wayfinding information needs to be provided in a hierarchy from general to specific. Other components of a successful wayfinding system include handheld and You-Are-Here maps, visual cues from buildings and landscaping, and signs containing information about accessibility.

- Parking facilities must be designed and maintained for safety, convenience, and accessibility. Parking structures and parking lots require good lighting, visibility, and effective signage at key decision-points and destinations.

- The Main Entrance area should appear welcoming, providing easy access to a Drop-Off area, weather protection, and attention to the needs of people with functional limitations. There should be room and accommodations for people waiting, effective signage and maps, and information about taxis and public transportation.

- The main Information Desk should be accessible and welcoming to all users, visually distinct from other counters and windows, with direct visual access to the Main Entrance area.

- The Admitting Department should provide for patients' visual and acoustical privacy and stress reduction. It should offer a comfortable place to wait and ample circulation space.

DISCUSSION QUESTIONS

1. What factors increase the difficulties of patients and visitors in locating a healthcare facility, finding their way to the Main Entrance, and proceeding to an Admitting Department?

2. What are some considerations in designing and locating an effective exterior sign system?

3. How can site layout and signage assist patients and visitors arriving by public transportation?

4. What are some requirements for a well-designed Main Entrance and Drop-Off area?

5. What factors contribute to the design of safe and navigable parking structures and parking lots?

6. What are some design considerations related to signage, parking, Main Entrance design, and first destinations for people with functional limitations?

7. What are some factors related to location, design, and staffing policies that can contribute to the effectiveness of Information Desks?

8. What are some primary patient needs related to the design of an Admitting area?

9. What is "invisible visitor syndrome," and what are some responses to this problem?

Design Review Questions

Traveling to a Healthcare Facility

Arriving by Public Transit

☐ Will a bus stop be located near (adjacent to or easily accessible from) the facility?

☐ Will a bus stop be visible from the Main Entrance?

☐ Will signs and maps (including audible and tactile messages) be available to assist patients and visitors in finding bus stops? (American Hospital Association, 1979; Harkness and Groom, 1976)

☐ Will there be a bus shelter?

☐ Will the bus shelter be comfortable, large enough, and weather-protected, with ample seating and effective lighting at night?

☐ Will bus schedules, route maps, and fare schedules be available to patients and visitors at the main Information Desk?

☐ Will phone numbers for local taxi services be posted near the Main Entrance and available at information desks?

Exterior Wayfinding

Exterior Signage

☐ Will destination messages be used consistently on exterior signs? (American Hospital Association, 1979; Marks, 1979)

☐ Will exterior sign messages be short so that drivers can read them quickly? (American Hospital Association, 1979; Marks, 1979)

☐ Will building names and other exterior sign messages be clear enough to be interpreted similarly by all users? (American Hospital Association, 1979; Follis and Hammer, 1979; Marks, 1979)

☐ Will sign messages be stated in positive terms whenever possible? (American Hospital Association, 1979; Marks, 1979)

☐ Will sign messages fit within a sixth-grade reading level? (American Hospital Association, 1979)

Design That Cares: Planning Health Facilities for Patients and Visitors, third edition, by Janet R. Carpman and Myron A. Grant. ©2016 by Jossey-Bass.

Exterior Sign Legibility

☐ Will exterior signs be oriented perpendicular to the flow of traffic? (American Hospital Association, 1979; Follis and Hammer, 1979)

☐ Will exterior signs be located so as to be within the viewer's 60-degree "cone of vision"? (Follis and Hammer, 1979)

☐ Will the color relationship between exterior sign text and background provide sufficient contrast? (American Hospital Association, 1979; Institute for Signage Research, 1979; Passini, 1977; Wechsler, 1979; Weisman, 1982)

☐ To accommodate people who are colorblind, will colors be used other than red and green? (American Hospital Association, 1979; Passini, 1977; Wechsler, 1979; Weisman, 1985)

☐ Will letter sizes on signs be large enough, and messages short enough, to be read by drivers traveling at posted speeds? (American Hospital Association, 1979)

☐ Will exterior signs be visible and legible at night as well as during the day?

Exterior Sign Messages

☐ Will the sign system be designed to give drivers different levels of information (from general to specific) at different points along the journey? (Selfridge, 1979)

☐ Will offsite trailblazer signs and directional signs direct drivers to the facility from nearby expressways and along major arrival routes? (Selfridge, 1979)

☐ Will directional signs direct drivers to parking and major destinations, including the Emergency Entrance? (Selfridge, 1979)

☐ Will pedestrian directional signs direct patients and visitors from parking to building entrances and back? (Selfridge, 1979)

Signs Related to Accessibility

☐ Will signage direct people with mobility limitations to accessible parking areas and accessible routes and Drop-Off areas?

☐ Will the international symbol of accessibility be used consistently?

Environmental Cues

☐ Will buildings and building entrances be distinctive and recognizable?

☐ Will landscaping allow unobstructed views to signs, intersections, and building entrances? (Carpman et al., 1985)

Design That Cares: Planning Health Facilities for Patients and Visitors, third edition, by Janet R. Carpman and Myron A. Grant. ©2016 by Jossey-Bass.

Exterior Handheld Maps

☐ Will handheld maps include an area map showing arrival routes from nearby expressways and major streets?

☐ Will handheld maps include a detailed map of the healthcare facility's site, showing buildings, parking structures and lots, adjacent streets, and major entrances?

☐ Will handheld maps include written directions to the healthcare facility?

Main Entrance and Drop-Off Area

☐ Will a Drop-Off area be located adjacent to the Main Entrance?

☐ Will sheltered access to the building be provided at the Main Entrance?

☐ Will the Main Entrance area be accessible to people with mobility limitations?

☐ Will smooth paving materials be selected so people using wheeled devices (such as wheelchairs, walkers, and strollers) can avoid a bumpy ride?

☐ Will an attendant be available to assist patients making their way between their cars and the building entrance?

☐ If the Main Entrance contains a confined canopy with poor air circulation, will an exhaust evacuation system be provided? (Cobb, 1990)

☐ In areas that experience snow and ice, will a snow-melting system be provided? (Cobb, 1990)

☐ Will the Drop-Off area be designed with ample room for cars dropping off and picking up patients and for those driving through?

☐ Will nearby parking be provided?

☐ Will a taxi stand be located nearby in a place that doesn't contribute to traffic congestion?

Parking

Valet Parking

☐ Will a valet parking service be provided? (Thames, 1987)

☐ Will valet parking attendants be trained in hospitality and customer experience? (Thames, 1987)

Parking Lots

☐ In parking lots with more than a few rows, will row identification signs be easy to read from a distance?

☐ At health facilities with multiple parking lots, will signs clearly identify the lot and the row? Will identification signs be placed frequently enough that drivers will see a sign no matter where they park?

☐ For facilities with large parking lots, will shuttle buses and lighted shuttle-bus shelters be available?

☐ Will emergency call devices be provided at shuttle-bus shelters and at other locations in parking lots?

Parking Structures

☐ Will patients' security needs in parking structures be assessed? (Speyer, 1987)

☐ Will a plan be in place for a parking-structure security system? (Speyer, 1987)

☐ Will provisions be made for maintenance and annual testing of the parking-structure security system? (Speyer, 1987)

☐ Will records be kept of security evaluations and protective measures? (Speyer, 1987)

☐ Will emergency intercoms or telephones be provided within parking structures at major entrances, exits, and lobby areas? (Kirkpatrick and Cudney, 1992)

☐ Will uniform illumination be provided throughout the parking structure? (Kirkpatrick and Cudney, 1992)

☐ Will lighting be used to highlight parking-structure destinations such as stairs and elevators? (Kirkpatrick and Cudney, 1992)

☐ Will sign colors be legible during the day and after dark? (Kirkpatrick and Cudney, 1992)

☐ Will wayfinding signs be located at key decision-points? (Kirkpatrick and Cudney, 1992)

☐ Will pedestrian and vehicular directional signs be provided?

☐ Will parking rows and parking structure levels be clearly identified? (Carpman, Grant, and Simmons, 1984)

☐ Will walls be whitewashed to reflect light and create a bright environment? (Kirkpatrick and Cudney, 1992)

☐ Will fire-protection elements be painted red for easy identification? (Kirkpatrick and Cudney, 1992)

☐ Will the parking-structure floor-to-ceiling height allow ambulance access to all areas?

☐ Will video cameras be available to provide surveillance of the parking area?

Park-and-Ride Options

☐ If patient and visitor parking is not within easy walking distance of the facility, will shuttle buses be available at frequent intervals?

☐ Will a comfortable, safe, weather-protected place with seating be available for those waiting for shuttle buses?

Long-Term Parking Rates

☐ Will the facility consider instituting reduced or free long-term parking fees? (Reizenstein et al., 1981)

Transition between Parking and the Main Entrance Area

☐ In health facilities with several public entrances, will pedestrian directional signs and You-Are-Here maps be located at strategic locations at the edges of parking lots?

☐ In parking structures that connect to buildings on more than one level, will there be information about exit floors? Will exit points be clearly identified?

☐ In parking structures that serve several buildings, will pedestrian directional signs and You-Are-Here maps be placed at pedestrian exits?

☐ Will effective illumination be provided along pedestrian routes from parking lots and parking structures to building entrances?

☐ Will building entrances be clearly identified?

The Main Entrance Area

☐ Will the Drop-Off and Main Entrance area provide effective weather protection?

☐ Will mud walk-off mats be provided?

☐ Will the Main Entrance area be spacious enough to minimize congestion?

Becoming Oriented

☐ Will wayfinding signs guide patients and visitors from parking and drop-off to the Main Entrance?

☐ Will exterior You-Are-Here (YAH) maps be available to orient patients and visitors to the layout of the site?

☐ Will directional signs and interior YAH maps be provided near the main Information Desk, at elevator lobbies, and at other potentially confusing interior areas?

☐ Will YAH maps be placed at pedestrian exits from parking areas?

☐ Will building names be clearly identified on YAH maps?

☐ Will YAH maps be oriented so that forward in space is "up" on the maps? (Levine, 1982)

☐ Will exterior YAH maps include memorable features of the environment? (Levine, 1982)

Access for People with Functional Limitations

☐ Will sidewalks be wide enough to allow two wheelchairs to pass easily? (American Hospital Association, 1979; English Tourist Board, 1983; Harkness and Groom, 1976; Kamisar, 1979)

☐ Will obstructions (such as grates) be eliminated so they don't catch wheels or crutches?

☐ Will benches or other street furniture that may make maneuvering difficult be kept away from the circulation path?

☐ Will curb cuts at street crossings be provided at a low enough grade to be accessible? (American Hospital Association, 1979; English Tourist Board, 1983; Harkness and Groom, 1976; Kamisar, 1979)

☐ Will grades be flat enough to allow easy movement? If grades must be greater than 5 percent, will handrails be provided?

☐ Will brick and other uneven paving materials be avoided so they don't create a bumpy ride for wheelchair users or hazards for people using walkers or pushing strollers?

☐ Will the Main Entrance area be accessible to people with mobility limitations and those with roller bags or strollers? (English Tourist Board, 1983; Harkness and Groom, 1976)

☐ Will the doorway be usable by people with mobility or vision limitations? (English Tourist Board, 1983; Harkness and Groom, 1976)

☐ Will automatic doors be provided at major entrances? (English Tourist Board, 1983; Harkness and Groom, 1976)

☐ Can doors be opened by people with little upper-body strength? (English Tourist Board, 1983; Harkness and Groom, 1976)

☐ If the force needed to open the door must exceed 8 pounds (to avoid having it blown open by the wind), will there be an automatic door? (English Tourist Board, 1983; Harkness and Groom, 1976)

☐ Will the Main Entrance area be free of obstructions? (English Tourist Board, 1983; Harkness and Groom, 1976)

☐ Will mud mats and pressure-sensitive mats be flush with the floor? (English Tourist Board, 1983; Harkness and Groom, 1976)

☐ Will newspaper machines, chairs, and other furniture be located out of the main circulation path? (English Tourist Board, 1983; Harkness and Groom, 1976)

☐ Will there be a place to store wheelchairs out of the flow of traffic? (English Tourist Board, 1983; Harkness and Groom, 1976)

☐ Will elevator lobbies be easily accessible? If there is a curb, will an access ramp be provided? (Harkness and Groom, 1976)

☐ Will elevators be wide enough to accommodate a wheelchair? Will they comply with ADA guidelines? (American Hospital Association, 1979; English Tourist Board, 1983; Harkness and Groom, 1976; Kamisar, 1979)

☐ Will elevator controls be within easy reach of someone who is seated? Will they comply with ADA guidelines? (American Hospital Association, 1979; English Tourist Board, 1983; Harkness and Groom, 1976; Kamisar, 1979)

Waiting in the Main Entrance Area

☐ Will ample space be provided in the Main Entrance area for patients and visitors to wait for transportation?

☐ Will patients and visitors have a view to the Drop-Off/Pick-Up area?

☐ Will comfortable places be provided for patients to sit? Will space be provided for patients' belongings?

☐ Will restrooms be available nearby?

☐ Will taxi phones and transit schedules be available?

☐ Will signs and maps be provided to direct people out of the facility, back to parking, and out to major roads?

First Destinations

Information Desk

☐ Will the Information Desk be in direct view from the Main Entrance?

☐ Will patients and visitors be able to distinguish the Information Desk from other counters or windows located in the Main Entrance area?

☐ Will the Information Desk be clearly identified?

☐ Will staff at the Information Desk have a clear view of the Main Entrance?

☐ Will there be ample space surrounding the Information Desk so the circulation area does not become congested?

☐ Will the Information Desk accommodate wheelchair users? (Harkness and Groom, 1976)

☐ Will staff be trained in direction-giving? (Olsen and Pershing, 1981)

Admitting or Registration

☐ Will there be a comfortable place for patients and companions to wait? (Valenta, 1981)

☐ Will interview areas in the Admitting Department be designed to ensure patients' acoustical privacy? (Valenta, 1981)

☐ Will interview areas be designed to facilitate conversation and self-disclosure? (Valenta, 1981)

☐ Will furniture be arranged so those having conversations can face one another and not be obstructed by equipment? (Valenta, 1981)

☐ Will electronic and written records be stored in ways that maintain patient confidentiality? (Valenta, 1981)

☐ Will staff and patients face each other at a comfortable conversational distance? (Valenta, 1981)

☐ Will accessible pathways be provided throughout the Admitting area? (Valenta, 1981)

☐ Will private offices, tall partitions, acoustic barriers, or spatial separations of work areas be provided to reduce noise and increase privacy? (Valenta, 1981)

☐ Will passageways be kept clear of obstructions? (Valenta, 1981)

☐ Will furniture be selected with safety in mind? (Valenta, 1981)

☐ Will chairs and other furnishings be stable? (Valenta, 1981)

☐ Will furniture with sharp or protruding edges not be selected? (Valenta, 1981)

☐ Will staff be able to control the temperature within the Admitting Department? (Valenta, 1981)

☐ Will staff be able to control lighting within the Admitting Department? (Valenta, 1981)

☐ Will natural lighting be available? (Valenta, 1981)

☐ Will the wayfinding system guide patients and their companions from the Admitting Department to other areas of the facility? (Valenta, 1981)

References

American Hospital Association. *Signs and Graphics for Health Care Facilities.* Chicago: AHA, 1979 [out of print].

Anderson, T. An interview with Tryst M. Anderson on "wayfinding" system for hospital parking structures. *Hospital Security and Safety Management* 15(7):12–18, November 1994.

Arneill, B., and Frasca-Beaulieu, K. Healing environments: Architecture and design conducive to health. In S. Frampton, L. Gilpin, and P. Charmel, editors. *Putting Patients First: Designing and Practicing Patient-Centered Care,* 163–90. San Francisco: Jossey-Bass, 2003.

Carpman, J. R., Grant, M. A., and Norton, C. Needs of the hearing impaired in a hospital setting. Unpublished research report No. 30, Patient and Visitor Participation Project, Office of the Replacement Hospital Program, University of Michigan, Ann Arbor, 1984.

Carpman, J. R., Grant, M. A., and Simmons, D. A. Hospital design and wayfinding: A video simulation study. *Environment and Behavior* 17(3):296–314, May 1985.

_____. No more mazes: Research about design for wayfinding in hospitals. Patient and Visitor Participation Project, Office of the Replacement Hospital Program, University of Michigan, Ann Arbor, 1984.

Chance, B. First impressions. *Health Facilities Management* 10(3):42–45, March 1997.

Cobb, A. Parking points out another serious problem: Where's the front door? *Health Facilities Management* 3(10):12–13, October 1990.

English Tourist Board. *Providing for Disabled Visitors.* London: English Tourist Board, 1983.

Follis, J., and Hammer, D. *Architectural Signing and Graphics.* New York: Watson Guptill, 1979.

Harkness, S. P., and Groom, J. N. *Building without Barriers for the Disabled.* New York: Watson Guptill, 1976.

Huelat, B. Wayfinding: Design for understanding. A position paper for the environmental standards council of the Center for Health Design. October 2007.

Institute for Signage Research. Technical and psychological considerations for sign systems in libraries. In D. Pollet and P. Haskel, editors. *Sign Systems for Libraries,* 229–41. New York: R. R. Bowker, 1979.

Kamisar, H. Signs for the handicapped patron. In D. Pollet and P. Haskel, editors. *Sign Systems for Libraries,* 99–103. New York: R. R. Bowker, 1979.

Kirkpatrick, S., and Cudney, G. Parking structure signage and safety improvements: A case study. *Parking Professional,* 13–22, February 1992.

Levine, M. You-Are-Here maps: Psychological considerations. *Environment and Behavior* 14(2):221–37, March 1982.

Marks, B. The language of signs. In D. Pollet and P. Haskel, editors. *Sign Systems for Libraries,* 89–97. New York: R. R. Bowker, 1979.

New hospital garage stresses perception of personal security. *Hospital Security and Safety Management,* 11–12, November 1996.

Olsen, R. V., and Pershing, A. Environmental evaluation of the interim entry to Bellevue Hospital. Unpublished report, Environmental Psychology Department, Bellevue Hospital, New York, 1981.

Passini, R. Wayfinding: A study of spatial problem-solving with implications for physical design. PhD dissertation, Pennsylvania State University, State College, 1977. [Available from ProQuest, 789 E. Eisenhower Parkway, Ann Arbor, MI 48108.]

Reizenstein, J. E., and Grant, M. A. Patient and visitor issues: Currently unmet needs and suggested solutions. Unpublished research report No. 4a, Patient and Visitor Participation Project, Office of Hospital Planning, Research and Development, University of Michigan, Ann Arbor, 1981.

Reizenstein, J. E., Grant, M. A., and Vaitkus, M. A. Visitor activities and schematic design preferences. Unpublished research report No. 4, Patient and Visitor Participation Project, Office of Hospital Planning, Research and Development, University of Michigan, Ann Arbor, 1981.

Rostenberg, B. Alternative health care facilities: Design reflects quality image. *Trustee* 40(4):15–18, April 1987.

Selfridge, K. M. Planning library signage systems. In D. Pollet and P. Haskel, editors. *Sign Systems for Libraries*, 49–67. New York: R. R. Bowker, 1979.

Shumaker, S., and Reizenstein, J. E. Environmental factors affecting inpatient stress in acute care hospitals. In G. W. Evans, editor. *Environmental Stress*, 179–223. New York: Cambridge University Press, 1982.

Speyer, R. Hospital parking facilities: How safe are they? *Hospitals* 61(20):38, October 20, 1987.

Thames, D. It's the little things that matter. *Texas Hospital* 43(1):27, January 1987.

Valenta, A. L. Human behavioral needs in hospital admissions management: Some architectural implications. PhD dissertation, University of Illinois at Chicago, Health Sciences Center, School of Public Health, 1981. [Available from ProQuest, 789 E. Eisenhower Parkway, Ann Arbor, MI 48108.]

Wechsler, S. Perceiving the visual message. In D. Pollet and P. Haskel, editors. *Sign Systems for Libraries*, 33–46. New York: R. R. Bowker, 1979.

Weisman, G. D. Way-finding and architectural legibility: Design considerations in housing environments for the elderly. University of Wisconsin-Milwaukee, School of Architecture & Urban Planning, 1985.

Zimring, C. M., Carpman, J. R., and Michelson, W. Designing for special populations: Mentally retarded persons, children, hospital visitors. In D. Stokols and I. Altman, editors. *Handbook of Environmental Psychology*, 919–49. New York: John Wiley and Sons, 1987.

CHAPTER 4

INTERIOR WAYFINDING AND THE CIRCULATION SYSTEM

Interior circulation systems typically consist of corridors, elevators, and stairways that connect the floors and areas of the facility, providing avenues for the movement of people and materials. Circulation areas are also places where patients and visitors spend time waiting, gathering information, and talking. They are places where equipment is stored. They are places where members of the medical staff confer. And they are also places where patients, visitors, and staff can become disoriented or lost (Carpman and Grant, 1989).

This chapter begins by examining how people find their way around large, complex buildings—the kinds of buildings that often house healthcare services. We will describe various components of a wayfinding system, such as floor numbering, sign terminology, and You-Are-Here (YAH) map design, and emphasize that these elements need to work in a mutually reinforcing way to make sense to first-time and other unfamiliar users. We then look at design features within the circulation system, discussing how corridors, stairways, and elevators can be designed to meet the needs of patients and visitors.

Finding One's Way through a Health Facility

For patients and visitors, time spent in a healthcare facility is often filled with anxiety. With the demands of illness or a family crisis occupying their minds, people may not be able to pay attention to their routes through the corridors of a complex environment. When patients and visitors are under stress and preoccupied with their own concerns, they cannot necessarily rely on previous knowledge

LEARNING OBJECTIVES
- Understand the challenges faced by patients and visitors as they find their way around a healthcare facility, as well as the costs—both direct and indirect—associated with disorientation and stress.
- Know the main components of an interior wayfinding system and how these can be planned and designed.
- Describe how decision-points can play a role in the design of an effective interior wayfinding system.
- Identify some design features that are part of interior circulation areas, including corridors, elevators, and stairways.

about how to make their way through an unfamiliar facility. Consequently, what might otherwise be considered annoying inconveniences, such as mazelike corridors, may tax the emotional strength of a patient facing surgery or a visitor concerned about a critically ill relative (Carpman, Grant, and Simmons, 1984; Shumaker and Reizenstein, 1982). (See also chapter 9.)

The term *wayfinding* refers to what people perceive, what they think about, and what they do to find their way from one place to another. Wayfinding involves five deceptively simple steps: knowing where you are, knowing your destination, knowing and following an effective route to your destination, recognizing your destination upon arrival, and finding your way back or on to your next destination (Carpman, 1991a, 1991b, 1991c).

Unfortunately, many healthcare environments are not designed for easy navigation by unfamiliar patients, visitors, and staff. Healthcare facilities are often housed in large, complex buildings. These are often built over time, with the inadvertent result that common patient and visitor destinations are not necessarily near one another. A single trip to see a physician, and its associated diagnostic tests, may seem like a tour of the entire medical complex.

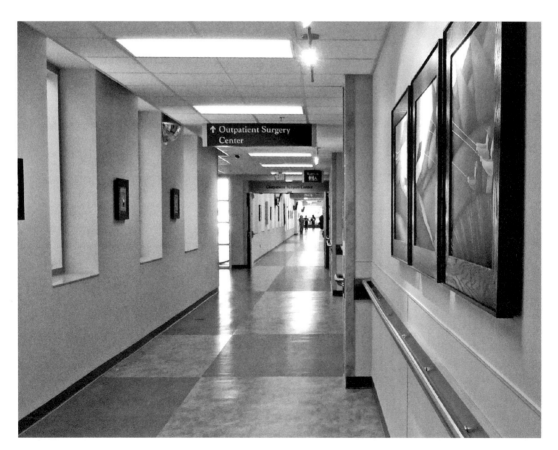

Wayfinding signs at decision-points, including intersections, will reassure unfamiliar patients and visitors that they are on the right path as they traverse long hallways.

Photo credit: Courtesy of St. Joseph Mercy Ann Arbor

Wayfinding difficulties may be made worse by the physical limitations of illness. Confusing signs that use unfamiliar medical terminology can make the customer experience even more challenging.

As unfamiliar patients and visitors make their way through a health facility, they will be hindered or helped by the availability of a variety of environmental cues. Effective wayfinding systems use a combination of signs, maps, directories, landmarks, artificial and natural lighting, and site and building layouts to help guide people to their destinations (Carpman, 1991a; Eubanks, 1989). The close proximity of common destinations, the availability of visual cues that provide landmarks (such as windows, plants, artwork, or changes in floor coverings), the use of easily understood terminology, clear systems for floor and room numbering, and the availability of understandable directions provided by well-trained staff, should all work together, along with wayfinding signs, as an integrated system (Carpman, 1991a; Weisman, 1982).

Costs of Unsuccessful Wayfinding

Successful wayfinding experiences—say, easily navigating from the main Information Desk to an inpatient room—are seldom thought about. On the other hand, when patients and visitors become disoriented or lost, they are likely to remember it, and not in a good way. When they are disoriented or lost, patients and visitors may take extra time to get places and may be late for appointments. In confusing buildings, work time may be lost when employees give directions or escort patients and visitors (Christensen, unpublished report; Carpman et al., 1984a; Corlett, Manenica, and Bishop, 1972; Zimring, 1982).

And there are other costs associated with disorientation. Disorientation is disruptive and causes stress: the amount depends on the individual's ability to cope with uncertainty and varies with specific situations, such as the need to be on time for an appointment (Best, 1967; Weisman, 1981; Wener and Kaminoff, 1983). Stress caused by disorientation may result in feelings of helplessness, raised blood pressure, headaches, increased physical exertion, and fatigue (Shumaker and Reizenstein, 1982). In addition, patients may be affected by the wayfinding troubles of their visitors who, because they became lost, may have less time to spend with patients. In one study of visitor stress, it was found that the largest source of stress for visitors was trying to find their way around the hospital (Reizenstein and Vaitkus, 1981; Wayfinding design research, 1987).

Wayfinding in healthcare facilities often requires unfamiliar patients and visitors to make complex, potentially confusing journeys comprising multiple steps, as in this example (St. Joseph's Health Care London, 2015):

- Enter from the Main Building's entrance.

- Walk into Main Lobby area (past Information Desk and General Store in centre).

- Take Elevator 1 or 2 (on the left) or Elevator 5 or 6 (on the right) up to Level 5.

- Exit elevator.

- From Elevator 1 or 2 turn right, from Elevator 5 or 6 turn left.

- Walk through double doors.

- Walk down this corridor.

- Pass two corridors on left.

- Check in at the nursing station at the end of the hall on the left.

Stress brought about by disorientation may lead to anger, hostility, discomfort, indignation, or even panic. Disorientation felt by those visiting a particular facility may surface as a generalized hostility toward the organization (Berkeley, 1973). Health facilities may even experience indirect wayfinding costs such as personnel turnover and absenteeism because of the stress brought about by employees continually trying to find their way (Christensen, unpublished report; Zimring, 1982). (See Research Box 4.1.)

RESEARCH BOX 4.1 HAVING THE MAP IN MIND

There are many wayfinding strategies, including following directions, reading signs, and using smartphone and tablet apps. One approach is to develop a mental image (cognitive map) of the building area. It's not necessary to have an exact mental replica of the physical space to be covered, but only one that's good enough to enable you to get from here to there.

In a study designed to investigate the development of such cognitive mapping abilities in a complex building, one researcher conducted three experiments to examine how everyday users picture the layout of a complex five-story hospital (Moeser, 1988). In the first experiment, 20 female student nurses, 10 with 4 months' experience and 10 with 25 months in the hospital, were asked to draw maps from memory of the four floors they commonly used. Although the more experienced students mapped significantly more locations correctly, none of the 20 maps resembled each other or accurate floor plans of the area. Eleven of the maps depicted landmarks as key elements and 9 delineated routes. Even at this rudimentary map-making level, the more experienced nursing students drew only about 30 percent of the rooms, elevators, and entrances correctly on any floor except one, on which 50 percent were located correctly.

To check whether these results stemmed from a deficiency in sketch-drawing ability, a second experiment asked 22 second-year students with 7 months' experience and 22 third-year student nurses with 21 months' experience to label modified floor plans of the four floors from an alphabetical list of rooms in the hospital. This time the groups did not significantly differ in the number of correct choices, but accuracy still remained well below 50 percent.

Because several students in the second experiment who claimed good knowledge of the floors complained that they could not understand the floor plans, a third experiment was devised to test nursing students' knowledge of the areas in the building.

In Experiment 3, 20 female student nurses with 22–26 months' experience overall and several months in each of several parts of the hospital were asked to complete standard direction-pointing and distance-estimation tasks on the first two floors. For comparison, the same tasks were given to 20 female second-year psychology students who were unfamiliar with the building. They received individual training of up to three hours memorizing the labeled map used in Experiment 2, followed two days later by a guided tour.

The results indicate that map reading was not the problem. The psychology students made fewer errors than the student nurses, pointing to 11 of the 12 locations tested, and better distance estimates on 10 of the 12 locations. The author notes that these results were obtained despite the fact that difficulty in securing nursing student volunteers meant that those who did participate were among the most confident among their peers with regard to their own wayfinding abilities.

If map-reading ability was not the problem and extended experience did not lead to more sophisticated cognitive wayfinding representations, what accounted for the disorientation? The author cites the building's complexity (layout) as the primary source of the nurses' difficulty in this study. She recommends that architects consider not only the functional needs in buildings, but also the burden that building complexity places on the average person's wayfinding-related cognitive abilities.

The researcher also emphasizes the importance of establishing standardized training to assist staff in acquiring a cognitive map before they actually traverse the building. Experience on the job would then combine, over time, with the initial memorization task to form a more distinctive image of the building structure, and with it, more successful and confident wayfinding.

For older patients and visitors, problems with spatial orientation may have a significant, long-term effect. One study suggests that problems with wayfinding may affect an older person's sense of control (Weisman, 1982). Special simulation techniques have been developed to familiarize older people about to move to a care facility with the layout of their new environment. The premise for this work is that having wayfinding information prior to moving may partially diminish the negative effects of relocation, such as increased incidence of illness and death (Hunt, 1984). Digital technology makes it relatively easy to develop images, maps, photos, and videos to assist with transitions to new and unfamiliar environments.

The importance of the link between stress and wayfinding is reinforced by additional empirical evidence. One study found that wayfinding aids, such as directional signs, decrease reported stress levels (Wener and Kaminoff, 1983). However, another study showed that large numbers of signs may be an indication of a confusing environment. In such cases, signs may be used as an attempt to remedy a fundamentally disorienting building (Weisman, 1979).

It's important to remember that simple buildings, as well as complex ones, can be confusing to unfamiliar users.

Building Layout and Landmarks

Navigating in complex buildings requires spatial problem-solving (Passini and Arthur, 1992). To find their way, people use previous experience in conjunction with directions and/or environmental cues. They make choices about where to turn and where not to turn, based on these cues (Downs, 1979; Kaplan, 1976; Weisman, 1981). However, to make the necessary choices, patients and visitors must be able to recognize where they are in relation to their destinations. Without this sense of location, they may become disoriented or lost.

It would be easy to assume that signs and directories are the most effective elements of a wayfinding system. But in a study of university buildings, the form of the building (including the number of corridors, the placement of decision-points, and the symmetry of the building) constituted the strongest predictor of successful wayfinding (Weisman, 1979). The availability of environmental cues and architectural features, such as visual distinctiveness, well-differentiated spaces, and easily recognized landmarks (plants, artwork, and furniture arrangements, for example), all provide useful information (Appleyard, 1969; Kaplan, 1976; Weisman, 1981). Instead of simply moving sequentially from one sign or spot along the path to another, with no idea of how it all connects, patients and visitors moving through a building with effective landmarks, views to the outside, and easily differentiated spaces can more easily understand the building's layout and how its spaces fit together. For example, one clinic made extensive use of columns, varied patterns in flooring, and natural lighting to direct patients and visitors from "public zones" to reception areas (Taylor, 1995). Another study showed that maps sent to patients and visitors before their arrival at a healthcare facility improved their ability to navigate to their destinations (Wright, Hull, and Lickorish, 1993).

General considerations for developing a coherent health facility wayfinding system include the following:

*   Consider first-time users as the "least common denominator" for wayfinding decision-making. They will be unfamiliar with every aspect of the setting and most likely to be disoriented. If the wayfinding system works for first-time users, it will work for all users (Baskaya, Wilson, and Özcan, 2004; Carpman et al., 1984a).

*   Keep in mind that the way to reduce the maze-like quality of healthcare facilities is not to rely on a single device such as signage, but instead to design or implement a mutually reinforcing group of aids to create a wayfinding *system*. Such a system may include the basic layout of the building and site, landscaping, architectural differentiation, interior and exterior landmarks, signs, maps, lighting, terminology, floor and room numbering, spoken directions, and technology (Weisman, 1982).

*   When possible, locate related functions (those that patients and visitors are likely to use during the same visit) in close proximity (for instance, Admitting, Laboratory, and Radiology) (Carpman et al., 1984a; Hauff, 1988).

*   When designing health facilities, consider the impact of the building's form and appearance on wayfinding for first-time users (Weisman, 1979). Consider corridor layout, views

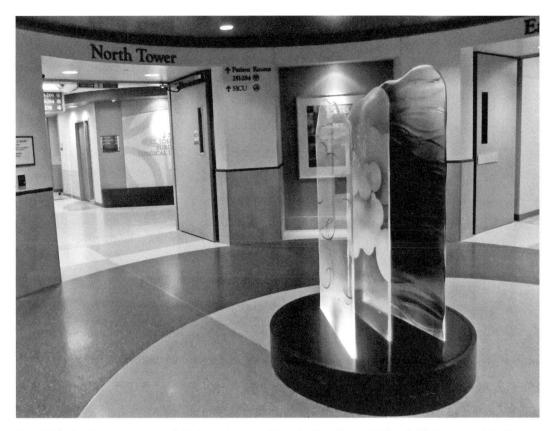

Noticeable landmarks, such as this internally lit glass sculpture, can help unfamiliar patients and visitors find their way around a health facility.

Photo credit: Courtesy of St. Joseph Mercy Ann Arbor

to the outside, location of decision-points such as corridor intersections, and interior design treatments.

- Develop interior landmarks by using such design elements as architectural details, lighting, color, texture, artwork, and plants to make different areas of the hospital unique, noticeable, and memorable (Carpman et al., 1984a).

Floor Numbering

To arrive at a healthcare facility, patients and visitors have had to negotiate city streets, parking areas, and pathways to the facility's entrance. For the most part, such exterior travel remains within the same plane; route decisions primarily involve which way to turn. But once people are inside the facility, an additional level of complexity is added: floor choice. Moreover, floor choice is made more complex when potential destinations are located below grade level, when buildings are linked by corridors or overhead walkways, and when floors are labeled in ways not understandable to first-time users. (See Research Box 4.2.)

From the user's point of view, finding the right floor may prove more troublesome than finding a destination on a particular floor. This was illustrated by a study of people trying to find their way in a town hall: the majority of wayfinding errors related to floor choice (Best, 1967). Similarly, studies have found getting off on the wrong floor to be a common and frustrating experience for older users (Devlin, 1980).

Floor number confusion can be reduced in several ways:

- Logically relate floor-number designations to the Main Entrance floor and indicate whether floors are above or below grade.

- Consider the relationship between floor numbers of buildings that are linked; avoid situations in which, for example, Floor 2 of one building links to Floor 4 of another (Carpman et al., 1984b).

- Plan floor-number designations that can be easily used in the room-numbering system (for example, rooms in Floor 5 could all begin with the number 5) (Carpman et al., 1984b).

- Begin room numbers on floors below the entrance level with a prefix likely to be widely understood by first-time users (Carpman et al., 1984b). (See Research Box 4.2.)

RESEARCH BOX 4.2 NUMBERING FLOORS IN A HEALTHCARE FACILITY

During the design phase for a new hospital at the University of Michigan Medical Center, a need arose to examine floor-numbering options and select the most effective one. The new hospital would have two floors below the Main Entrance level, one of which would continue into a new outpatient building. Given this spatial arrangement, the task was to develop a floor-numbering scheme that would be understandable to unfamiliar customers.

Researchers wanted to know which of several feasible and conventional floor-numbering alternatives would be most comprehensible to hospital patients, visitors, and staff (Carpman et al., 1984b). Because floor numbers would have to be abbreviated to fit on elevator buttons, they were limited to a maximum of four characters. The options tested were A and B, B1 and B2, Sub 1 and Sub 2, 1 and 2, and LL1 and LL2.

Participants were shown a set of graphics of a building with two floors below grade, one graphic for each option. They were asked about the clarity of

9	9	9	11	9
8	8	8	10	8
7	7	7	9	7
6	6	6	8	6
5	5	5	7	5
4	4	4	6	4
3	3	3	5	3
2	2	2	4	2
1	1	1	3	1
LL1	A	B1	2	SUB1
LL2	B	B2	1	SUB2

various options in relation to a simple wayfinding task. They rated each option with regard to its overall desirability and chose the "best" and "worst" options. The option most often interpreted clearly and preferred by patients and visitors was Sub 1 and Sub 2.

Sub 1 and Sub 2 gave users a clear point of reference and a clear distance to travel. To most people, the term *Sub* designated something that might be found *below;* Sub 1 meant one floor below entry, and Sub 2 meant two floors below entry. None of the other alternatives provided as clear a point of reference. With A and B, and with B1 and B2, users did not know which one was the lowest level; with LL1 and LL2, the participants found it difficult to interpret LL, and with 1 and 2, there was confusion about where floor counting began: at the lowest level or at the entry floor.

However, although staff saw wayfinding as an important patient and visitor criterion for deciding on a floor-numbering scheme, they also considered the image projected by the numbering options. Many of the staff reported that any alternative implying a basement location (that is, B1 and B2, and Sub 1 and Sub 2) produced a negative image. They felt that it might be demoralizing and feared that patients would not want to be treated in a basement.

It is important to consider that floor-numbering terminology can project an image. However, in selecting an alternative that seems to best meet the wayfinding needs of patients and visitors (for example, Sub 1 and Sub 2), some methods of moderating the "basement" image of the space need to be addressed.

Room Numbering

Once patients and visitors reach the appropriate floor, they continue to search for their destinations. Although some rooms will be identified by name (for example, the Surgery Waiting Area), patients, visitors, and staff may need to find a room or office with only a room number to guide them. The logic and placement of room numbers along a corridor facilitates their search. At corridor intersections, room numbers help patients and visitors decide whether to turn left or right or to go straight. Monitoring room numbers they pass by and watching for a specific room number lets them know when they have reached their destination.

Although there is no foolproof way to ensure the usefulness of room-numbering systems to first-time users, there are ways to make systems effective. Simplicity, consistency, flexibility, and visibility should be major criteria.

A numbering scheme should be simple. For instance, in buildings with a single long corridor, rooms could be numbered sequentially, beginning at one end of the facility and continuing to the other. In this example, odd numbers would be located on one side of the hall and even numbers on the other. Adjacent numbers such as 12 and 13 should be roughly across the hall from one another. Or in a building area with "racetrack" corridors, patient rooms could be numbered consecutively along the outside of the corridor, with staff rooms located along the inside of the corridor and having a different numbering system. Simplicity also suggests a correspondence between the room number and the floor number; for instance, all rooms on the fifth floor would begin with the number 5.

Another consideration related to simplicity is to avoid using a combination of letters and numbers to identify a space (such as NIB416), because complex sequences are difficult to read and remember. The letters *I, O, Q* should be avoided since they can cause confusion with the numerals 1 and 0.

Room-numbering schemes should be used consistently from floor to floor, especially when floors have similar layouts. Again, the system should begin with the lowest number at one end and should progress in the same direction on each floor.

One seemingly pervasive characteristic of health facilities is that they undergo frequent renovation (McLaughlin, 1976). A side effect of renovation is that corresponding room numbers come and go. Consequently, the room-numbering system needs to be flexible enough to allow for future renovation without unduly disrupting its logic. Leaving out ("skipping") a few numbers at planned intervals is one approach.

Efforts to create a room-numbering system that is simple, consistent, and flexible should be supplemented by attention to the visibility of the actual room numbers. For rooms that patients and visitors will identify primarily by number, numbers need to be large and should contrast well enough with the background so they can be easily recognized. It's important to keep in mind the needs of older users and people with vision limitations.

Room-numbering schemes for successful wayfinding cannot be a design afterthought, but should be planned from the earliest stages of the design process. When buildings are designed, rooms are labeled (numbered) on floor plans in order to keep track of each room during design, construction, and activation. The logic of these architectural numbering systems often has little to do with wayfinding clarity. Yet in the absence of other room-numbering schemes, clients often simply adopt these architectural room numbers as actual room numbers for wayfinding purposes. This practice can lead to wayfinding confusion. Patients and visitors are better served if the architectural numbering system is designed for its ultimate use as a wayfinding aid or, failing that, if owners understand that a separate wayfinding-related room-numbering system is needed. Wayfinding room-number planning is best dealt with before room numbers appear on architectural drawings. Changing room numbers after the building is activated is likely to be difficult and costly.

When developing a room-numbering system:

- Design the room-numbering system to be flexible enough to allow for future expansion and renovation without disrupting the sequence (Carpman et al., 1984a).

- Use the numbering system consistently on floors having similar uses and layouts (Carpman et al., 1984a).

- Within the numbering system, differentiate between the appearance of those numbers needed by patients and visitors (such as patient rooms and exam rooms) and those used only by staff. One way is to use a larger room number on signs indicating patient or visitor destinations (Carpman et al., 1984a).

- With the exception of inpatient rooms, provide a name and a number for rooms that are primary patient and visitor destinations. Use numbers alone or numbers and names for rooms used primarily by staff (Carpman et al., 1984a).

- Place inpatient room number signs so they are visible when the door is open.

- Avoid using a combination of letters and numbers to identify a space, such as NIB407.

- If letters and numbers must be used in the same sign, avoid letters that may be interpreted as numbers, such as *I*, *O*, and *Q* (Carpman et al., 1984a).

- Start numbering systems at one end or corner of a building and carry the system through to the other end (American Hospital Association, 1979).

- Whenever possible, use a simple numbering system, such as a continuous series with odd numbers on one side of the hall and even numbers on the other (American Hospital Association, 1979).

- Plan the room-numbering system to include skips in the number sequence at various locations along a floor, in order to allow for renovations or rooms that may be added in the future.

- In new construction projects, consider wayfinding-related room numbering before room numbers appear on architectural drawings.

- Consider coordinating inpatient room numbers and telephone numbers (Carpman et al., 1984a).

Sign Messages

Messages on wayfinding signs should be targeted to their audiences, but selecting wording is not always easy (Salmi, 2007). As described in chapter 3, many groups will use wayfinding signs in a health facility, including medical staff; patients; visitors; administrators; medical, nursing, and allied health students; and others. Users may not be literate, or may not read or speak English.

Healthcare facilities with significant numbers of customers speaking languages other than English should consider bilingual signs, translators, technology, and other ways to communicate. Health facilities that provide information in a customer's native language convey an important message of sensitivity and respect. This may be an important marketing strategy. In addition, the Department of Health and Human Services has stated that Title VI of the 1964 Civil Rights Act prohibits discrimination on the basis of having a primary language other than English (US Department of Health and Human Services, 1980). Research shows that the absence of limited English proficiency (LEP) services can create a barrier to care (Principles for Health Reform, 2015).

Signs that include more than one language will have more words per sign or more signs per location and will be more costly to produce (Selfridge, 1979). Some healthcare facilities employ or outsource interpreters to work with LEP and non-English-speaking patients and visitors, while others may offer incentives for assistance by employees who are proficient in additional languages (Derose and Baker, 2000).

Although wording used on wayfinding signs and in spoken directions represents an important way in which health facilities communicate with consumers, some technical and medical terms in the patient's own language may not be widely understood by patients and visitors (see Research Box 4.3). Problems stemming from use of technical terms are illustrated by the following anecdote:

An older woman was spotted in the hospital by a hospital staff member who thought she looked lost. He asked the woman where she was trying to go and she said, "Gerontology?" The staff member started to give detailed directions, but because the Institute of Gerontology was located several blocks away, he asked whether she was sure that this was her destination. "Oh, yes," she said, "I have it right here on this slip of paper." On the slip of paper was written "Gastroenterology."

RESEARCH BOX 4.3 SELECTING MESSAGES FOR WAYFINDING SIGNS

Little information was available to planners at the University of Michigan Medical Center to guide them in wording wayfinding signs. The Patient and Visitor Participation Project undertook studies that would shape the selection of wayfinding terminology (Carpman et al., 1984a). Medical terminology conventionally used for hospital departments and procedures (such as *Otorhinolaryngology* and *Cardiology*) was tested along with commonly used terminology (such as *Ear, Nose, and Throat* and *Heart*). Two-hundred-forty randomly sampled patients and visitors were interviewed about potential sign messages (terms).

Sixty-seven terms were tested to see whether there was a difference in the participants' understanding of lay terms versus technical or medical terms. Each term was tested in at least two ways: by presenting the respondent with the technical term and by giving the respondent a description or lay definition of the term. In the tests of technical terms, participants were shown the printed word (such as *Thoracic Surgery*) at the same time the interviewer clearly pronounced the term. Participants were then asked whether they knew what the term meant. If they said yes, they were asked what they thought of when they heard that term. For the second set of tests, involving lay terminology, participants were given a lay definition (such as "where people who do not need to be hospitalized receive medical care") and then were asked to suggest a term.

Overall, participants understood a greater number of the technical terms than the researchers had predicted. Participants didn't consistently favor either the technical or the lay terms.

The following terms were commonly understood:

· Admitting
· Dermatology

- Cardiology
- Diagnostic Radiology
- Intensive Care Unit (ICU)
- Ophthalmology
- Pediatrics
- Psychiatry

The following terms were commonly misunderstood:

- Ambulatory Care
- Internal Medicine
- Endocrine and Metabolism
- Neonatal
- Nuclear Medicine
- Otorhinolaryngology
- Walk-in Clinic

An unexpected finding of the research was that patients and visitors often thought they knew what a term meant when, in fact, they did not.

Confusion caused by misreading or misunderstanding technical or medical terminology increases the likelihood that some people, like the older woman in the earlier anecdote, may have a difficult time finding their way and wind up being late for, or even missing, appointments. Patients or visitors may refrain from asking questions because they think they understand a term when they really do not. Or the term may cause needless worry about their illness. For example:

A patient told one hospital staff member that earlier in his treatment he had been scheduled to go to Nuclear Medicine for some tests. He became so frightened at the thought of being bombarded with radiation that he almost canceled his appointment. To him, Nuclear Medicine meant radiation. He also assumed it meant that he had a terminal disease for which there would be little hope. To his surprise and joy, his fears on both counts were unfounded.

Patients interviewed in one study did not think there would be a difference in the quality of medical care at a hospital using lay terms as compared with one using medical terms. But they did say that the terminology used would influence their choice of a hospital. In other words, all things being equal, the majority of these patients said they would choose to go to a hospital that used lay terms on its wayfinding signs (Carpman et al., 1984a).

The following are some guidelines for selecting understandable messages on wayfinding signs:

• Use plain and simple wording in English and/or other languages when selecting terminology (Kearney, Rice, and Parks, 1987).

• Decide what wording will be used for naming each department or service and base these decisions on patients' and visitors' comprehension (Carpman et al., 1984a).

• Use consistent wording on signs and in written and verbal communications with patients and visitors (American Hospital Association, 1979; Marks, 1979).

• Develop messages that will be interpreted similarly by all users. Avoid using ambiguous wording, such as "Patient Access Center" for an admitting area.

• Use consistent wording on wayfinding signs throughout a health facility. For instance, avoid using "Imaging" on one sign and "Radiology" on another when these terms identify the same area (American Hospital Association, 1979; Marks, 1979).

• Avoid using words and phrases on signs that are beyond a sixth-grade reading level (American Hospital Association, 1979).

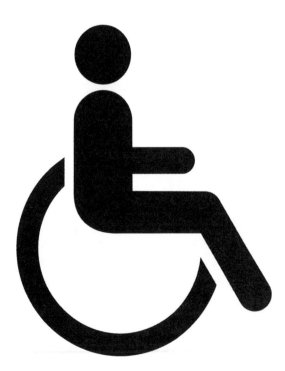

The universal symbol of accessibility identifies features of the environment—including routes, bathrooms, and parking areas—designed to accommodate everyone, regardless of ability or disability.

Symbols and Pictograms

Symbols (also known as icons or pictograms) are sometimes used in conjunction with written messages on wayfinding signs. Symbols for accessibility, male and female restrooms, and no-smoking areas are commonplace in most public buildings. They provide an easily recognizable form of information patients can use even if they don't read or have knowledge of a particular language. When a subject lends itself to graphic representation and when properly designed, symbols can make it easier for users to understand how to proceed.

However, pictograms don't always provide a benefit. Many health-facility terms cannot be easily translated into pictograms, and a pictogram system can quickly become contrived. In addition, pictograms used in conjunction with wording on directional signs can create complexity and diminish overall legibility. In order to be useful for wayfinding, pictograms need to make immediate, intuitive sense to the viewer.

Consider the following when choosing pictograms for health-facility wayfinding signs:

- Test pictograms for comprehension by patients and visitors (Carpman et al., 1984a).

- Evaluate the effect of pictograms on overall sign legibility.

- Coordinate pictogram design so styles, colors, shapes, and backgrounds are consistent (Follis and Hammer, 1979).

- Limit the number of pictograms used (Follis and Hammer, 1979).

- Unless pictograms are widely used and recognized, use them only as a supplement to written information (Follis and Hammer, 1979).

- Avoid using arrows for non-directional signs (Selfridge, 1979).

Sign Updating

Healthcare facilities, especially hospitals, undergo frequent renovations and relocations (McLaughlin, 1976). Such changes can wreak havoc with an otherwise finely-tuned sign system. When destinations move, related signs need to be changed.

There are several ways health facilities can approach sign updating. To facilitate consistency and accuracy, sign-related information and decisions should be the responsibility of a single staff member. Sign data (number of signs, location, messages, arrows, and the like) are typically part of a database. In this way, when a destination moves or its name changes, all signs that mention that destination can be easily identified, allowing the sign system to be proactively managed.

Signs can be designed so that individual messages can be altered or replaced easily. Healthcare facilities with in-house sign fabrication and installation will reduce out-of-pocket costs and turnaround time (MacKenzie and Krusberg, 1996). However, in order to mitigate unintentional damage or vandalism, signs should not be too easy to alter.

In order to ensure that the sign system continues to be functional, periodic evaluation is needed, similar to a regularly scheduled car tune-up. Each sign in the system needs to be inspected for accuracy, legibility, and condition.

Sign Spacing and Location

Patients, visitors, and staff attempting to make their way around an unfamiliar building require a great deal of information. They "read" the environment, not only in the literal sense of reading signs and maps, but also in terms of gathering information from other cues, including corridors, windows, stairways, doors, and lighting, among others. Patients and visitors use these visual cues to decide whether particular pathways are likely to lead to their destinations.

To the person trying to find a particular destination, everything on signs is critical: fonts, color, contrast between text and background, letter size, and wording. But no matter how good the sign is or how legible or clearly worded, the sign's usefulness is drastically diminished if it is not in the right location. Paying attention to the placement and spacing of signs is essential to reducing disorientation in health facilities.

In determining where signs should be placed, a common rule of thumb is to place them at decision-points: places along a path or corridor where users decide whether to continue in the same direction or turn (Daniel, 1979; Kamisar, 1979; Selfridge, 1979). The purpose of the study, reported in Research Box 4.4, was to determine where signs should be placed along hospital corridors and to develop a design-relevant definition of the concept of decision-point (Downs, 1979).

RESEARCH BOX 4.4 SPACING SIGNS IN A HEALTHCARE FACILITY

To simulate a typical health facility wayfinding experience, participants in a study at the University of Michigan Medical Center were asked to find a predetermined destination: the Cyclotron area (Carpman et al., 1984a). A 660-foot-long corridor in the existing hospital was selected, since the length of this corridor closely approximated the longest horizontal distance from entrance to destination that patients and visitors would traverse in the new hospital being designed. This study evaluated three schemes for locating directional signs along a hospital corridor. This illustration shows various environmental features along the study route and their distances from the starting point.

Although distance traveled was an important criterion in selecting the experimental setting, its complexity and the existence of alternative destinations were also important. The portion of the corridor used in the study started at the Physical Medicine and Rehabilitation Department, passed a major intersection, continued through

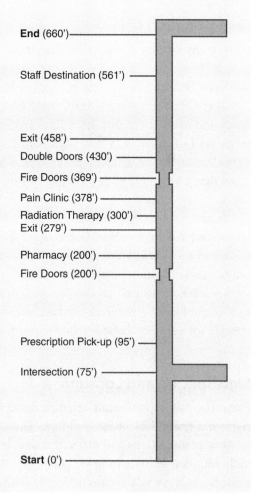

End (660')

Staff Destination (561')

Exit (458')
Double Doors (430')
Fire Doors (369')
Pain Clinic (378')
Radiation Therapy (300')
Exit (279')

Pharmacy (200')
Fire Doors (200')

Prescription Pick-up (95')

Intersection (75')

Start (0')

the Pharmacy and Radiation Therapy departments, passed the Pain Clinic, and ended with a right turn to the Cyclotron: the participants' destination. Randomly selected hospital visitors, who chose to participate in the study, were escorted to the Physical Medicine and Rehabilitation Department and told that their task was to find the Cyclotron.

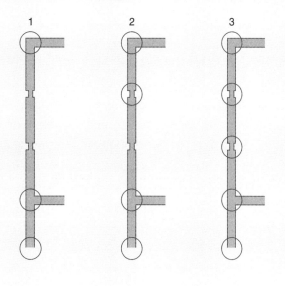

Because the study's objective was to determine ideal spacing and placement of signs, the number of signs strategically mounted along the corridor was systematically varied, to see whether people experiencing different conditions responded differently. As each participant walked along the corridor, the interviewer recorded the number of times he or she asked directions, made a wrong turn, or noticeably hesitated and the amount of time it took the participant to find the Cyclotron. After finding the destination, participants were asked to suggest locations for new signs and to report any stress brought about by this wayfinding task. This illustration shows the three schemes for locating directional signs along the hospital corridor. (The circles represent approximate sign locations.)

When participants' behaviors and attitudes were compared across conditions, it became obvious that the number of signs available at key decision-points had a significant effect. Overall, the greater the number of signs, the more likely the participant was to find the destination quickly and the less likely he or she was to request additional signs, hesitate or ask directions, or report an increased level of stress.

The results of this study make it clear that the basis for decisions about the location of signs should be not an arbitrary distance figure, but rather the identification of key decision-points. However, the significance of the study is in defining the nature of those key decision-points. The results indicated that directional signs are needed at intersections, at destinations, and where a single environmental cue or a series of such cues (such as changes in flooring material, changes in color scheme, or noticeable architectural features such as a fire door constriction in the hallway) conveys a message that the individual is moving from one area into another. If there are no key decision-points along a given route, the results indicate that signs should be placed approximately every 150–250 feet (~45.7–76.2 meters).

Consider the following guidelines for locating wayfinding signs in healthcare facilities:

◆ Coordinate sign location planning with the planning of mechanical and electrical fixtures (such as lights, sprinkler nozzles, and air vents) so that prime sign locations are not blocked (Carpman et al., 1984a).

◆ Place signs at decision-points. Decision-points are places along a corridor where people must decide whether to continue in the same direction or turn (such as at intersections or at destinations), or where a single environmental cue or a series of such cues indicates that they are moving into a new area (Carpman et al., 1984a).

◆ Consider placing reassurance signs 150–250 feet (~45.7–76.2 meters) after decision-points when another decision-point is not nearby (Carpman et al., 1984a; Downs, 1979).

◆ Locate directional signs, You-Are-Here maps, and identification signs consistently so people learn to look for signs in certain places (Levine, 1982; Wechsler, 1979; Weisman, 1982; Wilt and Maienschien, 1979).

◆ Locate directional signs perpendicular to the flow of foot traffic.

Interior You-Are-Here Maps

In chapter 3, we described ways in which exterior You-Are-Here (YAH) maps can help people orient themselves outside a building and find their way from one building to another. Similarly, interior YAH maps can help patients and visitors gain an overall understanding of a building's (or smaller area's) layout. However, the map must be well designed if it is to be a useful addition to the overall wayfinding system. (See Research Box 4.6 and Research Box 4.7.) People who use YAH maps should be able to locate themselves accurately in relation to their destinations and gain enough information from the maps to select an effective route.

Consider the following when designing interior You-Are-Here maps:

◆ Make sure map labels use terminology consistent with signs and other components of the wayfinding system (Levine, 1982).

◆ Align the map so that "forward is up" (that is, the direction the person is facing while looking at the map should be at the top of the map) (Aubrey and Dobbs, 1994; Levine, 1982).

◆ Incorporate landmarks into the map (Levine, 1982).

◆ Simplify the map area and highlight public corridors and destinations.

◆ If the map does not include the entire floor of the facility, provide an inset or some other graphic device to show the relation of the mapped portion of the building to the rest of the healthcare facility on that floor (Carpman and Grant, 1984).

◆ Draw the YAH arrow pointing in the direction and at the spot the viewer is facing while looking at the map (Levine, 1982).

RESEARCH BOX 4.6 DETERMINING ALIGNMENT OF YOU-ARE-HERE MAPS

Researchers at the State University of New York at Stony Brook conducted two experiments examining the effectiveness of alternative designs for YAH maps (Levine, Marchon, and Hanley, 1984). Both experiments looked at the use of YAH maps as a spatial problem-solving process.

Experiment 1

In a laboratory experiment, students examined a series of 16 slides depicting various YAH maps. The slides differed by where the YAH arrow pointed (that is, whether the YAH map was aligned so that "forward is up") and in the simulated destination participants were asked to find. After being shown each slide, participants were asked to indicate which direction they would travel in order to find their destination. In the second part of this experiment, participants were again shown slides, but this time they were first given a detailed explanation of how to read YAH maps and how to orient themselves using the YAH arrow.

Results from the two phases of the experiment were quite similar. When the YAH arrow was aligned so that "forward is up," participants gave correct direction-finding responses far more often than when the YAH arrow was aligned differently. Even when given explicit and detailed instructions on how to use the YAH map and arrow, participants consistently misread misaligned maps.

Experiment 2

In the second experiment, participants were asked to find a particular location within the university library. After being escorted to the starting point, participants were shown one of four library maps (two of the maps were properly aligned and two were misaligned) and asked to find a particular destination. Researchers recorded time spent examining the map and searching for the destination. Each participant completed the procedure twice: once after viewing an aligned map and once after viewing a misaligned map. Different destinations were assigned for the two trials.

Results were consistent with those of the first experiment. People viewing the aligned maps found their destinations significantly more often than those viewing misaligned maps. In addition, those given misaligned maps spent significantly more time viewing the map as well as more time searching for destinations than did those given aligned maps.

RESEARCH BOX 4.7   PLAN VIEW VERSUS PERSPECTIVE VIEW IN YOU-ARE-HERE MAPS

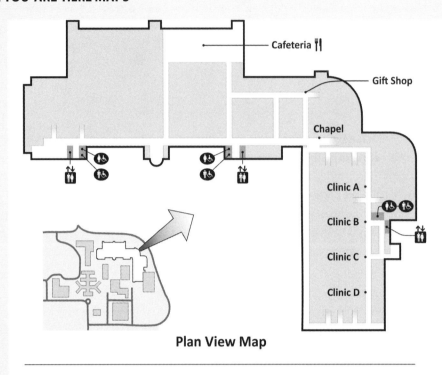

Plan View Map

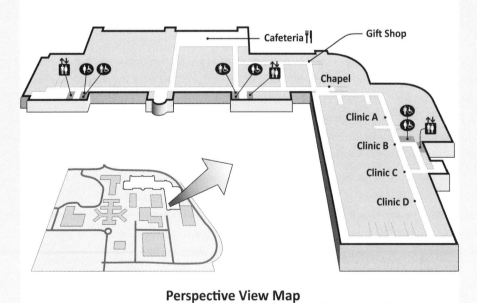

Perspective View Map

As part of a series of ongoing wayfinding studies, the Patient and Visitor Participation Project at the University of Michigan Medical Center undertook a study of interior YAH maps to examine two questions not previously addressed in the literature (Carpman and Grant, 1984). The first was whether hospital patients and visitors would prefer a plan-view graphic or a perspective (bird's-eye view) graphic as the way to represent the space where they were. The second was whether hospital patients and visitors would find it easier to understand a YAH map that included an inset depicting the location of the focal area in the context of the medical center campus, or a map without such an inset.

The plan-view and perspective- (bird's eye) view graphics of a hospital (shown on the previous page) are updated versions of the You-Are-Here map options studied. They contain insets showing the hospital's relation to the medical campus.

Seventy randomly selected patients and visitors were shown a series of YAH graphics and asked to express their preferences. Respondents were asked to choose among:

- Perspective view (no inset) versus plan view (no inset)
- Plan view (no inset) versus plan view (with inset)
- Perspective view (no inset) versus perspective view (with inset)
- Perspective view (with inset) versus plan view (with inset)

Although this research did not examine which map type was functionally superior in helping people find their way, it did show which map type people preferred. The results clearly showed that the perspective view was preferred over the plan view, whether presented with or without the inset. Maps with insets, whether plan view or perspective view, were preferred over those without.

Color Coding

Successful wayfinding depends, in part, on reading the physical environment as well as on reading and comprehending signs and other wayfinding cues. As individuals make their way, they will be helped or hindered by available cues.

In the past, colored lines on the floor were often used in hospitals as easy ways to guide patients and visitors to their destinations. Although this component of a wayfinding system was favored by patients and visitors, colored lines on floors or walls are no longer considered a good solution to wayfinding confusion in most facilities. In large healthcare facilities with many destinations, it is impossible to have colored lines leading to each patient-and-visitor destination without creating a multi-colored spaghetti of wall or floor lines. A system of floor lines might work in such facilities if they lead to only one or two destinations that are difficult to find using conventional wayfinding strategies. However, floor lines have some downsides, including sometimes being covered by carpeting, disappearing due to renovations, having colors that are hard to distinguish, having unclear starting and ending points, and the like. Similarly, lines on the wall may conflict with signs, artwork, doorways, or other design features (Shumaker and Reizenstein, 1982). (See Research Box 4.8.)

RESEARCH BOX 4.8 USING BANNERS AND COLORED LIGHTS TO AID WAYFINDING

In conjunction with the construction of a new entrance, designers at Bellevue Hospital in New York City developed their own orientation system (Olsen and Pershing, 1981). The design included carpeting, maps, color-coded neon lights and banners, and a numbering system to identify patient destinations.

Several months after the renovation, researchers evaluated the success of the new design. Overall, patients and visitors responded positively. They felt that the appearance of the entrance and corridor was much improved and that it showed that Bellevue "was doing something nice for them." Likewise, they noted that the attention paid to the orientation system showed that Bellevue cared about their comfort.

The orientation system itself received mixed reviews. The color-coded system of lights and banners seemed to be well understood: 81.7 percent of those interviewed were able to associate specific destinations with specific colors. Some respondents felt that the increased interest provided by the lights and banners along the corridor made the journey seem shorter than it actually was. However, patients and visitors found the use of numbered banners (indicating various service areas) and numbered windows (indicating specific locations, such as the screening nurse and the clinic registration area) confusing as destination markers. As a result of this evaluation, the researchers recommended that windows be renamed, using words instead of numbers.

Color coding is often wrongly thought to be an easy solution to wayfinding problems (Fusillo, Kaplan, and Whitehead, unpublished report). For example, in large, complex buildings there will be more floors and potential destinations than any simple color scheme can accommodate. Because many people (and certainly those under stress) may not be able to distinguish or remember a particular shade within a large number of colors, colored floor lines may add to, rather than mitigate, feelings of confusion.

Another drawback of color coding, even in relatively simple, small-scale facilities, is that it is not used solely for wayfinding purposes. Color may be used for decoration in the same area where it is supposed to have wayfinding meaning. If people cannot tell when color has meaning and when it does not, color is ineffective as a wayfinding cue.

Consider the following guidelines for color coding:

- When using colored floor lines, use highly contrasting colors. Use colored floor lines to lead to no more than two destinations.

- Avoid using color for decoration in the same way it is being used as a color-coded wayfinding cue (American Hospital Association, 1979; Reizenstein and Vaitkus, 1981).

Signage and the Americans with Disabilities Act

The Americans with Disabilities Act (ADA) was enacted to provide equal access, opportunities, and employment to Americans with disabilities. The ADA seeks to end discrimination against an estimated 54 million Americans (2008 American Community Survey, 2008). The most relevant sections related to wayfinding are contained within the ADA Standards for Accessible Design. (See chapter 9 for a general discussion of the ADA's requirements. Information may also be found at www.ada.gov.)

Directions Given by Staff

Some people need human reassurance regardless of the extent and quality of the overall wayfinding system. Although trained staff at Information Desks may be available, other staff and volunteers should be prepared to answer requests for directions (Carpman et al., 1984a). However, untrained staff may not have the skills necessary to give directions well. Large healthcare facilities should consider instituting an ongoing staff training program in giving consistent, accurate directions.

For example, before occupancy of more than 1 million square feet (~92,903 square meters) of new facilities, the University of Michigan Medical Center recognized the need to train its 800+ staff members about details of the new wayfinding system, with special emphasis on direction giving. Training sessions were designed for three groups:

- Staff whose duties involved giving directions, such as Information Desk attendants, diagnostic and treatment department receptionists, and inpatient unit clerks

- Staff whose duties involved traversing the facilities, including messengers, transporters, and phlebotomists

- Staff, such as maintenance and security personnel, whose duties involved quickly locating specific rooms (Carpman, unpublished reports, 1985; Carpman, 1985).

Wayfinding during Periods of Construction

During periods of construction or renovation, familiar circulation patterns are often interrupted, and patients, visitors, and staff cope with construction-related confusion. However, when mitigating wayfinding strategies are well planned, users should be able to find their way during periods of construction. Maintaining order in the face of significant change is challenging, possible, and necessary, as the following guidelines suggest:

- Keep alternative routes as simple as possible.

- Keep wayfinding instructions as simple as possible.

- Make sure that accurate wayfinding information is conveyed to patients and visitors.

- Use a good-humored approach to graphics and signage that acknowledges the user's experience of wayfinding challenges (Jacobson, 1986).

- Consider employing distinctive, noticeable graphics for wayfinding elements used during the construction period.

- Assign wayfinding-related management responsibilities to a single staff member during the construction period.

Wayfinding Technology

The technology revolution has reached the realm of wayfinding. Systems and devices that utilize sound, touch, and geographic sensing are available. They can help individuals select destinations, personalize selected routes, generate maps (and voice guidance) they can take with them, and provide constantly updated maps and directions en route. Interactive wayfinding, including websites, kiosks, and GPS capability in cars, handheld devices, smartphones, and tablets, is now common and can often assist first-time users and those with vision or hearing limitations to find their way (Baldwin, 2003). Although such wayfinding technology may not yet be affordable to all healthcare facilities, the availability of such systems highlights the need to consider a variety of wayfinding elements in addition to traditional signs and maps. Wayfinding technology will continue to evolve and be relied upon by an increasingly large segment of patients and visitors.

Corridor Functions and Amenities

Corridors in healthcare facilities are often long, with few distinctive or visually interesting features (Spivak, 1967). Since inpatients and others may need to get up and walk around for therapeutic reasons, corridors need to be safe and inviting.

Consider the following guidelines:

- Define wall and door boundaries by selecting door trim and baseboard colors that contrast with their surroundings.

- Create contrast between wall and floor surfaces of at least two digits on the gray scale.

- Use non-glare surfaces on walls. (Behar, unpublished paper)

Corridors with windows or other visual features are likely to attract more use than will plain hallways. However, the simple layout of the corridor should not be sacrificed in order to

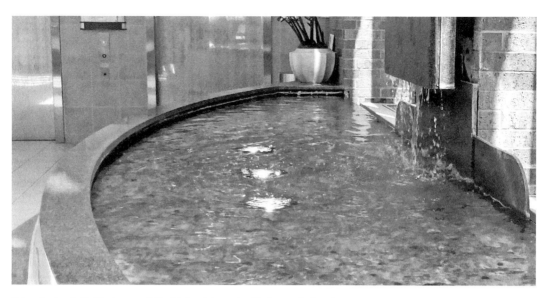

Unique landmarks that feature sound, like this fountain, can be effective wayfinding elements.
Photo credit: Courtesy of St. Joseph Mercy Ann Arbor

add visual complexity and richness (Weisman, 1982). (See also chapter 9.) Corridor interest can be increased in a number of ways:

- Create visual interest with artwork, such as posters, photographs, paintings, and murals. Artwork may also function as wayfinding landmarks (D'Alessio, 1986; Weisman, 1982).

- Consider placing art on the ceiling at particular locations, such as staff elevator lobbies, to provide focal points for patients on gurneys (Shaw, 1976).

- Provide views to the outside along corridors, providing respite and a focus for attention and wayfinding (Bobrow and Thomas, 1976; Calderhead, 1975).

- Locate windows along corridors rather than at the ends of corridors, in order to avoid glare.

Carpeting

Carpeted corridors and patient rooms are a way to soften a harsh-seeming healthcare environment. In general, carpeting is considered more comfortable and psychologically warm than hard-surface flooring and has even been associated with longer visits by family and friends (Cheek, Maxwell, and Weisman, 1971; Counsell et al., 2000; Eagle, 2010; Harris, 2000). Carpeting has also been found to reduce ambient noise levels and injuries from falls (Philbin and Gray, 2002; Pierce, 1973; Spivak, 1967; Willmott, 1986). Due to infection-control concerns, carpet must be carefully selected and maintained. With proper care, carpeting should pose no microbiological hazard to the typical patient (Lankford et al., 2006; Simmons, Reizenstein, and Grant, 1982; Skoutelis et al., 1994). In 1985, the Centers for Disease Control lifted their recommendations against use of carpets in patient-care areas, stating that "there is no epidemiologic evidence to show that carpets influence the nosocomial infection rate in hospitals" (Selhulster et al., 2004; Wise, 1994).

Along with its benefits, carpeting in corridors has a few drawbacks. Carts, beds, gurneys, diagnostic equipment, and wheelchairs are more difficult to move on carpeted surfaces than on hard floors, although special casters and a low-pile, unpadded carpet can alleviate the problem (Deschambeau, 1965). The ADA mandates a maximum pile height of ½ inch, as measured from the bottom of the tuft (US Department of Justice, 2010). Carpeting specifications that need to be carefully considered include fire safety, stain resistance, static-electricity resistance, friction resistance, and the presence of a permanent antimicrobial finish (Conductive Carpet Tile, 2013; Facility Guidelines Institute, 2010; Gulwadi and Calkins, 2008; Odell, 2007).

Consider the following guidelines when selecting carpeting and other floor coverings:

- Select a resilient carpet for ease of wheelchair handling. Specify a pile height of less than ½ inch (~0.64 centimeter) (less than ¼ inch [~0.32 centimeter] for people with less than normal strength), with an uncut or tip-sheer high-density pile, so that wheelchairs are not pulled in another direction by the carpeting.

- Choose a stain-resistant carpet with an added biological guard to prevent bacterial growth and resulting odors.

- Consider static-resistant carpet or treat carpet to be static resistant to reduce electrical interference for people with hearing aids.

- Permanently install area rugs, if they are used at all, in order to reduce patient falls.

- Select floor colors that contrast with the colors of walls and furniture.

- Limit contrast between adjacent carpet areas so that the carpet seams are not mistaken for stairs.

- Avoid cushioned floors because they can be permanently dented and are not durable for high-traffic use.

- Avoid using paving materials, such as brick, that produce an irregular surface.

- Avoid using flooring materials that may cause tripping (Behar, unpublished paper).

Lighting

Lighting can significantly influence the overall ambience of corridors and the effectiveness of a variety of wayfinding elements. The use of task and mood lighting is hardly new, but lighting can serve a number of other functions, especially in areas where the accurate assessment of patients' skin tones is less important. Corridors should be illuminated in a way that facilitates safe and comfortable movement. For example, lighting can be used to signal changes such as the beginning of a ramp or a different floor surface. Variations in corridor illumination can also become an element of the wayfinding system when the variations indicate turns, distinguish the circulation path from other spaces, and highlight meaningful spaces and important information along the way. Lighting can also help define areas along a hallway and visually break up a long corridor into segments, helping to avoid a tunnel effect.

Consider the following guidelines for improving corridor lighting:

- Avoid over-lighting the corridor. One approach is to use a continuous band of low-intensity light rather than periodic bright lights, which can cause glare (Facility Guidelines Institute, 2010; Hayward, 1982; Souhrada, 1989).

- Avoid corridor lighting that shines in patients' eyes as they are transported on gurneys. This can be accomplished by using linear fluorescents mounted on one side of the ceiling or wall (Facility Guidelines Institute, 2010; Hayward, 1982; Souhrada, 1989).

- Mitigate a tunnel effect by mounting linear fluorescents on opposite sides of the corridor, at regular intervals. Switch sides at corridor intersections, but no more frequently than approximately every 75–100 feet (~23–30.5 meters) (Facility Guidelines Institute, 2010; Hayward, 1982; Souhrada, 1989).

- Use special lighting color or intensity to highlight meaningful spaces, such as reception areas, nursing stations, or major intersections (Fong, 2003; Hayward, 1982).

- Use conventional fluorescent fixtures or specially designed lights to illuminate ceiling-hung signs (Fong and Nichelson, 2006).

- Plan, locate, and direct lighting so as to effectively illuminate wayfinding signs and You-Are-Here maps (Facility Guidelines Institute, 2010; Hayward, 1982; Souhrada, 1989).

- In situations where directional signs, YAH maps, or identification signs are dimly lit, provide spot lighting or additional ambient lighting along the corridor (Facility Guidelines Institute, 2010; Hayward, 1982; Souhrada, 1989).

Handrails and Seating

For some patients, a walk down the hall may feel like a major expedition. Frail from surgery, illness, or age, some patients (and some visitors) need physical support while walking and places to sit and rest along the way. Handrails positioned along a corridor can give patients and visitors the psychological and physical support they need to get up and walk. Patients unsure of their strength may be encouraged to venture down a hallway when handrails are available. Strategically placed benches or seating alcoves provide needed rest stops for patients and visitors.

In some facilities, handrails are incorporated into the design of wall bumper guards. Although this allows one design feature to serve two purposes, it is important to make sure that these bumper guards perform effectively as handrails. To ensure that patients and visitors can firmly grasp handrails, the handrail portion of the bumper guard should be rounded to fit a hand, with a sizable indentation on the back to allow the fingers to grip. It should be ~1¼–1½ inches (~3.2–3.8 centimeters) in diameter. The handrail should be mounted ~1½ inches (~3.8 centimeters) from the wall and ~32–34 inches (~81.3–86.4 centimeters) from the floor. This clearance allows gripping without the chance of a person's arm becoming lodged between the wall and the handrail in the event of a fall (American National Standards Institute, 1980; Carpman and Grant, 1983; Harkness and Groom, 1976).

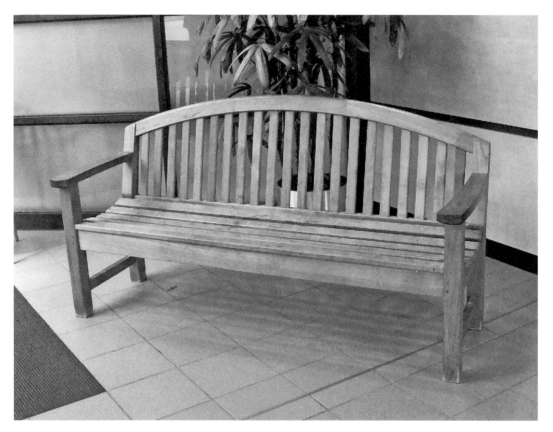

Patients and visitors appreciate being able to sit along corridors in a health facility. Benches featuring armrests and space under the seat make it easier for customers to sit and rise.

Photo credit: Courtesy of St. Joseph Mercy Ann Arbor.

Traveling from Floor to Floor

Just as corridors are used to get from one part of the same floor to another and from one building to another, elevators and stairways are used to travel from floor to floor. In many ways, the related design and behavioral issues are similar: patients and visitors need to travel comfortably and safely and they need to find their way without difficulty.

Elevators

Patients and visitors need to be able to easily enter elevators, reach elevator control panels, and understand how to use them. Consider the following guidelines:

- Install elevators with doors wide enough to accommodate a stretcher and associated personnel and equipment.

- Because elevators are used by patients who may move and respond slowly, adjust doors to close slowly.

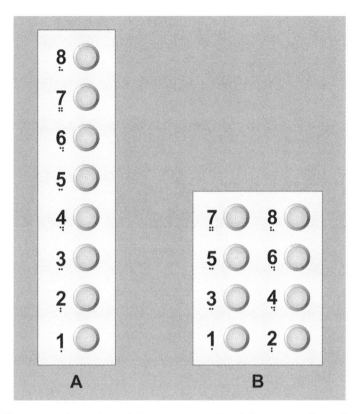

Inside elevator cabs, call buttons are easier to understand when they are arranged vertically, to represent floor-to-floor relationships (as in option A), rather than horizontally (as in option B).

- Indicate elevator floor designations with raised numerals and Braille, as required by ADA or other regulations (Harkness and Groom, 1976).

- Consider placing small signs on the control panel to provide redundant cues for certain call buttons, such as Cafeteria, Floor 1 (Main), and so on.

- When call buttons inside elevator cabs use letters to identify floors, display easily understood explanations next to the buttons: for example, the word *Mezzanine* next to MZ and the words *Plaza Level* next to PL.

- Use understandable pictograms and words to indicate buttons used for door opening, door closing, and emergency (Carpman and Grant, 2012).

- Arrange call buttons vertically inside elevator cabs to reflect floor-to-floor relationships.

- Install elevator controls within the easy reach of wheelchair users, as required by ADA and other regulations (Harkness and Groom, 1976).

- Provide an understandable and easy-to-read display that indicates the present floor location.

- Design elevator lighting to minimize reflective glare on the floor-number display.

- Use materials in the elevator cab that resist unintentional damage and vandalism.

- Locate floor-number identification in the elevator lobby, opposite the elevator and in clear view of those exiting the elevator.

- Provide metal tactile numbers for floor designations on each floor, ~60 inches (~1.5 meters) above the floor on the fixed point at the open side of the elevator door or, when center-opening doors are used, on both sides, or as required by code (Michigan Department of Labor, 1985).

- Outside the elevator, provide call buttons with understandable symbols or pictograms indicating Up and Down.

- Provide easily understood indicators in each elevator lobby, showing the direction an elevator is moving.

- Provide an elevator directory located near the call buttons, listing major destinations on each floor served by the elevator.

- Provide a smaller version of the elevator directory inside the elevator cab.

- In elevator lobbies, provide a place for patients and visitors to sit while waiting for the elevator.

- In large hospitals, consider designating certain elevators for the public and outpatients, and others for staff and inpatients.

Stairways

In 1974, the US Consumer Product Safety Commission called stairs the most hazardous consumer product. Eight years later, it estimated that there were over twice as many injuries resulting from stairway use as from the next-greatest hazard, bicycles, and that about 4,000 people die each year as a result of stair-related injuries. A later study indicates that older people account for 85 percent of those deaths (Hunt and Ross, 1989).

In hospitals, stairways are potentially dangerous places. Frail patients under the influence of medication, distracted visitors, and rushing staff are potential victims of stairway accidents that can result in anything from bumps and bruises to broken bones and fatal injuries.

Yet in addition to their usefulness in emergencies, when elevators are not in use, stairways fill a necessary role as a vertical circulation alternative to slow or crowded elevators. Stairs can also provide exercise. One study showed that the inclusion of "motivational" signage and music may successfully attract more stair users, but may also pose safety risks (Hölscher et al., 2006; Kerr et al., 2004).

According to reviews of stairway accident research, safety researchers in several countries have videotaped the successes and failures of tens of thousands of stair users in many types of public settings (Archea, 1985; Pauls, 1985; Templer and Archea, 1983).The goal of the research was to determine optimal stairway design characteristics. Researchers found that successful stair use depends on navigating the first two or three steps, that is, on making the transition from a level surface to the circumscribed foot placement necessary to go down or up. In descent, where most accidents occur, users make a series of rapid visual and kinesthetic tests, first estimating where to place their feet and then verifying that estimate by getting a feel of the treads. In this context, stair accidents occur when the user's testing process is disrupted. Distractions—such as other people, noise, loose handrails, and visual changes in stair and wall placement or design—often cause accidents. Unanticipated hazards such as trash or loose treads are other typical causes of falls on stairs (Templer and Archea, 1983).

A singular and unambiguous indication of the edge of each tread is essential information for users as they look down (or up) a flight of stairs (Archea, 1985). Treads should not seem to merge together like a ramp; rather, adjoining treads should contrast with one another through the use of contrasting colors or lighting (Hunt and Ross, 1989).The chances of overstepping are increased when the design of stair coverings uses repetitive, random, or geometric patterns with vivid colors, stripes running parallel to the tread edge, or subtle dimensional irregularities and three-dimensional textures, which can all obscure the visual information needed to distinguish the edge of each tread (Pauls, 1985).

Consider the following guidelines with regard to stairway coverings such as carpeting, in order to achieve maximum clarity:

- Provide contrast with walls and other vertical surfaces.

- Provide effective contrast between stair treads and risers.

- In order to clearly differentiate floor and wall surfaces at stairways, use a band of color that contrasts with both floor and wall colors (Hunt and Ross, 1989).

One researcher notes that codes and standards in the United States do not always conform well to human ergonomics. For example, stairwells may be so wide and handrails placed so low that users in the center area of any stair cannot reach the handrail if they happen to stumble. Similarly, one study analyzing videotaped accidents found that the maximum effective stair-riser height should be 6 inches (~15.2 millimeters), not the commonly used 7-inch (~17.8 centimeters) standard (Pauls, 1985).

Given the needs of healthcare facility users, it is important to optimize these sorts of dimensions, rather than just meeting minimum criteria. As a starting point for effective stairway design, researchers offer three conditions for creating safe stair use: steps should be readily visible, treads should be large enough to provide effective footing, and handrails should be easily reached and grasped.

Consider the following guidelines for safe stairway design:

- Avoid obscuring tread edges with optical illusions or "visual noise," such as vivid floral or geometric patterns, stripes running parallel to the tread edge, and three-dimensional textures that may create visual confusion (Archea, 1985).

- Provide visual cues that accentuate and correspond with the conditions on a stairway. All colors, edges, lines, alignments, patterns, and textures should interact to produce a true representation of the extent and position of the treads (Archea, 1985).

- Provide easily discernible tread edges by using surface and edge to create a figure–ground relationship where each tread edge appears as a figure and the riser surface below appears as the background (Archea, 1985).

- Use light to clarify the tread edge, but plan lighting locations carefully to prevent shadows, which may be mistaken as the edge of a tread (Archea, 1985).

- Provide a strong, easily grasped, and easily seen handrail, as many people use handrails to pull themselves up from one tread to the next and also as compensation for vision limitations (Archea, 1985).

- Avoid stairs with protruding treads or open risers because they are difficult to navigate by people with vision or mobility disabilities (Harkness and Groom, 1976).

- Consider round handrails (~1¼–1½ inches, ~3.2–3.8 centimeters in diameter) with sufficient clearance between the handrail and the wall (~1½ inches, ~3.8 centimeters). These can be easily gripped without the chance that a person's arm will become lodged in the gap, in the event of a fall (Harkness and Groom, 1976).

- Consider placing handrails at a height that allows users to glide from elbow to wrist, thus using the arm as a "third foot" for better stability and greater mobility (Hiatt, 1991).

- Provide handrails for short inclines (one- to three-step differences) (Baier and Shumaker, 1989).

- Provide handrails on both sides of a staircase (Harkness and Groom, 1976).

- Extend handrails beyond the first and last steps of a staircase (Harkness and Groom, 1976).

- Avoid constructing stairways out of slippery materials (Harkness and Groom, 1976).

- Avoid the simultaneous change of several environmental factors (such as lighting, view, floor surface) on a stairway (Templer, Mullet, and Archea, 1978).

- Provide effective illumination in stairways. Eliminate glare and shadows so that patients and visitors with vision disabilities are not hindered (Templer, Mullet, and Archea, 1978).

- Provide visual cues that distinguish stairway treads from risers (Templer, Mullet, and Archea, 1978).

- Consider providing artwork in stairwells to make them visually interesting and to encourage their use.

Unplanned Uses of Corridors, Elevators, and Stairways

Corridors, elevators, and stairways are often the unclaimed territories of a health facility. They are not always attended to by departmental managers and may receive less day-to-day attention than they need. Circulation areas may become ad hoc storage areas for wheelchairs, linens, and gurneys; impromptu conference rooms for physicians and other medical personnel; and informal waiting areas for patients and visitors. With all of their unplanned uses, corridors can become cluttered and noisy.

These unplanned uses affect patients, visitors, and staff by reducing privacy and creating a poor image of the facility. When staff members confer in hallways or elevators, patient information may be overheard by unauthorized people. Not only may this breach the standard of confidentiality, it may also cause unnecessary alarm in those overhearing the information.

Although it is probably unrealistic to assume that all unplanned corridor use can be eliminated, clutter and noise can often be reduced. Constructing alcoves and other storage areas, providing ample conference room space, and designing comfortable waiting areas and lounges can go a long way toward solving the problem.

Summary

- ○ Healthcare facilities are typically large and complex, with numerous patient/visitor destinations often widely separated. Patients and visitors may be preoccupied and physically and/or emotionally stressed, making it difficult for them to navigate. Spatial disorientation adds to stress, can take extra time and cause patients to be late for or miss appointments. It can produce feelings of helplessness, anger, and even panic, as well as generalized hostility toward the institution. Disorientation may also have physiological effects, such as increased heart-rate. Staff, as well as patients and visitors, can experience negative effects of disorientation.

- ○ Well-placed and easy-to-read signage must be supplemented by other components of a wayfinding *system* such as building layout, architectural differentiation, landmarks like plants and artwork, lighting, maps, terminology, room and floor numbering, spoken directions, and technology.

- ○ When possible, related functions should be located close to one another.

- ○ Decision-points occur on a given route when a person is moving from one area into another, as at intersections or destinations. Decision-points also occur at places where environmental features indicate changes in lighting, flooring, color schemes, and the like. Signs should be located at these decision-points, rather than at arbitrary intervals along the path. If there are no key decision-points along a route, reassurance signs should be placed approximately every 150 to 250 feet (~45.7–76.2 meters).

- ○ Avoid creating corridors that are uninviting and disorienting by incorporating design features such as well-defined wall and door boundaries, non-glare surfaces, views to the outdoors, and visual interest from artwork. Lighting and carpeting should facilitate safe and comfortable movement. Handrails can provide psychological and physical support. Strategically placed seating offers needed rest stops.

- ○ For movement from floor to floor, elevators must be designed so that patients and visitors are able to enter easily, reach elevator control panels, and understand how to use them.

- ○ Stairways—necessary but potentially dangerous places—need to be designed to facilitate the transition from level surface to circumscribed tread by a complete, correct, and consistent pattern of cues, and by handrails that are easily reached and gripped.

DISCUSSION QUESTIONS

1. What are some factors that make successful wayfinding particularly challenging for patients and visitors in a healthcare facility?

2. What can be some costs, both direct and indirect, of unsuccessful wayfinding experiences in a healthcare facility?

3. What other environmental clues can be employed, along with signage, to form a mutually reinforcing wayfinding system?

4. What factors should be considered when designing a successful floor-numbering system in order to avoid floor-number confusion, including the special problems of linking buildings and below-grade locations?

5. What factors should be considered when designing an effective room-numbering system?

6. What are important considerations when selecting wording (messages) for signage, maps, and other wayfinding information?

7. What are some characteristics of effective signage with regard to color, design, and flexibility?

8. What is meant by the term *decision-point,* and how should the concept be employed in the location of signage?

9. What are some of the factors that should be considered during the design of corridors, elevator lobbies, and stairs?

Design Review Questions

Finding One's Way through a Health Facility

Building Layout and Landmarks

☐ Will the wayfinding system be designed to satisfy the orientation needs of first-time users? (Carpman et al., 1984a; Hauff, 1988)

☐ Will the wayfinding system include such components as the basic layout of the building and site, interior and exterior landmarks, views to the outside, signs, wording, floor numbers, room numbers, spoken directions, You-Are-Here maps, handheld maps, directional signs, identification signs, directories, and technology? (Weisman, 1982)

☐ Will related healthcare-facility functions be located close to one another? (Carpman et al., 1984a; Hauff, 1988)

☐ If a new healthcare facility is being designed, will decision-makers consider the impact of the building's appearance and form on wayfinding? (Weisman, 1979)

☐ Will interior landmarks include architectural details, lighting, color, texture, artwork, and plants? (Carpman et al., 1984a)

Floor Numbering

☐ Will floor-number designations relate to the Main Entrance floor and indicate whether floors are above or below ground?

☐ Will floor-number relationships between linked buildings be considered so that, for example, Floor 2 of one building does not link to Floor 4 of another? (Carpman et al., 1984b)

☐ Will floor numbers be used in the room-numbering system (for example, rooms on Floor 5 would all begin with the number 5)? (Carpman et al., 1984b)

Room Numbering

☐ Will room numbers on the floors below the entrance level begin with a prefix likely to be understood by first-time users? (Carpman et al., 1984a)

☐ Will the room-numbering system be designed to facilitate wayfinding ease?

☐ Will the room-numbering system provide gaps in the numbering sequence to allow for future expansion and renovation? (Carpman et al., 1984a)

☐ Will the room-numbering system be used consistently on floors having similar uses and layouts? (Carpman et al., 1984a)

Design That Cares: Planning Health Facilities for Patients and Visitors, third edition, by Janet R. Carpman and Myron A. Grant. ©2016 by Jossey-Bass.

☐ Will room numbers on signs be legible to patients and visitors? (Carpman et al., 1984a)

☐ Will the appearance of room numbers on signs identifying patient and visitor destinations (such as patient rooms and exam rooms) be differentiated from room numbers on signs identifying staff destinations? (Carpman et al., 1984a)

☐ With the exception of inpatient rooms, will patient and visitor destinations be clearly identified by common-language names as well as numbers? (Carpman et al., 1984a)

☐ If the number of a room is its primary means of identification by patients and visitors, will the numbers be legible? (Carpman et al., 1984a)

☐ Will patient room-identification signs be visible when doors are open?

☐ Will combinations of letters and numbers, such as NIB407, be avoided?

☐ If letters and numbers must be combined to create a room number, will letters be avoided that may be interpreted as numbers (such as *I*, *O*, and *Q*)? (Carpman et al., 1984a)

☐ Will the room-numbering system begin at one end or corner of a floor and flow sequentially through to the other end? (American Hospital Association, 1979)

☐ Will a simple room-numbering system be used, such as a continuous series with odd numbers on one side of the hall and even numbers on the other? (American Hospital Association, 1979)

☐ In new construction projects, will wayfinding-related room numbering be considered early in the design process, prior to showing room numbers on architectural plans?

☐ Will patient room numbers and telephone numbers be coordinated? (Carpman et al., 1984a)

Sign Messages

☐ Will plain and simple wording in English and/or other languages be used? (Kearney, Rice, and Parks, 1987)

☐ Will wayfinding wording be tested for comprehension by patients and visitors? (Carpman et al., 1984a)

☐ Will consistent wayfinding wording be used throughout the facility? (American Hospital Association, 1979; Marks, 1979)

☐ Will ambiguous wording be avoided? (Follis and Hammer, 1979; Marks, 1979)

☐ Will each department use consistent wayfinding wording on its signs and in written and verbal communications with patients and visitors? (American Hospital Association, 1979; Marks, 1979)

☐ Will wayfinding wording be within a sixth-grade reading level? (American Hospital Association, 1979)

Symbols and Pictograms

☐ Will symbols and pictograms under consideration—other than those universally used—be tested for comprehension by patients and visitors? (Carpman et al., 1984a)

☐ Will the effect of symbols and pictograms on sign legibility be evaluated?

☐ Will symbol and pictogram styles, colors, shapes, and backgrounds be used consistently? (Follis and Hammer, 1979)

☐ Unless they are widely recognized, will symbols and pictograms be used only to supplement verbal information? (Follis and Hammer, 1979)

☐ Will arrows be used only as direction indicators? (Selfridge, 1979)

Sign Updating

☐ Will there be a staff member responsible for managing and maintaining the wayfinding system?

☐ Will there be a database developed to catalogue wayfinding signs and their locations and messages?

☐ Will the sign system be managed proactively?

☐ Will the design of wayfinding signs allow easy wording changes without inviting unintentional damage or vandalism?

☐ Will the wayfinding sign system be regularly reviewed for damage, as well as wording accuracy and consistency?

Sign Spacing and Location

☐ Will overhead sign locations be planned in conjunction with mechanical, electrical, and lighting fixtures so views to prime sign locations are not obstructed? (Carpman et al., 1984a)

☐ Will signs be placed at decision-points? (Carpman et al., 1984a)

☐ Will reassurance signs be placed approximately 150–250 feet (~45.7–76.2 meters) after major decision-points if another decision-point has not already occurred? (Carpman et al., 1984a; Downs, 1979)

☐ Will wayfinding signs and You-Are-Here maps be placed in consistent locations? (Levine, 1982; Wechsler, 1979; Weisman, 1982; Wilt and Maienschien, 1979)

☐ Will directional signs be located perpendicular to the flow of foot traffic?

Interior You-Are-Here Maps

☐ Will the wording used to identify destinations on YAH maps be consistent with wording used on directional and identification signs? (Levine, 1982)

☐ Will YAH maps be oriented so that "forward is up" (that is, the direction the person is facing while viewing the map is at the top of the map)? (Levine, 1982)

☐ Will distinctive architectural or interior design elements, such as landmarks, be incorporated into YAH maps? (Levine, 1982)

☐ Will YAH maps be kept simple by emphasizing public corridors and destinations and by deemphasizing staff areas?

☐ Will an inset be used on YAH maps to show the relation of the mapped portion of the building to the rest of the facility? (Carpman and Grant, 1984)

☐ Will the You-Are-Here arrow be drawn so it points in the direction and at the spot the viewer is facing while looking at the map? (Levine, 1982)

Color Coding

☐ If a system of colored floor lines is used as part of an overall wayfinding system, will it consist of contrasting colors leading to no more than two destinations?

☐ If color coding is necessary, will it be used logically and consistently throughout the facility? (American Hospital Association, 1979; Reizenstein and Vaitkus, 1981)

☐ If color is used as a wayfinding cue, will it be used only in that way and not also "for decoration"? (American Hospital Association, 1979; Reizenstein and Vaitkus, 1981)

Wayfinding during Periods of Construction

☐ Will alternative routes be as simple as possible?

☐ Will wayfinding instructions be as simple as possible?

☐ Will all information be accurately conveyed to patients and visitors?

☐ Will construction-related signs and graphics use a good-humored and empathetic approach? (Jacobson, 1986)

☐ Will a distinctive, noticeable graphic image be considered for wayfinding elements used during construction?

☐ Will wayfinding-related responsibilities be assigned to a single staff member during the construction period?

Wayfinding Technology

☐ Will wayfinding technology be considered as a way to supplement essential elements of the wayfinding system, such as directional signs and You-Are-Here maps?

Corridor Functions and Amenities

☐ Will wall and door boundaries be defined by door trim and baseboard colors that contrast with their surroundings?

☐ Will the color of adjacent wall and floor surfaces provide contrast of at least two digits on the gray scale?

☐ Will walls have non-glare surfaces?

☐ Will artwork be used to create visual interest? (D'Alessio, 1986; Weisman, 1982)

☐ Will artwork be located on the ceiling in places where patients wait on gurneys? (Shaw, 1976)

☐ Will corridors have outside views? (Bobrow and Thomas, 1976; Calderhead, 1975)

☐ In order to avoid glare, will windows be provided along corridors, rather than at the ends?

Carpeting

☐ Will the following carpet attributes be considered: fire safety, stain resistance, static-electricity resistance, friction resistance, and the presence of a permanent antimicrobial finish?

☐ Will resilient carpet be selected with a very short pile height for ease of wheelchair handling? (Behar, unpublished; U.S. Department of Justice, 2010)

☐ Will stain-resistant carpet be selected with features that prevent bacterial growth and resulting odors? (Behar, unpublished; Lankford et al., 2006; Skoutelis et al., 1994)

☐ Will static-resistant carpet be considered in order to reduce electrical interference for people with hearing aids? (Behar, unpublished)

☐ If area rugs will be used, will they be permanently installed? (Behar, unpublished)

Design That Cares: Planning Health Facilities for Patients and Visitors, third edition, by Janet R. Carpman and Myron A. Grant. ©2016 by Jossey-Bass.

☐ Will floor colors be selected to contrast with walls and furniture? (Behar, unpublished)

☐ Will contrast be limited between adjacent carpets so they are not mistaken for stairs? (Behar, unpublished)

☐ Will cushioned floors be avoided in high-use areas, since they can become permanently dented and are not durable? (Behar, unpublished)

☐ Will irregular paving and flooring materials not be selected? (Behar, unpublished)

Lighting

☐ Will over-lighting be avoided? (Facility Guidelines Institute, 2010; Hayward, 1982; Souhrada, 1989)

☐ Will corridor lighting be designed so it does not shine in the eyes of patients on gurneys? (Facility Guidelines Institute, 2010; Hayward, 1982; Souhrada, 1989)

☐ Will a lighting "tunnel effect" be avoided? (Facility Guidelines Institute, 2010; Hayward, 1982; Souhrada, 1989)

☐ Will special lighting color or intensity be used to highlight meaningful spaces? (Fong, 2003)

☐ Will light fixtures be used to illuminate ceiling-hung wayfinding signs? (Fong and Nichelson, 1976)

☐ Will lighting be planned, located, and directed to effectively illuminate wayfinding signs and You-Are-Here maps? (Facility Guidelines Institute, 2010; Hayward, 1982; Souhrada, 1989)

☐ In situations where directional signs, YAH maps, or identification signs will not be effectively lit by standard corridor lighting, will spot lighting or additional ambient lighting be provided? (Facility Guidelines Institute, 2010; Hayward, 1982; Souhrada, 1989)

Handrails and Seating

☐ Will handrails or bumper guards with incorporated handrails be used along corridors? (American National Standards Institute, 1980; Carpman and Grant, 1983; Fong, 2003)

☐ Will the handrail (or the handrail portion of a bumper guard) be rounded on top and behind to fit a hand and designed to be ~1¼–1½ inches (~3.2–3.8 centimeters) in diameter? (American National Standards Institute, 1980; Carpman and Grant, 1983; Fong, 2003)

☐ Will the handrail be mounted ~1½ inches (~3.8 centimeters) from the wall? (American National Standards Institute, 1980; Carpman and Grant, 1983; Fong, 2003)

☐ Will the handrail be mounted ~32–34 inches (~81.3–86.4 centimeters) from the floor? (American National Standards Institute, 1980; Carpman and Grant, 1983; Fong, 2003)

☐ Will benches and seating alcoves be provided where inpatients and outpatients need them? (American National Standards Institute, 1980; Carpman and Grant, 1983; Fong, 2003)

Traveling from Floor to Floor

Elevators

☐ Will elevator doors be wide enough to accommodate a stretcher and the associated personnel and equipment?

☐ Will elevator doors close slowly?

☐ Will floor designations be indicated with raised numerals and Braille, as required by ADA or other regulations? (Harkness and Groom, 1976)

☐ On control panels inside elevator cabs, will redundant cuing (such as a label for Cafeteria) be used for related call buttons?

☐ If call buttons use letters to identify floors, will easily-understood explanations be displayed next to the buttons?

☐ Will understandable symbols (pictograms) and words be used on call buttons for door opening, door closing, and emergency?

☐ Will call buttons in elevator cabs be arranged vertically, in order to reflect floor-to-floor relationships?

☐ Will elevator controls be installed within easy reach of wheelchair users, as required by ADA and other regulations? (Harkness and Groom, 1976)

☐ Will elevator lighting be designed so as not to cause reflective glare on the floor number display?

☐ Will there be an understandable and easy-to-read display indicating the present floor location?

☐ Will the elevator cab be constructed of damage-resistant materials?

☐ Will floor number signs be placed in the elevator lobby, directly opposite the elevator and in clear view of those exiting the elevator?

☐ Will metal tactile floor numbers be installed on each floor, 60 inches (~1.5 meters) above the floor on the fixed point at the open side of the elevator door or, when center-opening doors are used, on both sides, or as required by code? (Michigan Department of Labor, 1985)

Design That Cares: Planning Health Facilities for Patients and Visitors, third edition, by Janet R. Carpman and Myron A. Grant. ©2016 by Jossey-Bass.

☐ Will call buttons in elevator lobbies use understandable symbols or pictograms indicating Up and Down?

☐ Will elevator directories be provided near call buttons in elevator lobbies?

☐ Will downsized versions of elevator directories be provided inside elevator cabs?

☐ Will there be a place for patients and visitors to sit while waiting for the elevator?

☐ Will elevators for the public and outpatients be separate from elevators for staff and inpatients?

Stairways

☐ Will stair treads be large enough, front to back, to provide effective footing? (Pauls, 1985)

☐ Will protruding stair treads or open risers be avoided? (Harkness and Groom, 1976)

☐ Will stairway treads be constructed of non-slippery materials? (Harkness and Groom, 1976)

☐ Will visual cues such as colors, edges, lines, alignments, patterns, and textures interact to make stair treads and risers clear? (Archea, 1985)

☐ Will stairway carpeting contrast with walls and other vertical surfaces? (Hunt and Ross, 1989)

☐ Will a band of color that contrasts with both floor and wall colors be used to clearly differentiate floor and wall surfaces at stairways? (Hunt and Ross, 1989)

☐ Will stair-tread edges be free from optical illusions, such as vivid floral or geometric patterns, stripes running parallel to the tread edge, or three-dimensional textures? (Archea, 1985)

☐ Will stair-tread edges be easily discernible from adjacent risers through figure–ground relationships where the edge appears as a figure and the riser below appears as the background? (Archea, 1985)

☐ Will there be effective illumination (without glare or shadows) in and around stairways? (Templer, Mullet, and Archea, 1978)

☐ Will lighting be used effectively to clarify stair-tread edges and prevent shadows? (Archea, 1985)

☐ Will handrails in stairways and along corridors be strong and easy to see, reach, and grasp? (Archea, 1985)

☐ Will handrails be provided on short (one- to three-step) stairways? (Templer et al., 1978)

☐ Will handrails be ~1¼–1½ inches (~3.2–3.8 centimeters) in diameter and mounted ~1½ inches (~3.8 centimeters) from walls and ~32–34 inches (~81.3–86.4 centimeters) from the floor? (Harkness and Groom, 1976)

☐ Will handrails be provided on both sides of staircases? (Harkness and Groom, 1976)

☐ Will handrails extend beyond the first and last steps of staircases? (Harkness and Groom, 1976)

☐ Will handrails be located at a height that allows users to glide from elbow to wrist, using one arm as a "third foot" for better stability and greater mobility? (Hiatt, 1991)

☐ Will artwork be provided in stairwells to encourage use and make them visually interesting?

☐ Will the situation be avoided in which several environmental factors (such as illumination, view, or floor covering) change simultaneously on the stairway? (Templer et al., 1978)

Unplanned Uses of Corridors, Elevators, and Stairways

☐ Will effective, easily accessible storage areas be planned so corridors will not be cluttered with equipment?

☐ Will ample conference room space be provided where physicians and other medical personnel can hold impromptu meetings?

☐ Will a sufficient number of consultation rooms be provided in which medical staff can meet privately with families?

References

American Hospital Association. *Signs and Graphics for Health Care Facilities.* Chicago: AHA, 1979. [Out of print.]

American National Standards Institute. American National Standards Specifications for Making Buildings and Facilities Accessible to and Usable by Physically Handicapped People (A117.1–1980). New York: ANSI, 1980.

Appleyard, D. Why buildings are known: A perspective tool for architects and planners. *Environment and Behavior* 1(2):131–56, December 1969.

Archea, J. C. Environmental factors associated with stair accidents by the elderly. *Clinics in Geriatric Medicine* 1(3):555–69, August 1985.

Aubrey, J., Li, K., and Dobbs, A. Age differences in the interpretation of misaligned "You-Are-Here" Maps. *Journal of Gerontology* 49 (1): 29–31, January 1994.

Baier, S., and Shumaker, M. Z. *Bed Number 10.* Boca Raton, FL: CRC Press, 1989.

Baldwin, D. Wayfinding technology: A road map to the future. *Journal of Visual Impairment and Blindness* 97 (10):612–20, 2003.

Baskaya, A., Wilson, C., and Özcan, Y. Wayfinding in an unfamiliar environment: Different spatial settings of two polyclinics. *Environment and Behavior* 36(6): 839–67, November 2004.

Behar, S. Attractive products for independence. Unpublished paper. [No further information available.]

Berkeley, E. P. More than you want to know about the Boston City Hall. *Architecture Plus* 1(1):72–77, 98, February 1973.

Best, G. Direction-finding in large buildings. Master's thesis, University of Manchester, Manchester, England, 1967.

Bobrow, M. L., and Thomas, J. Achieving quality in hospital design. *Hospital Forum* 19(4):4–6, September 1976.

Calderhead, J., ed. *Hospitals for People.* London: King Edward's Hospital Fund for London, 1975.

Carpman, J. R. Creating hospitals where people can find their way. Joint Commission on Accreditation of Healthcare Organizations Plant, Technology, and Safety Management Series, No. 1, 1991 series, pp. 25–29. Oakbrook Terrace, IL: JCAHO, 1991a.

_____. Wayfinding in health care: Six common myths. *Health Facilities Management* 4(5):24, 26, 28, May 1991b.

_____. Wayfinding: The sign of the times. *Group Practice,* 42–44.[3], July–August 1991c.

_____. Description of the wayfinding training program for the new University of Michigan Hospital and Health Care Center. Unpublished report, Ann Arbor, October 1985.

_____. *You Can Get There from Here: Wayfinding System for the New University Hospital and Health Care Center.* Ann Arbor: Office of Planning and Marketing, Office of Human Resource Development, University of Michigan Hospitals, November 1985.

Carpman, J. R., and Grant, M. A. *Directional Sense: How to Find Your Way Around.* Boston: Institute for Human Centered Design, 2012.

_____. Executive summary: Color, cubicle curtains, handrails. Unpublished research report No. 23, Patient and Visitor Participation Project, Office of Hospital Planning, Research and Development, University of Michigan, Ann Arbor, 1983.

_____. Executive summary: Design of interior "You-Are-Here" maps. Unpublished research report No. 29, Patient and Visitor Participation Project, Office of the Replacement Hospital Program, University of Michigan, Ann Arbor, 1984.

_____. Lost in space. *ID/Industrial Design*, 66–67, 88, January–February 1989.

Carpman, J. R., Grant, M. A., and Simmons, D. A. No more mazes: Research about design for wayfinding in hospitals. Patient and Visitor Participation Project, Office of the Replacement Hospital Program, University of Michigan, Ann Arbor, 1984a.

_____. Wayfinding in the hospital environment: The impact of various floor numbering alternatives. *Journal of Environmental Systems* 13(4):353–64, May 1984b.

Cheek, F. E., Maxwell, R., and Weisman, R. Carpeting the ward: An exploratory study in environmental psychology. *Mental Hygiene* 55(1):109–18, January 1971.

Christensen, K. An impact analysis framework for calculating the costs of staff disorientation in hospitals. Unpublished report, University of California at Los Angeles, n.d.

Conductive carpet tile cannot meet NFPA 99 healthcare standard. *Staticworx.* Static Electricity Professionals Blog. 2013. http://static-electricity-blog.typepad.com/static_electricity_profess/2011 /10/conductive-carpet-tile-cannot-meet-nfpa-99-healthcare-standard.html.

Corlett, E. N., Manenica, I., and Bishop, R. P. The design of direction-finding systems in buildings. *Applied Ergonomic* 3(2):66–69, June 1972.

Counsell, S. R., Holder, C. M., Liebenauer, L. L., Palmer, R. M., Fortinsky, R. H., Kresevic, D. M., et al. Effects of a multicomponent intervention on functional outcomes and process of care in hospitalized older patients. *Journal of the American Geriatrics Society* 48(12):1572–81, 2000.

D'Alessio, A. Marshall Erdman's art program: Art as medicine. *Group Practice,* 72–80, September–October 1986.

Daniel, E. H. Signs and the school media center. In D. Pollet and P. Haskell, editors. *Sign Systems for Libraries,* 127–35. New York: R. R. Bowker, 1979.

Derose, K., and Baker, D. Limited English proficiency and Latinos' use of physician services. *Medical Care Research and Review* 57(1):76–91, March 2000.

Deschambeau, G. L. More effort needed to move cart on carpet than tile study finds. *Modern Hospital* 105(1):30, July 1965.

Devlin, A. Housing for the elderly: Cognitive considerations. *Environment and Behavior* 12(4):451–66, December 1980.

Downs, R. Mazes, minds, and maps. In D. Pollet and P. Haskell, editors. *Sign Systems for Libraries,* 17–32. New York: R. R. Bowker, 1979.

Eagle, A. Rolling it out. *Health Facility Management* 23(5):32–34, May 2010.

Eubanks, P. Wayfinding: More than just putting up signs. *Health Facilities Management* 2(6):20, 22, 25, June 1989.

Facility Guidelines Institute. *Guidelines for Design and Construction of Health Care Facilities,* 2010 edition. Chicago: ASHE (American Society for Healthcare Engineering of the American Hospital Association), 2010.

Follis, J., and Hammer, D. *Architectural Signing and Graphics.* New York: Watson Guptill, 1979.

Fong, D. B. Illuminating thoughts: Devising lighting strategies for clinical spaces. *Health Facilities Management,* 24–29, July 2003.

Fong, D. B., and Nichelson, K. Evidence-based lighting design. *Healthcare Design* 6(5): 50–53, September 2006.

Fusillo, A. E., Kaplan, S., and Whitehead, B. Human environmental considerations in health facility design. Unpublished report, Systems Science Institute, University of Louisville, Louisville, KY, n.d.

Gulwadi, G. B., and Calkins, M. P. *The Impact of Healthcare Environmental Design on Patient Falls.* Concord, CA: The Center for Health Design, 2008.

Harkness, S. P., and Groom, J. N. *Building without Barriers for the Disabled.* New York: Watson Guptill, 1976.

Harris, D. D. Environmental quality and healing environments: A study of flooring materials in a healthcare telemetry unit. Doctoral dissertation, Texas A&M University, College Station TX, 2000. [Available from ProQuest, 789 E. Eisenhower Parkway, Ann Arbor, MI 48108.]

Hauff, W. Physical plant efficiency: Evaluating the use of space. *Health Progress,* 19–20, November 15, 1988.

Hayward, D. G. Working notes, Office of Hospital Planning, Research and Development, University of Michigan, Ann Arbor, 1982.

Hiatt, L. Breakthroughs in long term care design. *Journal of Health Care Interior Design* 3:205–15, 1991.

Hölscher, C., Meilinger, T., Vrachliotis, G., Brösamle, M., and Knauff, M. Up the down staircase: Wayfinding strategies in multi-level buildings. *Journal of Environmental Psychology* 26:284–299, 2006.

Hunt, M. Environmental learning without being there. *Environment and Behavior* 16(3):307–34, May 1984.

Hunt, M. E., and Ross, L. E. Stairway carpet design: A simple preconstruction evaluation approach. *Journal of Applied Gerontology* 8(4):481–91, December 1989.

Jacobson, J. Patient relations program eases construction's inconvenience. *Health Progress,* 101, December 1986.

Kamisar, H. Signs for the handicapped patron. In D. Pollet and P. Haskell, editors. *Sign Systems for Libraries,* 99–103. New York: R. R. Bowker, 1979.

Kaplan, S. Adaptation, structure, and knowledge. In G. Moore and R. Golledge, editors. *Environmental Knowing: Theories, Research and Methods,* 32–45. Stroudsburg, PA: Dowden, Hutchinson and Ross, 1976.

Kearney, M., Rice, J., and Parks, D. Creating hospital signs—practical design tips. *Hospital Guest Relations Report* 2(4):10–12, April 1987.

Kerr, N., Yore, M., Ham, S., and Dietz, W. Increasing stair use in a worksite through environmental changes. *American Journal of Health Promotion* 18(4):312–15, March, April 2004.

Lankford, M. G., Collins, S., Youngberg, L., Rooney, D. M., Warren, J. R., and Noskin, G. A. Assessment of materials commonly utilized in health care: Implications for bacterial survival and transmission. *American Journal of Infection Control* 34(5):258–63, 2006.

Levine, M. You-Are-Here maps: Psychological considerations. *Environment and Behavior* 14(2):221–37, March 1982.

Levine, M., Marchon, I., and Hanley, G. The placement and misplacement of You-Are-Here maps. *Environment and Behavior* 16(2):139–57, March 1984.

MacKenzie, S., and Krusberg, J. Can I get there from here? Wayfinding systems for healthcare facilities. *Leadership,* 42–46, September/October, 1996.

Marks, B. The language of signs. In D. Pollet and P. Haskell, editors. *Sign Systems for Libraries*, 89–97. New York: R. R. Bowker, 1979.

McLaughlin, H. The monumental headache: Overtly monumental and systematic hospitals are usually functional disasters. *Architectural Record* 160(1):118, July 1976.

Michigan Department of Labor. *Barrier-Free Design Codes.* Lansing: Michigan Department of Labor, 1985.

Moeser, S. D. Cognitive mapping in a complex building. *Environment and Behavior* 20(1):21–49, January 1988.

Odell, S. Finish line: Selecting attractive and hygienic interior surfaces. *Health Facilities Management*, 25–30, January 2007.

Olsen, R. V., and Pershing, A. Environmental evaluation of the interim entry to Bellevue Hospital. Unpublished report, Environmental Psychology Department, Bellevue Hospital, New York City, 1981.

Passini, R., and Arthur, P. *Wayfinding: People, Signs, and Architecture.* New York: McGraw-Hill, 1992.

Pauls, J. L. Review of stair-safety research with an emphasis on Canadian studies. *Ergonomics* 28(7): 999–1010, 1985.

Philbin, M. K., and Gray, L. Changing levels of quiet in an intensive care nursery. *Journal of Perinatology* 22(6):455–60, 2002.

Pierce, G. Carpeting cuts maintenance costs. *Canadian Hospital* 50(4):55–60, April 1973.

Principles for Health Reform and Language Access. 2015. www.socialworkers.org/advocacy/healthcare reform/documents/language access and health reform principles.pdf.

Reizenstein, J. E., and Vaitkus, M. A. Hospital visitors and environmental stress. Patient and Visitor Participation Project, Office of the Replacement Hospital Program, University of Michigan, Ann Arbor, 1981.

Salmi, P. Wayfinding design: Hidden barriers to universal access. *Implications* 5(8):1–6, 2007. www .informedesign.org.

Selfridge, K. M. Planning library signage systems. In D. Pollet and P. Haskell, editors. *Sign Systems for Libraries*, 49–67. New York: R. R. Bowker, 1979.

Selhulster, L. M., Chinn, R. Y., Arduino, M. J., Carpenter J., Donlan, R., Ashford, D., et al. *Guidelines for Environmental Infection Control in Healthcare Facilities.* Recommendations from CDC and the Healthcare Infection Control Practices Advisory Committee. Chicago: American Society for Healthcare Engineering/American Hospital Association, 2004.

Shaw, H. Anti-stress art. *Nursing Times* 72(25):960–61, June 24, 1976.

Shumaker, S., and Reizenstein, J. E. Environmental factors affecting inpatient stress in acute care hospitals. In G. W. Evans, editor. *Environmental Stress*, 179–223. New York: Cambridge University Press, 1982.

Simmons, D. A., Reizenstein, J. E., and Grant, M. A. Considering carpets in hospital use. *Dimensions in Health Service* 59(6):18–21, June 1982.

Skoutelis, A. T., Westenfelder, G. O., Beckerdite M., and Phair, J. P. Hospital carpeting and epidemiology of Clostridium difficile. *American Journal of Infection Control* 22(4):212–17, 1994.

Souhrada, L. Lighting decisions affect image, morale, efficiency. *Health Facilities Management* 2(5):19–27, May 1989.

Spivak, M. Sensory distortions in tunnels and corridors. *Hospital and Community Psychiatry* 18(1): 12–18, January 1967.

St. Joseph's Health Care London. 2015. www.sjhc.london.on.ca/your-visit/parkwood-hospital/program -and-service-detailed-directions/. Accessed November 2015.

Taylor, K. Wayfinding. *Health Facilities Management* 8(8):66–69, August 1995.

Templer, J., and Archea, J. *Stairway Design for Reducing Fall Injuries in Industry*. Atlanta: Georgia Institute of Technology, Pedestrian Research Lab, 1983.

Templer, J. A., Mullet, G. M., and Archea, J. *An Analysis of the Behavior of Stair Users*. Springfield, VA: National Technical Information Service, 1978.

2008 American Community Survey. 2008. http://factfinder.census.gov.

US Department of Health and Human Services. 45 Fed. Reg. 82972 (December17, 1980) (Notice). Quoted in Chen, A. H., Youdelman, M. K., and Brooks, J. The legal framework for language access in healthcare settings: Title VI and beyond. *Journal of General Internal Medicine* 22(Supplement 2):362–67, November 2007. Published online October 24, 2007. doi:10.1007/s11606–007–0366–2. www.ncbi .nlm.nih.gov/pmc/articles/PMC2150609/.

US Department of Justice. *2010 Standards for Accessible Design*, Chapter 3 Building Blocks, 302.2 Carpet. September 15, 2010. www.access-board.gov/ada-aba/comparison/chapter3.htm.

Wayfinding design research: Respecting the needs of patients and visitors. *Signs of the Times*, October 1987, pp. 58–60.

Wechsler, S. Perceiving the visual message. In D. Pollet and P. Haskell, editors. *Sign Systems for Libraries*, 33–46. New York: R. R. Bowker, 1979.

Weisman, G. D. Wayfinding and architectural legibility: Design considerations in housing environments for the elderly. In V. Regnier and J. Pynoos, editors. *Housing for the Elderly: Satisfaction and Preferences*, 441–64. New York: Garland, 1982.

Weisman, G. D. Wayfinding in the built environment. *Environment and Behavior* 13(2):189–204, March 1981.

Weisman, G. D. Way-finding in the built environment: A study in architectural legibility. PhD dissertation, University of Michigan, Ann Arbor, 1979. [Available from ProQuest, 789 E. Eisenhower Parkway, Ann Arbor, MI 48108.]

Wener, R. E., and Kaminoff, R. D. Improving environmental information: Effects of signs on perceived crowding and behavior. *Environment and Behavior* 15(1):2–20, January 1983.

Willmott, M. The effect of vinyl floor surface and a carpeted surface upon walking in elderly hospital patients. *Age and Aging* 15:119–120, 1986.

Wilt, L., and Maienschien, J. Symbol signs for libraries. In D. Pollet and P. Haskell, editors. *Sign Systems for Libraries*, 105–13. New York: R. R. Bowker, 1979.

Wise, K. O. Carpet choices for healthcare facilities. *Journal of Healthcare Materiel Management* 12(7):34–39, July 1994.

Wright, P., Hull, A., and Lickorish, A. Navigating in a hospital outpatients' department: The merits of maps and wall signs. *Journal of Architectural and Planning Research* 10(1):76–89, Spring 1993.

Zimring, C. M. The built environment as a source of psychological stress: Impacts of buildings and cities on satisfaction and behavior. In G. W. Evans, editor. *Environmental Stress*, 151–78. New York: Cambridge University Press, 1982.

CHAPTER 5

RECEPTION AND WAITING AREAS

Patients and visitors are likely to spend considerable time waiting when they visit a healthcare facility. Patients wait to be admitted, wait to see a physician or other caregiver, and wait to receive test results. Visitors wait for progress reports and a chance to see patients. All this waiting takes place in a variety of spaces throughout the facility: in departments, in the Main Lobby, in dedicated waiting areas, in patient rooms, and in hallways. Some of these spaces are little more than small rooms with chairs, others are associated with a reception area, and still others, such as the Main Lobby, serve a number of functions.

Long, tedious hours of waiting are an unfortunate fact of life in most healthcare facilities, but good design can help mitigate some of the negative aspects of this experience. This chapter looks at design and behavior issues related to dedicated reception and waiting areas. While waiting, patients and visitors need to know that they have not been forgotten by those in charge; they need to be physically comfortable; they need to be close to amenities such as restrooms, food service, and drinking fountains; they need to have things to do, watch, or read (including accessing their digital devices); and they need to be able to choose whether to interact with others or keep to themselves.

Entering a Reception and Waiting Area

When they arrive at a reception and waiting area, patients and visitors need information: they need to know where they should go to wait and what will happen next. This information can come from staff, as well as from features of the designed environment, including interior architecture, furnishings, and signage.

One study of waiting behavior in an Admitting Department found that without effective wayfinding information, patients often had difficulty finding their destinations (Nelson-Shulman, 1983–84). Once they were inside the Admitting Department, the lack of available information caused confusion and congestion. Not knowing that they should register so that paperwork could be started, for instance, patients simply stood around waiting to be called. Patients' waiting experiences were eased by having ready access to information (such as signs directing them to restrooms and the cafeteria), a brochure explaining Admitting Department procedures, and a welcome sign with directions for registration.

Some healthcare facilities have streamlined the arrival process to such a degree that the patient simply presents a bar code and is then scanned in, at which point all relevant information and directions can be relayed in a personalized manner (Scalise, 2005). Other facilities, such as those following the Planetree model, encourage Information and Registration staff to be proactive by greeting and directing incoming patients as if they were expected. Such hospitality appears to reduce patient stress (Arneill and Frasca-Beaulieu, 2003).

Consider the following suggestions for designing the entry/exit area of reception and waiting areas:

- Make the entrance visually distinct from the corridor and other nonpublic destinations by using color, floor materials, and landmarks (Petersen, 1981b).

- Use signage and other wayfinding aids to direct patients and visitors to the waiting area.

- Provide an identification sign in clear view of patients and visitors approaching the area to let them know they have arrived at their destination.

- Provide patients with information about policies and procedures before they are seen in Outpatient Clinics and Admitting Departments.

- Place directional signs in the corridor opposite the entrance to the waiting and reception area or in direct view from the entrance area (Nelson-Shulman, 1983–84).

Reception Areas

Healthcare facilities sometimes seem like impersonal places where patients are processed rather than being treated with special care. Such an assembly-line atmosphere is neither necessary nor desirable, and the reception area can play an important role in projecting a more caring image. The circulation pattern providing access to the reception desk, nearby seating and carpeting, the reception desk's proximity to other spaces, as well as the interior design of the reception and waiting area all influence the image projected. For example, themed artwork depicting natural, calming scenes may help create a warmer atmosphere than would bare white walls. Features such as fountains, sculptures, and other visual elements may also contribute to a more caring ambience. For instance, one health facility in metropolitan Washington, DC utilized a Potomac River theme on the walls of its main reception area that not only provided pleasing visual stimulation, but also functioned as a wayfinding landmark (Huelat, 2007).

In diagnostic and treatment areas, the Reception Desk often provides the strongest cue to patients or visitors that they have arrived at their destination. When locating and orienting a Reception Desk, consider the following:

•   Position the desk so it faces the majority of incoming patients and their companions.

•   Place the desk so that a queuing line does not infringe on waiting or circulation areas.

•   To ensure patients' acoustical privacy, make sure that the queuing line forms a distance away—approximately 4 feet (~1.2 meters)—from the counter. (Petersen, 1981b)

The reception area is a focal point of the waiting area. In addition to functioning as a greeting, information-exchange, and registration area, it provides a sense of security for those waiting. (See Research Box 5.1.)

Being able to see and be seen by staff at the Reception Desk reassures patients and companions that they have not been forgotten. Those who are ill can see that help is available.

RESEARCH BOX 5.1 PROVIDING INFORMATION IN RECEPTION AREAS AND ADMITTING

Waiting can be stressful for patients, and a lack of information can aggravate the situation. To test the effect of providing information, a study was conducted in the Admitting Department of an urban hospital (Nelson-Shulman, 1983–84).

The study compared two groups of patients: those who were given the typical amount of information and those who were provided a number of additional information aids, including orientation signs, a brochure explaining hospital policies, a letter answering frequently-asked questions, and a welcome sign describing registration procedures. While they waited in the Admitting Department, participants in the study were observed for 5-minute intervals. Patients were interviewed at the end of the admitting process, before being escorted to their rooms. The interview concerned such topics as attitudes toward the hospital, perceived waiting time, and knowledge about the admitting process.

Patients given increased information expressed significantly greater knowledge and familiarity with the admitting process, relied significantly more on signs rather than on asking hospital staff for assistance, initiated approximately half as many contacts with Registration-Desk staff, and were more likely to believe that something had been done by the hospital to ease their wait, than did the group not receiving additional information. Although the study did not examine the effectiveness of different types of information or different ways of presenting information, it did show that providing information could significantly ease the stress of the waiting experience.

In reception and waiting areas, patients' and visitors' sense of security can be enhanced by design:

- Position the Reception Desk so staff members have a clear view of people entering the reception and waiting area.

- Position the Reception Desk so staff members have a clear view of the entire waiting area. (Petersen, 1981b)

The design of Reception Desks can affect patient comfort and perceived privacy. For example, at the time of registration, patients often carry purses, briefcases, and other personal belongings. They appreciate having a place to put these items while they talk with clerks and fill out papers. Seniors and people with vision limitations, who may have a hard time seeing where the form ends and the counter begins, would benefit from completing their paperwork on a counter with a surface color that contrasts with the clinic's forms. Surfaces and lighting that prevent glare are also useful. In addition, as they register, patients may need to discuss personal matters with staff. Reception-counter design should provide some acoustical privacy.

The desk itself also influences a patient's image of a healthcare facility. A desk that is sterile and uninteresting, bare of anything but signs and registration forms, may seem institutional; and a cluttered desk, stacked high with noisy equipment and paperwork, may seem unapproachable. A desk may seem friendlier when staff members have room to display a few personal items and where unnecessary equipment is out of sight. One study suggests that facilities avoid sliding glass windows that physically and symbolically separate staff from visitors (Pennachio, 2003).

Consider these suggestions to help make a Registration Desk and Reception area more appealing to patients and visitors:

- Design and position the Reception Desk, seating, and circulation areas so patients and companions can readily see where to go (Petersen, 1981b).

- Construct Reception and Registration desks and counters of non-glare material. Avoid creating sharp edges (Petersen, 1981b).

- Select countertop colors to contrast with the forms patients fill out (Petersen, 1981b).

- Provide non-glare task lighting (Petersen, 1981b).

- Allow Reception and Registration staff to personalize their spaces with a few photos and knickknacks (Petersen, 1981b).

- Provide wide counters or shelf space to hold patients' personal items while they are registering (Petersen, 1981b).

- Provide visual and acoustical screening between patient registration stations using partitions or booths (Keenan and Goldman, 1989; Petersen, 1981b).

- Make sure Reception and Registration Desks accommodate wheelchair users and others who may need to sit, providing ample space for legs and counter space at an appropriate height (see ADA guidelines).

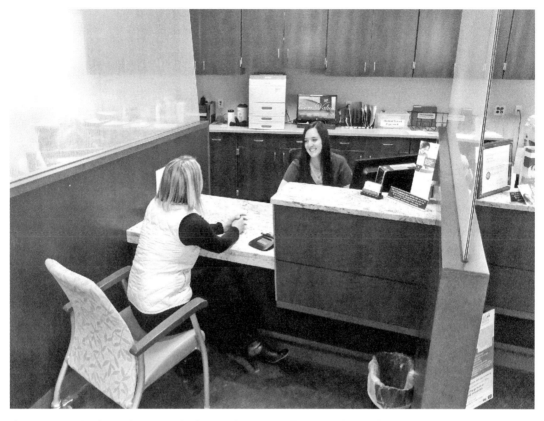

These Registration booths provide some visual and acoustical privacy, as well as room underneath for the patient's legs.
Photo credit: Courtesy of St. Joseph Mercy Chelsea

- Provide chairs for those who need to sit (Petersen, 1981b).
- Provide coat storage (Petersen, 1981b).

Waiting Areas

Healthcare facilities contain waiting areas for a variety of functions and locations: the Main Lobby, treatment waiting, diagnostic-test waiting, Surgery waiting, Emergency Room waiting, Intensive Care Unit waiting, inpatient unit waiting, and others. Although family members and friends who find themselves in these waiting areas will have different design-related needs, some issues are common to all of them (Pendell, Coray, and Veneklasen, 1975). We will discuss these common needs first, and focus on particular types of waiting areas.

Size and Location

A waiting area that is constantly crowded, necessitating that some patients and visitors stand or move into the hallway, is likely to increase stress and general discomfort. On the other hand, a waiting area that is oversized or underused wastes space and resources. It is important to properly gauge the size of waiting areas to their use, carefully balancing the need to accommodate peak loads with the need to conserve space. (See Research Box 5.2.) Although space-allocation estimates are often imprecise, a rule of thumb is to provide approximately 15 net square feet (~1.4 square meters) per person during peak load periods (Petersen, 1981b).

A waiting area's location matters. A waiting area hidden down a remote hallway, away from amenities like restrooms or vending machines, may seem too isolated. A waiting area in a hallway or one that is not much more than an alcove off a busy corridor would not be very comfortable and may indicate to patients and visitors that the facility does not care enough to provide well-located, well-designed space.

When locating waiting areas, consider the following:

- Place waiting areas so that they are separate from, but near, a corridor.

- Make sure patients and visitors in a diagnostic or treatment waiting area can see and be seen by staff.

- Locate waiting areas adjacent to restrooms, drinking fountains, vending machines, designated cell-phone areas, and other amenities. (Petersen, 1981b)

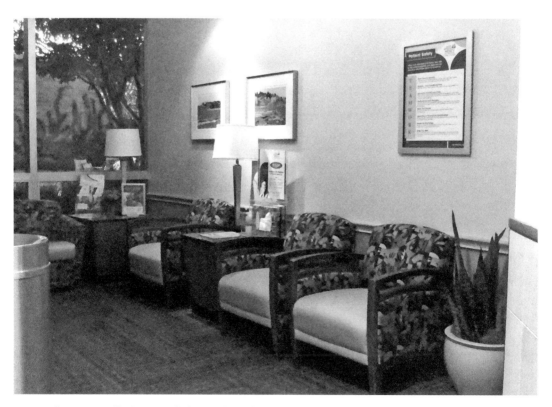

Even a small waiting area, like this one, can be functionally, comfortably, and attractively designed for patients and visitors.

Photo credit: Courtesy of St. Joseph Mercy Chelsea

RESEARCH BOX 5.2 WAITING-AREA DESIGN, PERCEIVED WAIT TIMES, AND QUALITY OF CARE

A study conducted under the auspices of The Center for Health Design's Pebble Project found a correlation between a waiting area's attractiveness, perceived wait time, and quality of care. Seven outpatient clinics were selected and ranked according to the "attractiveness of the physical environment." Data from nearly 1,000 patients were obtained through observation and survey. Participants were asked about the amount of wait time, perceived appropriateness of the amount of wait time, and wait-time activities.

The results indicate a direct correlation between the attractiveness of the waiting area and perceived quality of care, reduced anxiety, and positive interaction with staff members. That is, higher attractiveness of a waiting area was correlated with lower perceived wait time, greater perception of quality of care, and fewer feelings of anxiety. Reductions in feelings of anxiety were a direct result of perceived quality of care, which in turn was itself a result of the comfort and pleasing nature of the waiting environment. Moreover, the study noted that an attractive waiting area resulted in a lower perceived wait time, regardless of actual wait time (Becker and Douglass, 2006).

Waiting-Area Activities and Television

People using waiting areas differ in age, gender, physical limitations, and preferences for how they spend their time while waiting. Some like to people-watch; others want to read quietly or talk with friends or relatives; still others prefer to use digital devices, watch television, listen to music, work on crafts, or play with their children. Yet even though the stress created by waiting can be reduced when people are given choices about what to do with their time, many waiting areas do not accommodate this wide range of activities (Petersen, 1981a). The key is to provide environmental supports for as many different activities as possible. Create distinct activity areas by incorporating features into waiting-area design that draw people to them. (See Research Box 5.2.) A number of design features (for example, aquariums, mobiles, paintings, posters, plants, televisions, lighting, and reading material) can create such areas (Petersen, 1981b; Swartz, 1989).

Interior and exterior windows provide important focal points for activity, because many people enjoy looking out onto a pleasant scene. Windows also help patients and visitors feel less isolated. Visitors who must wait for long periods can benefit from being at least visually connected to peripheral activity. In one study, when visitors were shown a three-dimensional model of a typical waiting area and asked to choose between a solid wall and a glass wall for the separation between the waiting area and the hallway, the vast majority preferred the glass wall (Reizenstein, Grant, and Vaitkus, 1981). The glass wall would make the visitors feel a part of what was going on and also provide interesting views.

People may find it preferable to catch a glimpse of the activity in a waiting area or to be able to see into it before entering. For both patients and visitors, previewing waiting-area activity eases the transition from a corridor, where they are relatively anonymous, to the seemingly intimate group setting of a waiting area. Previewing enables them to decide whether to go in at all, making unnecessary what otherwise might be an awkward exit. It also gives users an opportunity to decide in advance about where to sit and place their belongings.

Many health facilities provide televisions in waiting areas, to serve as a positive distraction and to help pass the time. However, one study highlights the potential negative effects of television on patients and visitors. Researchers found that blood donors exposed to regular daytime programming on television experienced greater stress than patients in a room where the television was turned off. These researchers also compared videotapes of nature scenes and urban scenes. Televisions displaying nature settings were associated with lower stress than televisions showing more stimulating urban scenes (Ulrich, Simons, and Miles, 2003). Thus, the type of programming provided on televisions in waiting areas is an important consideration.

In Britain, there has been organized protest against televisions and piped-in music in hospitals (PipeDown, 2008). Over the course of almost two years, more than 900 signatures were collected on a petition to ban the use of televisions, radios, and music systems in hospitals and doctors' waiting areas (Rodgers, 2007). To our knowledge, this type of organized protest has not happened in the United States.

Not only might TVs increase stress levels, but the noise may be disruptive to others present in waiting areas. Moreover, TVs and other distractions may cause visitors to sense that they are in for a long wait (Pennachio, 2003). Nevertheless, people should be given the choice of whether or not to listen to television and music.

If television is installed, administrators should consider muting it, offering closed-captioning, and/or providing headphones with individual volume control. Another option is a wireless headphone system; however, it is important to choose a wireless system that will not interfere with medical equipment. Another strategy is to screen the television's sound and view from other activity areas in the waiting area (Reizenstein and Grant, 1981 [unpub. No. 6]). Dividers and alcoves can break up a waiting area into smaller activity areas. Plants also help divide the space into smaller areas and provide both a degree of visual privacy and something pleasant to look at.

Seating Arrangements

People in waiting areas tend to congregate in groups of different sizes. Since some people prefer to be alone, others want to be with one or two people, and some come in larger groups, it is important to offer seating that accommodates groups of different sizes.

Seating arrangements also affect patients' and visitors' abilities to converse comfortably. Many people prefer to sit at angles to one another or face to face (Mehrabian and Diamond, 1970, 1971; Sommer, 1961). The typical fixed-seating arrangement, with people sitting side by side, is not conducive to conversation. An inward-facing seating arrangement, with some clusters of chairs around tables, is more likely to facilitate conversation (Carmichael and Agre, 2002).

Research has also shown that some visitors prefer couches, so as to be able to sit nearer loved ones. Couches and loveseats have their drawbacks, however, as such unobstructed proximity is not desirable for most strangers, and seats without ample arm support are difficult for sitting and rising (see Research Box 5.3) (Lowes, 1998; Pennachio, 2003).

Patients and visitors may also like to have access to information, including books and other materials, as well as online resources. Some health facilities devote specific space within or adjacent to waiting areas for these learning areas, so that such resources are available, even if they are not always utilized (Arneill and Frasca-Beaulieu, 2003; Carmichael and Agre, 2002).

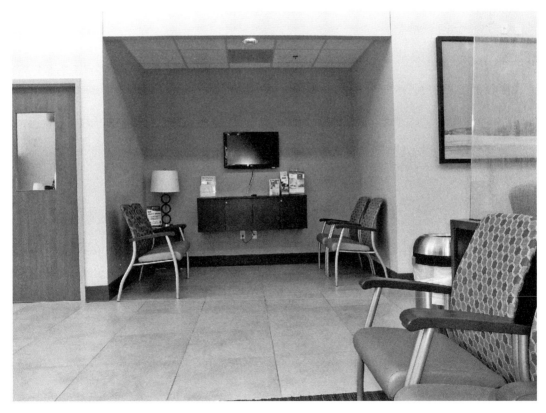

A small alcove set into a larger waiting area can provide some visual and acoustical privacy for families.
Photo credit: Courtesy of St. Joseph Mercy Chelsea

Waiting areas need to accommodate wheelchair users. When movable seating is provided, the area can be adjusted to make room for a person in a wheelchair *within* the seating arrangement, as opposed to isolating that person in a special area.

The following recommendations may be helpful in making decisions about seating arrangements in waiting areas:

- Provide seating that enables people to arrange themselves in groups of different configurations and sizes, as they wish (Arneill and Frasca-Beaulieu, 2003; Lowes, 1998; Pennachio, 2003; Reizenstein and Grant, 1981 [unpub. No. 6]).

- Provide seating that enables people to position their bodies comfortably for conversation, with regard to both the distance from one seat to another and the angle at which one person can face another (Lowes, 1998; Mehrabian and Diamond, 1970, 1971; Pennachio, 2003; Sommer, 1961).

- Select chairs that are easy to move or provide wheelchair space among the seats.

Seating Comfort

Comfortable seating is particularly important because patients and visitors may spend hours in waiting areas. For visitors of inpatients, the hours may turn into days. Seating must accommodate people of different heights and weights, including those who cannot easily rise from low, conventional seating or who cannot sit for long periods of time on backless chairs. Comfortable seating gives effective back and arm support and does not cut off leg circulation (see Research Box 5.3). Firm cushion support, padded arms, and a space to place the feet under the body's center of gravity are other ways seating design can accommodate users' needs. Armrests also help give patients and visitors a sense of separation from others in a crowded waiting area. (See chapter 9.)

Consider the following guidelines for providing comfortable seating:

- Provide seating that accommodates a wide range of users, including children; pregnant women; heavy, short, or tall people; seniors; and those who are frail or weak (Petersen, 1981a).

- Whenever possible, provide seating with backs and arms that support thighs, lower back, and upper back (Carpman and Grant, 1983 [unpub. No. 22], 1984 [unpub. No. 25], 1984 [unpub. No. 27]).

- Avoid seating with sharp edges (Carpman and Grant, 1983 [unpub. No. 22], 1984 [unpub. No. 25], 1984 [unpub. No. 27]).

- Select seating material that is comfortable, neither scratching users nor causing them to perspire (Carpman and Grant, 1983 [unpub. No. 22], 1984 [unpub. No. 25], 1984 [unpub. No. 27]; Ellis, 1988).

- As an aid in rising and sitting, provide seating with firm support at the front edge, room for the sitter's feet to tuck under the front of the chair, and arms that extend out to or slightly past the front edge of the seat. Avoid low seating (Carpman and Grant, 1984 [unpub. No.27]).

- Provide seating with armrests, so that when seats are placed next to each other, armrests give people a sense of separation from their neighbors (Carpman and Grant, 1984 [unpub. No. 27]; Lowes, 1998; Swartz, 1989).

RESEARCH BOX 5.3 EVALUATING WAITING-AREA SEATING

One way to learn about waiting-area seating is to have patients and visitors assess different types of chairs in actual waiting areas. To this end, a study was conducted to evaluate patients' and visitors' detailed impressions about the comfort of 18 different seats being considered for the University of Michigan Medical Center (Carpman and Grant, 1984 [unpub. No. 27]). The information collected in this study, combined with cost, availability, and departmental wishes, was used in seating selection.

Respondents sat in test chairs for varying periods of time (10 minutes or less, 11 to 20 minutes, 21 to 30 minutes, and 30 minutes or more). Some questions focused on specifics of chair comfort, including ease of getting into and out of the chair and provision of thigh, lower-back, upper-back, and arm support. Other questions focused on chair size, stability, and appearance. Patients and visitors were also asked about sitting in close proximity to others, a common situation in waiting areas.

An important finding of this study was the difference in perceived comfort related to the presence or absence of armrests. Thus, when waiting-area seats need to be placed next to each other, as is often necessary in order to maximize the number of people who can be seated, it is important to use a seat with armrests in order to give people some sense of their own territory and some sense of separation—if only symbolic—from their immediate neighbors. Armrests also provide assistance as people sit and rise.

The study also suggested that special attention be given to seating for older patients and visitors. Seating design features related to back, thigh, and arm support, as well as ease of sitting and rising, are especially important for this group.

Flooring, Wall Coverings, and Lighting

Attention to the design of floors, walls, and ceilings can help create a comfortable and safe waiting environment. Interior-design details such as floor coverings, artwork, and lighting can make a big difference, especially to patients and visitors waiting for long periods of time.

Patients and visitors should not have to worry about their safety inside a health facility, and nonskid floor surfaces are one way to alleviate this problem. Flooring for a waiting area must also suit people with mobility limitations, dampen noise, and be visually appealing. The consensus of researchers seems to be that carpeting with very low pile, used without a pad, is functional if it can be negotiated by wheelchair users (Pennachio, 2003; Simmons, Reizenstein, and Grant, 1982). Other types of surfaces, such as stone or tile, can also be used in high-traffic areas as long as they don't cause bumpy rides or have raised areas that can cause tripping (Lowes, 1998).

Seniors and people with vision limitations may have trouble distinguishing between floors and walls, especially at edges. Contrasting colors or intensities and even textures can be helpful.

Noise can be an issue in health facilities as a result of hard surfaces, conversation, music, digital devices, and equipment. Flooring materials, along with acoustic ceiling materials, can help dampen noise.

Lighting also affects the ambience and comfort of waiting areas. Bright, cool fluorescent lighting is often considered institutional, while warm fluorescent or incandescent lighting is considered friendlier. Table lamps create a softer, warmer, and generally more inviting atmosphere, while providing effective task lighting for most activities (Lowes, 1998; Pennachio, 2003). Whenever possible, natural lighting should be incorporated into design, as it is both easier to look at than artificial lighting and seems more calming to many patients and visitors (Arneill and Frasca-Beaulieu, 2003). Lighting design is particularly critical for seniors, who need higher intensities of light than do younger people, but whose eyes cannot tolerate glare. Consequently, illumination levels, distribution, color, and the manner in which light interacts with other design features are all important considerations:

- Select nonskid floor surfaces in hallways (Simmons et al., 1982).

- Select flooring and ceiling materials to help reduce noise (Simmons et al., 1982).

- Select floor and wall colors that provide visual contrast (Hayward, 1982).

- Design lighting to be intense enough for reading, and yet not overly bright or glaring (Hayward, 1982).

- Consider indirect lighting and other non-institutional lighting such as table lamps and recessed spotlights for waiting areas (Fong and Nichelson, 2006).

- Consider the interaction among lighting, flooring, and other surfaces in order to avoid glare (Brainard, 1995; Fong and Nichelson, 2006).

- Avoid lighting that produces excessive heat (Hayward, 1982).

- Incorporate natural light wherever possible (Hayward, 1982).

- Consider lighting color when selecting fluorescent or LED lights (Hayward, 1982).

Waiting-Area Amenities

Waiting is not a one-dimensional activity; patients' and visitors' lives do not stop once they enter a waiting area. People may still need to use a restroom, look after their children, work, use digital devices, learn more about their illness, or get something to eat. The availability of amenities satisfying these needs helps ease the stress of the waiting experience.

Restrooms

Patients and visitors need convenient access to restrooms. Because they often feel tied to the waiting area, afraid that if they leave they may miss an important message, restrooms should be located nearby.

Restrooms should not be too close to waiting areas, however. Although waiting areas are public areas, patients and visitors do not consider them thoroughfares for people who just need to use the restroom. In one study, three-fourths of the visitors interviewed preferred that restrooms not be located inside a waiting area. Instead, they felt that restrooms should be accessed from the hallway just outside a waiting area (Reizenstein, Grant, and Vaitkus, 1981). In addition to cutting down on traffic, visitors felt that they would have a higher level of acoustical and visual privacy by using restrooms located outside a waiting area.

The design of a restroom is also important. Even though restrooms are one of the few places in healthcare facilities devoted to purely personal activities, many are not designed to handle related activities such as changing clothes, personal grooming, diapering, or nursing a baby. For waiting areas where visitors may spend the night, nearby restrooms need to accommodate personal grooming or dressing. Many of these needs can be facilitated without much difficulty. In addition to meeting the needs of people with functional limitations, the following conditions should be met:

- Provide access to public restrooms from hallways rather than from waiting areas (Reizenstein et al., 1981).
- Provide unobstructed counter space for diapering in both men's and women's public restrooms.
- Provide electrical outlets (for electric shavers and hair dryers) in both men's and women's public restrooms.
- Provide clothes hooks in each restroom.
- If space permits, provide a comfortable chair.

Places for Belongings

Many people enter health facilities with belongings—purses, backpacks, briefcases, bags, books, and assorted paraphernalia. During the winter months, hats, coats, gloves, and other cold weather gear add to the load. In addition, hospital visitors often bring flowers, gifts, food, and other items for patients. In the absence of planned places for people to store belongings, they place them on adjoining seats, removing potential seating space. Because personal belongings need to be accommodated, each waiting area should contain some coat hooks and tables or other places for people to temporarily place their things. Security should be considered when planning temporary storage accommodations (Petersen, 1981a).

Refreshments

Eating is a common way of passing time while waiting. For visitors or outpatients who must wait for several hours, snacks can tide them over until they have a chance to get a meal. Inpatient visitors may appreciate having access to coffee without having to leave the patient floor. Even though many people do not like the quality of food available in vending machines, they value the convenience of these machines and would like them available near waiting areas (Reizenstein and Grant, 1981 [unpub. No. 6]). It is also important to provide readily accessible water fountains.

Food and drink can lead to litter and spills. Providing wastebaskets may limit this problem, but increased housekeeping attention will probably be needed to keep waiting areas clean.

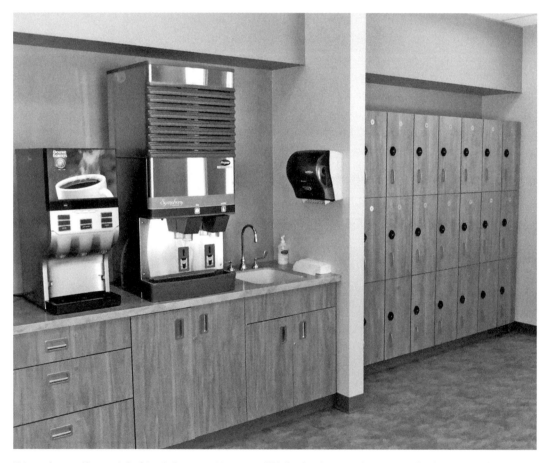

Visitors who spend long periods of time in Surgery waiting areas will likely take advantage of amenities such as beverages and lockers.
Photo credit: Courtesy of St. Joseph Mercy Ann Arbor

Consider the following guidelines for making refreshments available to patients and visitors who are waiting:

* Provide vending machines close to waiting areas, perhaps in an out-of-the-way alcove (Petersen, 1981b; Reizenstein and Grant, 1981 [unpub. No. 6]).

* Stock vending machines with nutritious foods that have good eye appeal (Petersen, 1981b).

* Provide hot water, tea, cocoa, and coffee. This is particularly important in high-stress waiting areas (Petersen, 1981b).

* Provide trash receptacles (Petersen, 1981b).

* Install water fountains that can be reached by wheelchair users and by short people (including children) (Petersen, 1981b).

Play Areas

When people go to a physician's office for a brief examination, to the Emergency Department with an injured friend, or to the hospital for a diagnostic test, they may be accompanied by children, whether or not the facility officially welcomes them. The predictable presence of children in waiting areas creates special design requirements. The environment needs to enable parents and children to wait comfortably while not bothering other adults (Alcock et al., 1985).

Accommodating children in some waiting areas need not cause dramatic changes in facility design or policy. The first step is to decide which waiting areas in adult-oriented facilities are most likely to be visited by children. Waiting areas for physicians' offices, outpatient departments, diagnostic areas, emergency departments, and main lobbies are top candidates.

Next comes the question of which environmental design features are desirable. One expert recommends providing children's play spaces that are physically identifiable and have an ambience of their own. These play spaces should be protected from major circulation paths, and play materials should be displayed. These spaces can be small and should be located so that they can be easily monitored from the reception desk and from some of the waiting-area seats. Children in these play spaces need to be observed and supervised by both parents and staff (Olds, 1978).

Because children at play tend to be noisy, it's wise to provide space and sound-attenuating materials between the children's play area and the rest of the waiting area. Most waiting-area seats should be oriented away from the play area and separated by a barrier of some sort, so that others who are waiting do not have to become involved with children's play. Another alternative is to provide children's game tables. These could also contain quiet electronic games appealing to both younger and older children (Olds, 1978).

When designing small play spaces for children within adult waiting areas, consider the following:

- Create a play area in the most protected part of the room, out of the circulation flow.
- Place the play area within good visual and acoustical range of the reception area, so staff can act as tacit supervisors.
- Use sound-attenuating materials in the waiting area.
- Place some adult seating clusters facing the play area and some directed away from it.
- Provide play materials that are sturdily constructed, have some inherent complexity, and, if possible, can be used by more than one child at a time.
- Avoid selecting toys with small pieces that are easily lost or swallowed.
- Provide some multi-person seating without arms, like couches, to enable a parent to comfort or hold a child.
- Provide some small tables containing board games or quiet electronic games. (Olds, 1978)

Music

Patients awaiting treatment may be interested in listening to music, since music provides positive distraction and can have a calming effect (see Research Box 5.4). One literature review of 12 studies of music and patients in hospitals found that music reduced anxiety in patients in short-term waiting areas for Day Surgery. The majority of the studies reviewed showed significant improvements in self-reported anxiety measures, while more than half reported improvements in physiological measures (for example, blood pressure, heart rate, respiratory rate, blood pressure, or cortisol levels) (Cooke, Chaboyer, and Hiratos, 2005). As with any research, differences in sample populations and study designs limit the ability to make sweeping conclusions about the effects of music on all kinds of patients. (For a discussion of the therapeutic effects of music for people with dementia, see chapter 9.) Also, variation in the delivery of healthcare services may influence the effects of music in other settings and under different conditions.

Visitors, as well as patients, can benefit from listening to music while waiting. One study reported lower self-reported anxiety for visitors who listened to music while they waited than for visitors without access to music. In this study, a CD-player, amplifier, and speaker system were installed in the waiting area. The majority of visitors were waiting for patients undergoing surgery, while others were waiting to see or hear updates about patients in intensive care. Music with a tempo between 60 and 80 beats per minute was chosen, since these tempos are believed to induce relaxation (Routhieaux and Tansik, 1997). Visitors were less stressed and more relaxed when the music was playing.

Music can be an easy, affordable, and effective intervention for reducing anxiety in patients awaiting treatment. However, an important consideration is the effect of piped-in music versus individual listening devices such as smartphones, MP3 players, iPods, and the like. To some people, piped-in background music can be irritating or perceived as adding to noise levels (Brown and Theorell, 2005; Webber, 2008). And for people with hearing limitations, piped-in music can make it harder to hear and participate in conversations.

Given these negative responses, if patients and visitors do not bring along their own music, providing individual listening devices and a selection of soothing music may be preferred over piped-in music.

RESEARCH BOX 5.4 USING MUSIC TO REDUCE ANXIETY

In a study of the relationship between music and anxiety, one researcher examined the effects of a music intervention on anxiety, heart rate, and blood pressure for patients awaiting cardiac catheterization (Hamel, 2001). Patients were randomly assigned to two groups: a control group that received treatment as usual, and a test group that received 20 minutes of music intervention via a CD-player with headphones.

The researcher preselected the music "Trance-Zendance" by Halpern, New Age music designed for relaxation that has been used in other studies in clinical settings. The tempo, 70–80 beats per minute, similar to the human heart rate, is thought to be soothing (Hamel, 2001).

Measures of self-reported anxiety using the State-Trait Anxiety Inventory (STAI), blood pressure, and heart rate were taken when patient-respondents arrived. The test group then listened to the Halpern piece for 20 minutes, while the control group waited without music. Measures were taken again prior to the time when patient-respondents left the unit for the cardiac catheterization.

The results indicated that patients who listened to this music while waiting experienced a greater decrease in STAI scores than did the control group. Within the music group, STAI scores were significantly lower after the intervention than before the intervention. While not statistically significant, heart rate and systolic blood pressure also dropped in the music group. A statistically significant increase in heart rate and blood pressure was found for the control group after the waiting period.

The results of this study are consistent with other studies demonstrating anxiety reduction in patients exposed to New Age or slow rhythmic music while waiting (Haun, Mainous, and Looney, 2001; Hayes et al., 2003; Szeto and Yung, 1999; Yung et al., 2002). The author recommends providing patients with a choice of soothing music and suggests further research examining the effects of music on perceived wait times.

Patient and Family Information

One way of reducing stress for some patients and visitors is to provide medical information. Medical procedures and equipment can be frightening and stress-inducing, particularly in

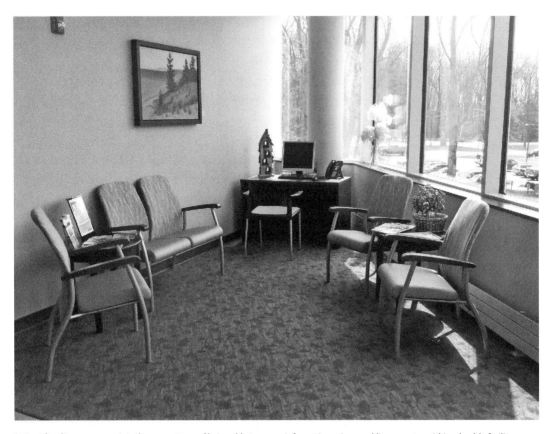

Patient families may appreciate the convenience of being able to access information using a public computer within a health-facility waiting area.

Photo credit: Courtesy of St. Joseph Mercy Chelsea

such departments as Cardiology, Nuclear Medicine, Radiation Therapy, and MRI. If space and budgets allow, an area devoted to patient information could be provided within these departments and others where pretreatment orientation would be helpful. A patient information area should enable a healthcare professional to talk with patients and companions in a comfortable, private setting (Carmichael and Agre, 2002). Digital devices with internet access could be provided along with a guide to online resources.

Clocks

Time is a concern in waiting areas. Patients and visitors wonder how much longer they will have to wait, when they will be done, whether they will have time to run errands on their way home, or whether their parking meter has expired. Even though they may wear a watch or can get the time from their cell phone, clocks still reassure some patients and visitors and free others from having to ask the time. Clocks should have legible numerals and be placed so that they can be seen from most seats in the waiting area (Petersen, 1981b).

Main Lobby

The Main Lobby is a special waiting area: the most visible and public space in the facility. It serves both tangible and symbolic functions. A number of activities take place within it, including talking, reading, people-watching, resting, and child-watching, as well as necessities such as using digital devices and obtaining information. Main lobbies tend to be heavily used by a variety of people: inpatients well enough to walk a bit for a change of scene, visitors who want to get away from the waiting areas on inpatient floors, children accompanying visitors, staff, and others who have business in the facility. Main lobbies can also be used for all types of entertainment.

As with any diverse public group, there will be lobby users with particular requirements, including seniors and people with functional limitations. The lobby will make a symbolic statement about the health facility in its visual image and especially in its function. Ideally, the lobby will project an image of a competent, professional healthcare facility sensitive to the needs of its users (Arneill and Frasca-Beaulieu, 2003).

One of the functions of the Main Entrance is to ease the process of picking up and dropping off companions. People should be able to stay warm and dry inside the lobby and still be able to see their ride approaching. (See also chapter 3.)

Many people in the Main Lobby like to watch people going by without putting themselves in the middle of the traffic. For this and other reasons, the main corridor should be functionally separate from the lobby but visually connected to it. A variety of seating options and arrangements can cater to the diversity of patients and visitors in the Main Lobby.

Previously stated guidelines for waiting areas also apply to main lobbies. In addition:

- Arrange lobby seating so those waiting inside the lobby can see cars driving up outside in the Drop-Off and Pick-Up area.

- Provide an attractive way of displaying newspapers, brochures, and other reading materials.

- Ensure that a dedicated space is provided for wheelchair storage, near the Main Entrance, but out of the circulation path.

- Consider how the lobby can be rearranged, on occasion, to accommodate entertainment for waiting patients and visitors: provide a performance area with dedicated lighting, space for a grand piano, and electrical outlets for equipment, and make sure furniture is moveable.

Well-designed main lobbies and waiting areas give patients and visitors a number of ways to reduce stress. Unfortunately, lobbies do not always meet this objective. For example, in one study of three hospital lobbies in Canada, researchers evaluated design based on interviews with visitors and staff, as well as a checklist of physical features. Common problems included overcrowding, the need for furniture to be flexibly arranged into conversation groups, noise, conflicting circulation paths, lack of privacy in the admitting area, poor signage and lack of other wayfinding aids, and too few nearby restrooms. Other problems included the presence of unattended children, poor illumination, low levels of security, and excessive distance between the lobby and the parking lot (Hamilton, unpublished report).

Main Lobby design also needs to consider maintenance and housekeeping criteria. It is important that lobbies be well maintained so they can meet patient and visitor needs over time.

High-Stress Waiting Areas

Family and friends of patients in Emergency Departments, surgical areas, and Intensive Care Units experience more stress than other visitors do because they are concerned with patients who may be experiencing health crises. They tend to behave differently than do visitors in less stressful situations.

For example, these visitors tend to keep vigils in the waiting area, which may be as close as they can get to the patient's bedside. They spend long hours—sometimes days and weeks—in what is often a confined and isolated waiting space. Many times, large numbers of family and friends gather to support the patient and each other. In order to accommodate large groups, high-stress waiting areas need to be larger than others, with the flexibility to be split up into several areas. For family members who want to be physically close, couches and other forms of comfortable multiple seating should be provided. For some people, the vigil goes on around the clock. Furnishings that are comfortable to sleep on and policies that allow staff to provide pillows and blankets can add greatly to visitors' comfort. An alcove where hot coffee and tea can be made adds to the facility's symbolic message of caring and thoughtfulness.

Patients' families and friends are not the only ones who make use of high-stress waiting areas. Patients may find themselves in various waiting or holding areas in both outpatient and inpatient healthcare facilities. One study examined the patient experience of a surgical holding area and determined that several environmental factors may contribute to patient anxiety, stress, or discomfort: staff having personal conversations in their presence, the physical environment of the holding area, and lack of acoustical privacy. Study findings also indicated the importance of providing positive distractions and reassurance from staff that patient families would be updated about their patient's condition (Bailey, McVey, and Pevreal, 2005).

Consider the following guidelines when designing high-stress waiting areas:

- Locate waiting areas close to high-stress units. It is best if the waiting area is visible from the reception desk or nurses' station (Clipson and Wehrer, 1973; Task Force on Guidelines of the Society of Critical Care Medicine, 1988).

- Provide ample waiting spaces (one-and-a-half to two seats per patient bed) that contain a number of separate family-sized "territories" (Task Force, 1988).

- Provide couches, chairs, and other furnishings that can be arranged to enable family and friends to be comfortable for long periods of time (Clipson and Wehrer, 1973).

- Provide couches and other furnishings that offer comfortable sleeping surfaces.

- Provide an intercom or telephone connection between the nurses' station and the high-stress waiting area.

- Provide a place where coffee and tea can be made.

- Provide lighting, finishes, artwork, and accessories that create a warm, intimate, non-institutional atmosphere.

- Provide access to music. (See "Music" section earlier in this chapter.)

- Provide restrooms adjacent to family waiting areas, with counters and electrical outlets that will allow visitors to freshen up.

- Provide Wi-Fi and outlets for charging devices.

- Provide bulletin boards with information about nearby accommodations, public transportation, and other amenities (Liddle, 1988).

- Provide pamphlets or online resources within the waiting area for family members to learn more about the patient's illness (Clipson and Wehrer, 1973).

- Provide a comfortable and private place for family members to consult with medical personnel or to grieve (Clipson and Wehrer, 1973).

Summary

○ Patients and visitors arriving in a reception and waiting area need to know how to proceed with the Registration or Admitting process and what will happen next. The Reception Desk should be positioned for easy visibility for both patients and staff. It should be physically accommodating with regard to height, provide non-glare surfaces and space for personal belongings, and provide for visual and acoustical privacy.

○ Patients and visitors need to be comfortable while they wait and know that they have not been forgotten. Waiting areas should be carefully sized and located near a major circulation path. Seating arrangements should accommodate wheelchair users and allow for groups of various sizes.

○ Waiting areas should accommodate a wide range of activities, as well as offering amenities to ease the waiting process. Coat racks and space for storing belongings, restrooms, food services, and drinking fountains should be close by. Things to do, watch, and read should be available. As needed, there should be areas that allow children and parents to wait comfortably, without bothering other adults.

○ The Main Lobby area should be designed for frequent use by a wide variety of patients and visitors. Nearby seating, out of the main traffic pattern, should offer good visibility of the Drop-Off and Pick-Up area, as well as opportunities for people-watching.

○ High-stress waiting areas such as those in Emergency Departments, surgical areas, and Intensive Care Units need to accommodate proportionally larger numbers of people for longer times than do other waiting areas. Accommodating privacy, comfort, and convenience will convey a health facility's image of caring and thoughtfulness.

DISCUSSION QUESTIONS

1. What kinds of information do patients and visitors need as they arrive at a Registration Area or Admitting Department?

2. What are the requirements for effective design and positioning of a Reception Desk?

3. What are important considerations in locating waiting areas?

4. What factors should be considered with regard to television and music in waiting areas?

5. What important considerations are related to waiting-area seating?

6. What accommodations should be made for children in waiting areas?

7. What special considerations apply to the design and location of a Main Lobby waiting area?

8. What are some needs of patients and visitors in high-stress waiting areas?

Design Review Questions

Entering a Reception and Waiting Area

☐ Will an identification sign be legible as patients and visitors approach the waiting area?

☐ Will the entrance to the waiting or reception area be distinct from the corridor? (Petersen, 1981b)

☐ Will signage and other wayfinding aids be used to direct patients and visitors to the waiting area?

☐ Will directional signs be placed in the corridor opposite or in direct view from the entrance to the reception and waiting area?

☐ Will patients in outpatient Admitting Departments be given information about policies and procedures? (Nelson-Shulman, 1983–84)

Reception Areas

☐ Will the Reception Desk be positioned so it faces incoming patients and visitors?

☐ Will the Reception Desk be positioned so a queuing line can be formed without causing congestion? (Petersen, 1981b)

☐ To ensure the patient's acoustical privacy, will the queuing line form approximately 4 feet (~1.2 meters) from the counter? (Petersen, 1981b)

☐ Will the Reception Desk be configured and positioned so staff members have a clear view of people entering? (Petersen, 1981b)

☐ Will the Reception Desk be positioned so staff members have a clear view of the waiting area? (Petersen, 1981b)

☐ Will the Reception Desk, seating, and circulation areas be designed and positioned so patients and companions can readily see where to go? (Petersen, 1981b)

☐ Will the colors of the counters where patients will be writing contrast with the colors of the forms they fill out?

☐ Will Reception and Registration Desks and counters be constructed of non-glare material without sharp edges? (Petersen, 1981b)

☐ Will non-glare task lighting be provided? (Petersen, 1981b)

☐ Will Reception staff be able to personalize their spaces? (Petersen, 1981b)

☐ Will Reception Desks be designed with wide counters or shelf space for patients' belongings? (Petersen, 1981b)

Design That Cares: Planning Health Facilities for Patients and Visitors, third edition, by Janet R. Carpman and Myron A. Grant. ©2016 by Jossey-Bass.

☐ Will Registration partitions or booths be designed to provide visual and acoustical privacy? (Keenan and Goldman, 1989; Petersen, 1981b)

☐ Will the Registration or Reception Desk accommodate wheelchair users and others who may need to sit and write? Will these desks also provide ample leg room and counter space? (Petersen, 1981b)

☐ Will a chair be provided for those who need to sit? (Petersen, 1981b)

☐ Will there be a place to store coats? (Petersen, 1981b)

Waiting Areas

Size and Location

☐ Will the waiting area be sized to accommodate approximately 15 net square feet (~1.4 square meters) per person during peak periods? (Petersen, 1981b)

☐ Will waiting areas be separate from, but adjacent to, a corridor? (Petersen, 1981b)

☐ Will patients and visitors in waiting areas be able to make visual contact with the receptionist? (Petersen, 1981b)

☐ Will restrooms, drinking fountains, vending machines, and other necessary amenities be available near waiting areas? (Petersen, 1981b)

Waiting-Area Activities and Television

☐ Will interior and exterior windows be provided? (Reizenstein et al., 1981)

☐ Will patients and visitors be able to see into the waiting area before entering it?

☐ If television is available, will headphones be provided? Will the television be installed so its sound and view are screened from other activity zones in the waiting area? (Reizenstein and Grant, 1981 [unpub. No. 6])

Seating Arrangements

☐ Will seating and other furnishings be provided so people can arrange themselves in different-sized social groups and participate in different activities? (Reizenstein and Grant, 1981 [unpub. No. 6])

☐ Will seating enable people to position themselves comfortably for conversation? (Mehrabian and Diamond, 1970, 1971; Sommer, 1961)

☐ Will wheelchair spaces be provided among the seats?

Seating Comfort

☐ Will seating accommodate a wide range of users? (Petersen, 1981b)

☐ Will seating have backs and arms and support patients' thighs, lower backs, and upper backs? (Carpman and Grant, 1983 [unpub. No. 22], 1984 [unpub. No. 25], 1984 [unpub. No. 27])

☐ Will seating with sharp edges be avoided? (Carpman and Grant, 1983 [unpub. No. 22], 1984 [unpub. No. 25], 1984 [unpub. No. 27])

☐ Will seating material be comfortable? (Carpman and Grant, 1983 [unpub. No. 22], 1984 [unpub. No. 25], 1984 [unpub. No. 27])

☐ Will seating provide firm support at the front edge, room for the patient's feet to tuck under the front of the chair, and arms that extend out to or slightly past the front edge of the seat? Will seating be high enough to facilitate easy rising? (Carpman and Grant, 1984 [unpub. No. 27])

☐ Will armrests be included on seats located next to each other? (Carpman and Grant, 1984 [unpub. No. 27]; Swartz, 1989)

Flooring, Wall Coverings, and Lighting

☐ Will a nonskid floor surface be used? (Simmons et al., 1982)

☐ Will flooring and ceiling materials help reduce noise? (Simmons et al., 1982)

☐ Will flooring and wall colors provide visual contrast? (Hayward, 1982)

☐ Will lighting be effective for reading, yet not overly bright or glaring? (Hayward, 1982)

☐ Will indirect and other non-institutional lighting be used, such as table lamps or recessed spotlights? (Hayward, 1982; Fong and Nichelson, 2006)

☐ Will the interaction among lighting, flooring, and other surfaces be planned and arranged to avoid glare? (Brainard, 1995; Hayward, 1982; Fong and Nichelson, 2006)

☐ Will floor and wall colors provide visual contrast? (Hayward, 1982)

☐ Will natural lighting be incorporated wherever possible?

☐ Will lighting not produce excessive heat? (Hayward, 1982)

☐ Will the color of lighting be considered? (Hayward, 1982)

Waiting-Area Amenities

Restrooms

☐ Will restrooms be accessed from hallways rather than from inside waiting areas? (Reizen-stein et al., 1981)

☐ Will both men's and women's restrooms contain a diapering area?

☐ Will outlets be provided for electric shavers and hair dryers?

☐ Will clothes hooks be available?

☐ If space permits, will a comfortable chair be provided?

Places for Belongings

☐ Will waiting areas contain tables, coat hooks, or other means for storing belongings? (Petersen, 1981b)

Refreshments

☐ Will vending machines be available near waiting areas? (Petersen, 1981b; Reizenstein and Grant, 1981 [unpub. No. 6])

☐ Will vending machines be stocked with nutritious foods that have good eye appeal? (Petersen, 1981b)

☐ Will hot drinks be available nearby? (Petersen, 1981b)

☐ Will trash receptacles be provided? (Petersen, 1981b)

☐ Will water fountains accommodate children, short adults, and wheelchair users?

Play Areas

☐ Will adult waiting areas be able to accommodate children, as needed? (Olds, 1978)

☐ Will play areas be located in the most protected part of each waiting space, out of the circulation flow? (Olds, 1978)

☐ Will play areas be located so children in them can be seen and heard from the reception area? (Olds, 1978)

☐ Will sound-attenuating materials be used in the waiting area? (Olds, 1978)

☐ Will some adult seating clusters face the play area? (Olds, 1978)

☐ Will some adult seating clusters face away from the play area? (Olds, 1978)

☐ Will play materials be provided that are sturdily constructed, have some inherent complexity, and can be used by more than one child at a time? (Olds, 1978)

☐ Will toys with small pieces be avoided? (Olds, 1978)

☐ Will some multi-person seating without arms be provided? (Olds, 1978)

☐ Will some small game tables be provided? (Olds, 1978)

Music

☐ Will patients awaiting surgery have a choice about listening to music?

☐ Will soothing music choices be available? (Routhieaux and Tansik, 1997)

☐ Will visitors in the waiting area have a choice about listening to music?

☐ Will individual listening devices be available?

Patient and Family Information

☐ Will a patient and family information area be provided adjacent to the waiting area in departments that perform invasive procedures?

☐ Will the patient and family information area be equipped with digital devices and/or materials that explain medical procedures?

Clocks

☐ Will waiting areas contain clocks with legible numbers? (Petersen, 1981b)

Main Lobby

☐ Will seating be arranged so people waiting can see cars arriving in the Drop-Off and Pick-Up area?

☐ Will the main corridor be functionally separate from, yet visually connected to, the Main Lobby?

☐ Will there be a display rack for reading material?

☐ Will space be provided for wheelchair storage near the main entrance, but out of the circulation path?

☐ Will the Main Lobby accommodate entertainment, including an impromptu stage area with dedicated lighting, space for a grand piano, electrical outlets for equipment, and moveable furniture?

High-Stress Waiting Areas

☐ Will high-stress waiting areas be located close to related units?

☐ Will the waiting area be visible from the reception desk or nurses' station? (Clipson and Wehrer, 1973; Task Force, 1988)

☐ Will large waiting areas be sized to allow for 1½ to 2 seats per patient bed and contain separate family-sized "territories"? (Task Force, 1988)

☐ Will couches, chairs, and other furnishings enable family and friends to gather closely?

☐ Will waiting-area furniture be comfortable for long periods of time? (Clipson and Wehrer, 1973)

☐ Will couches and other furnishings accommodate sleeping?

☐ Will there be an intercom or telephone between the nurses' station and the family waiting area?

☐ Will coffee and tea be available within the waiting area?

☐ Will lighting, finishes, artwork, and accessories lend a warm, non-institutional feeling to the waiting area?

☐ Will patients and visitors have opportunities to choose from and listen to music provided by the facility?

☐ Will restrooms be located adjacent to family waiting areas, and contain counters and outlets?

☐ Will Wi-Fi and electrical outlets for charging digital devices be available?

☐ Will bulletin boards and the facility's website offer information about nearby accommodations, public transportation, and other amenities? (Liddle, 1988)

☐ Will pamphlets or other materials be provided within the waiting area for family members to learn more about the patient's illness? (Clipson and Wehrer, 1973)

☐ Will a comfortable and private place be provided for family members to grieve? (Clipson and Wehrer, 1973)

Design That Cares: Planning Health Facilities for Patients and Visitors, third edition, by Janet R. Carpman and Myron A. Grant. ©2016 by Jossey-Bass.

References

Alcock, A., Goodman, I., et al. Environment and waiting behaviors in emergency waiting areas. *Children's Health Care: Journal of the Association for the Care of Children's Health* 13(4):174–80, Spring 1985.

Arneill, B., and Frasca-Beaulieu, K. Healing environments: Architecture and design conducive to health. In S. Frampton, L. Gilpin, and P. Charmel, editors. *Putting Patients First: Designing and Practicing Patient-Centered Care,* 163–90. San Francisco: Jossey-Bass, 2003.

Bailey, J., McVey, L., and Pevreal, A. Surveying patients as a start to quality improvement in the surgical suites holding area. *Journal of Nursing Care Quality* 20(4):319–26, October–December 2005.

Becker, F., and Douglass, S. The ecology of the patient visit: Attractiveness, waiting times, and perceived quality of care. *Healthcare Design,* 12–19, November 2006.

Brainard, G. The future is now: Implications of the effect of light on hormones, brain, and behavior. *Journal of Healthcare Design* 7:49–56, 1995.

Brown, S., and Theorell, T. The social uses of background music for personal enhancement. In S. Brown and U. Volgsten, editors. *Music and Manipulation: On the Social Uses and Social Control of Music,* 126–60. New York: Berghahn Books, 2005.

Carmichael, J., and Agre, P. Preferences in surgical waiting area amenities. *Association of Operating Room Nurses* 75(6):1077–83, June 2002.

Carpman, J. R., and Grant, M. A. Evaluation of waiting room seating. Unpublished research report No. 27, Patient and Visitor Participation Project, Office of Hospital Planning, Research and Development, University of Michigan, Ann Arbor, 1984.

_____. Hospital patient room furnishings mock-ups. Unpublished research report No. 25, Patient and Visitor Participation Project, Office of Hospital Planning, Research and Development, University of Michigan, Ann Arbor, 1984.

_____. Outdoor seating evaluation. Unpublished research report No. 22, Patient and Visitor Participation Project, Office of Hospital Planning, Research and Development, University of Michigan, Ann Arbor, 1983.

Clipson, C. W., and Wehrer, I. I. *Planning for Cardiac Care: A Guide to the Planning and Design of Cardiac Care Facilities.* Ann Arbor, MI: Health Administration Press, 1973.

Cooke, M., Chaboyer, W., and Hiratos, M. Music and its effect on anxiety in short waiting periods: A critical appraisal. *Journal of Clinical Nursing* 14(2): 145–55, February 2005.

Ellis, M. Everyday aids and appliances: Choosing easy chairs for the disabled. *British Medical Journal* 296(6623):701–2, March 5, 1988.

Fong, D. B., and Nichelson, K. Evidence-based lighting design. *Healthcare Design* 6(5):50–53, September 2006.

Hamel, W. J. The effects of music intervention on anxiety in the patient waiting for cardiac catheterization. *Intensive and Critical Care Nursing* 17(5): 279–85 October 2001.

Hamilton, D. N. Lobby study. Unpublished report No. 2-A, Saskatoon Hospital Evaluation Project, University of Saskatchewan, Canada, n.d.

Haun, M., Mainous, R. O., and Looney, S. W. Effect of music on anxiety of women awaiting breast biopsy. *Behavioral Medicine* 27(3):127–32, Fall 2001.

Hayes, A., Buffman, M., Lanier, E., Rodahl, E., and Sasso, C. A music intervention to reduce anxiety prior to gastrointestinal procedures. *Gastroenterology Nursing* 26(4):145–49, 2003.

Hayward, D. G. Working notes, Office of Hospital Planning, Research and Development, University of Michigan, Ann Arbor, 1982.

Huelat, B. Wayfinding: Design for understanding. A position paper for the environmental standards council of the Center for Health Design. October 2007.

Keenan, L., and Goldman, E. Positive imaging: Design as marketing tool in diagnosis centers. *Administrative Radiology* 8(2):36–41, February 1989.

Liddle, K. Reaching out . . . to meet the needs of relatives in intensive care units. *Intensive Care Nursing* 4(4):146–59, December 1988.

Lowes, R. Is your waiting room a practice builder—or a holding pen? *Medical Economics* 75(13):132–34, July 13, 1998.

Mehrabian, A., and Diamond, S. G. Effects of furniture arrangement, props and personality on social interaction. *Journal of Personality and Social Psychology* 20(1):18–30, October 1971.

_____. Seating arrangements and conversation. *Sociometry* 34:281–89, 1970.

Nelson-Shulman, Y. Information and environmental stress: Report of a hospital intervention. *Journal of Environmental Systems* 13(4):303–16, 1983–84.

Olds, A. Psychological considerations in humanizing the physical environment of pediatric outpatient and hospital settings. In E. Gellert, editor. *Psychosocial Aspects of Pediatric Care*, 111–44. New York: Grune and Stratton, 1978.

Pendell, S. D., Coray, K. E., and Veneklasen, W. D. Architectural/behavioral correlates of hospital lobbies. Architectural Psychology Symposium, Rocky Mountain Psychological Association, Salt Lake City, May 1975.

Pennachio, DL. Create a first-rate first impression. *Medical Economics* 80(21):47–48, November 2003.

Petersen, R. W. Behavioral design in OPD architecture: Considerations for reception and waiting areas. In *Proceedings of the Symposium on Pediatric Clinic and Emergency Architecture*, Chicago: American Academy of Pediatrics, June 26–28, 1981a.

_____. Behavioral design criteria: Patient and companion needs for reception and waiting areas. Unpublished report, R. W. Petersen and Associates, McMinnville, OR, July 31, 1981b.

PipeDown. Petition against hospital Muzac grows. 2008. www.pipedown.info/index.php?id=16&cmd =news.

Reizenstein, J. E., and Grant, M. A. Patient activities and schematic design preferences. Unpublished research report No. 2, Patient and Visitor Participation Project, Office of Hospital Planning, Research and Development, University of Michigan, Ann Arbor, 1981.

_____. Spontaneous design suggestions by patients and visitors. Unpublished report No. 6, Patient and Visitor Participation Project, Office of Hospital Planning, Research and Development, University of Michigan, Ann Arbor, 1981.

Reizenstein, J. E., Grant, M. A., and Vaitkus, M. A. Visitor activities and schematic design preferences. Unpublished report No. 4, Patient and Visitor Participation Project, Office of Hospital Planning, Research and Development, University of Michigan, Ann Arbor, 1981.

Rodgers, N. Against forced music in hospitals. February 28, 2007. www.gopetition.com/petitions /against-forced-music-in-hospitals.html.

Routhieaux, R., and Tansik, D. The benefits of music in hospital waiting rooms. *Health Care Supervisor* 16(2):31–40, December 1997.

Scalise, D. Where the patient and technology meet. *Hospitals and Health Networks* 79(8):34–38, August 2005.

Simmons, D. A., Reizenstein, J. E., and Grant, M. A. Considering carpets in hospital use. *Dimensions in Health Service* 59(6):18–21, June 1982.

Sommer, R. The distance for comfortable conversation: A further study. *Sociometry* 25:111–16, 1961.

Swartz, J. The doctor's office: Poor design may cost you patients. *Canadian Medical Association Journal* 140:320–21, February 1989.

Szeto, C., and Yung, P. Introducing a music programme to reduce preoperative anxiety. *British Journal of Theatre Nursing*, 9:455–59, 1999.

Task Force on Guidelines of the Society of Critical Care Medicine. Recommendations for critical care unit design. *Critical Care Medicine* 16(8):796–806, 1988.

Ulrich, R. S., Simons, R. F., and Miles, M. A. Effects of environmental simulations and television on blood donor stress. *Journal of Architectural and Planning Research* 20(1):38–47, Spring 2003.

Webber, J. The campaign for freedom from piped music. June 2, 2008. www.pipedown.info/.

Welch, P. Hospital emergency facilities: Translating behavioral issues into design. Report. Cambridge, MA: Harvard University, Department of Architecture, 1977.

Yung, P., Chui-Kam, S., French, P., and Chan, T. A controlled trial of music and pre-operative anxiety in Chinese men undergoing transurethral resection of the prostate. *Journal of Advanced Nursing* 39(4:352–59, August 2002.

CHAPTER 6

DIAGNOSTIC AND TREATMENT AREAS

Diagnostic and treatment areas take on many forms. In a private physician's office, patients typically proceed from the waiting and reception area directly to an examination room, where they undress, wait, are examined by a physician, undergo treatment, and put on their clothes. The entire examination and treatment process takes place within one room. In an outpatient clinic or other large facility, patients may move from an outer waiting and reception area to a dressing room, to a gowned-waiting area, and finally to one of a number of diagnostic or treatment rooms.

No matter the number of spaces involved, the basic behavior remains the same: patients move from an initial waiting area, change clothes, find a place to store their clothes, strive to maintain a sense of dignity while wearing a patient gown, undergo treatment or examination, and then reverse the process. Some patients bring a companion along for assistance or to make the experience more pleasant.

This chapter explores issues involved in a visit to a diagnostic or treatment area. We focus on certain scenarios, such as a visit to a hospital outpatient clinic, in order to consider a range of design and behavior issues. (Design issues relating to patients' and visitors' use of reception and waiting areas are discussed in chapter 5.) Even when examination and treatment spaces are small, such as in a physician's office, these design and behavior issues still need to be accommodated.

Of course, the processes and procedures that occur within diagnostic and treatment areas are not all the same. For instance, the needs of patients undergoing dialysis will differ from those being treated with radiation therapy. In each case, special equipment or protective shielding may

LEARNING OBJECTIVES
- Understand the emotional and physical needs of patients in diagnostic and treatment areas.
- Learn ways in which a healthcare facility can provide for patient comfort and privacy in changing and examination rooms.
- Become familiar with design features of diagnostic and treatment areas that reduce patient anxiety and provide optimum conditions for diagnosis and treatment.
- Be able to describe the needs of patients and companions for psychological comfort, convenience, and safety during the diagnostic and treatment process.

need to be factored into design requirements. Since space does not permit us to develop design criteria for every type of diagnostic and treatment area, this chapter will focus on generic diagnostic and treatment areas and issues pertaining to most patients and companions.

Accommodating Patients' Needs in Diagnostic and Treatment Areas

Patients seek examination, diagnostic, and treatment services for a variety of reasons, such as an annual physical examination, minor surgery, or long-term treatment of a life-threatening disease. Depending on the circumstances, their emotional states and physical conditions may differ dramatically. They may come to the facility alone or accompanied by family and friends. Depending on past experience with the facility, they may be very familiar or totally unfamiliar with examination and treatment processes. Consequently, the facility must be flexible enough to accommodate a wide range of patients' physical, emotional, and information needs.

Patients may be unfamiliar with, and intimidated by, medical procedures. Even a patient coming in for a simple procedure or examination may be fearful of disease, machinery, and procedures. The facility can do a great deal to ease this anxiety.

Policies as well as design can accommodate patients in a way that limits unnecessary interaction with the more frightening aspects of medical procedures. For example, for patients who will be involved in complex or unfamiliar protocols, the facility might provide an online information video that would allow patients to preview various features of their examination or treatment.

For many patients and visitors, the diagnostic and treatment area represents an unfamiliar and somewhat frightening environment. Medical terminology may be confusing, and patients may find the physical layout complex. (Interior wayfinding is discussed in chapter 4.) Finding their way from one place to another may seem challenging.

Patients may have a number of destinations: dressing room, gowned-waiting, restroom, treatment room, physician's office, and checkout area. If each destination within the diagnostic area is located in sequence, patients can easily move from space to space. This arrangement eliminates backtracking, saves time, and reduces the chances of patients becoming lost (Conway et al., 1977; Green, 1976; Kebart, 1974; Simple, efficient departmental design, 1977). It is important to provide clearly identified examination and treatment rooms, so patients who leave to use the restroom can find their way back on their own. Providing an understandable wayfinding system not only helps avoid confusion, but also lessens the frequency of lost patients inadvertently entering staff areas.

Undressing and Dressing

Many procedures and examinations require patients to wear hospital gowns. In some settings, such as a private physician's office, patients undress in the examination room. In larger outpatient clinics, patients disrobe in a separate dressing room or cubicle before moving to the treatment area. In either case, patients remove some clothes and don a hospital gown.

Although the process of dressing for treatment seems routine, preparing for treatment or examination also has psychological implications. In giving up street clothes, the individual begins to take on the role of "patient." The design of the dressing room indicates to patients how the facility views this role transformation. In the process of gowning, patients are usually put into a less modest situation than when wearing ordinary street clothing. With attention to design details, the facility has an opportunity to show respect for the patient's dignity:

- When planning changing rooms, consider providing a lockable door for patient security and privacy (Ringoir, 1980).

- If a dressing room door cannot be locked, install an indicator on the outside that shows whether or not the room is occupied (Conway et al., 1977).

- When planning a group-changing area with dressing cubicles, provide curtains or doors that provide visual privacy.

- For gowned patients, provide bathroom facilities and water fountains out of public view (Lindheim, 1971; Ringoir, 1980).

- Locate changing rooms close to procedure rooms in order to maximize patients' privacy (Keenan and Goldman, 1989).

- Locate the circulation path from dressing rooms to gowned-waiting and examination or treatment rooms out of public view.

Patients, and in some instances their companions, spend varying amounts of time in the dressing area. Some patients with functional limitations may take a great deal of time to change clothes. The design of the dressing area will influence how comfortably this time is spent and whether a variety of related activities (dressing and undressing, waiting, grooming, communicating with others) can be accommodated:

- Provide at least one dressing area large enough to accommodate two people or a wheelchair user and a companion (Lindheim, 1971).

- If dressing areas are also used as waiting spaces, provide chairs and enough space for patients to wait comfortably.

- Provide comfortable chairs and a small stool or other piece of furniture for patients who have difficulty bending over to tie their shoes (Burgun, 1976; Lindheim, 1971).

- Keep dressing areas slightly warmer than the rest of the facility (Burgun, 1976; Lindheim, 1971).

- Provide a mirror that can be seen by short people, tall people, and wheelchair users.

- Provide carpeting on dressing-area floors to keep bare feet warm.

- Install hooks and shelves in easily reached places for hanging clothes and storing personal items.

- Provide effective lighting.

- Avoid isolating patients; provide some mechanism for patients to communicate with staff (Lindheim, 1971).

If patients leave the dressing room or if the dressing room is to be used by another patient, some provision needs to be made for storing belongings. Unless the dressing room can be locked, unattended belongings create potential security challenges. In the absence of secure, locked spaces, patients must carry valuables through diagnostic procedures and spaces where they may be misplaced. One study showed that given a choice, most patients prefer leaving their belongings in a locker rather than taking them along in a bag (Lindheim, 1971; Reizenstein, Grant, and Vaitkus, 1981 [unpub.]). With either system, there are management issues and design issues to consider. Lockers need to be durable and easy to operate by patients with varying physical abilities. Lockers should be located in a place where they can be monitored directly by staff or by closed-circuit camera. If bags are used to store belongings, they need to be durable and easily stored out of the way in treatment rooms. Staff may need to help patients keep track of their bagged belongings.

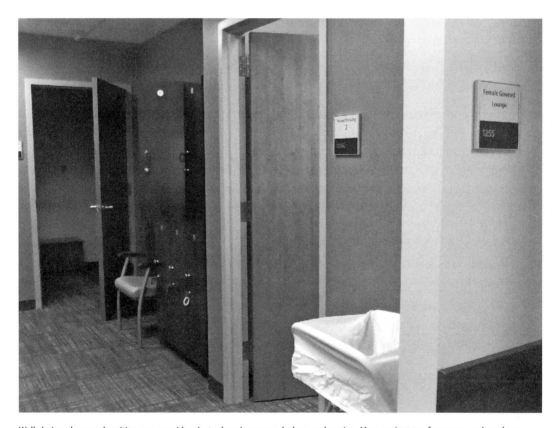

Well-designed gowned-waiting areas provide private changing rooms, lockers, and seating. Many patients prefer women-only and men-only areas when they are gowned.
Photo credit: Courtesy of St. Joseph Mercy Chelsea

Waiting While Wearing a Hospital Gown

Jokes about the revealing nature of hospital gowns are legion, but the reality is that wearing a gown is considered embarrassing by many patients (Reizenstein and Grant, 1981a [unpub.]). What may seem sufficient cover while waiting in an examination room with some visual privacy may seem too exposed in a group waiting area. As one study showed, if they must wear a typical hospital gown, many patients prefer to wait in single-gender areas (Lindheim, 1971).

If a less-revealing gown is provided, concerns over modesty are somewhat alleviated and patients feel more comfortable waiting in a mixed-gender area (Reizenstein and Grant, 1981a [unpub.], 1981b [unpub.]). By providing less-revealing gowns or by providing robes, health facilities can show respect for patients' dignity and will not necessarily have to provide separate male, female, and gender-neutral waiting areas. A more modest gown or a robe also enables patients to feel more comfortable in a waiting area where others are both dressed and gowned, so companions can more comfortably accompany patients throughout the process. (A detailed discussion of waiting areas can be found in chapter 5.)

Maintaining Privacy

Because patients are partially or fully undressed during many procedures, it is important to maintain bodily privacy and reduce the chance of unintentional exposure. Room layout and privacy curtains in examination and treatment rooms can help prevent exposure to people looking in from the hallway. In obstetrics and gynecology examination rooms, for example, it is important to avoid situating examination tables with the patient's feet toward the doorway.

Some patients have refused parts of a physical examination due to lack of privacy (Barlas et al., 2001). However, privacy includes being able to control what patients can see and hear of others as well as what others can see or hear about them. A situation in which one patient accidentally sees another patient disrobed may embarrass both people.

Acoustical and other informational privacy must be provided. Some patients have reported withholding important medical history information because they were afraid of being overheard by others (Barlas et al., 2001; Malcolm, 2001; Olsen and Sabin, 2003). And it may be as disturbing to overhear a discussion between a physician and another patient as it is to know that one's personal conversations can be overheard. Moreover, any healthcare information that is processed, stored, transmitted, or received electronically is subject to HIPAA, the American Insurance Portability and Accountability Act of 1996 (American Health Insurance, 1996; Dubbs, 2003). Among other provisions, closed-circuit monitors and digital-device screens with patient information must be kept out of view by unauthorized personnel.

A general understanding of the issues, coupled with good planning, can enable staff to avoid compromising patients' visual, acoustical, and bodily privacy. Consider these guidelines:

- Design examination and treatment rooms so patients are not exposed when a door is opened (Burgun, 1976).

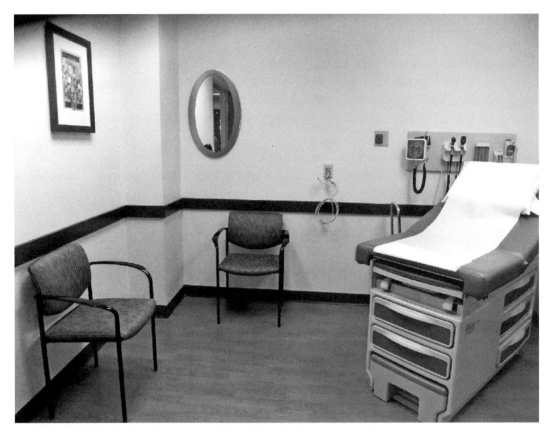

This exam room features artwork and a mirror for the patient, as well as seating for a companion.
Photo credit: Courtesy of St. Joseph Mercy Chelsea

- Design the layout of furnishings in examination and treatment rooms to provide optimum visual and acoustical privacy for patients undergoing the procedures typically performed in these rooms.

- Provide privacy curtains in examination and treatment rooms and encourage staff to use them.

- Where technicians observe patients on a closed-circuit monitor in a control room, position the monitor so it cannot be viewed by passersby (American Health Insurance, 1996; Conway et al., 1977; Dubbs, 2003). The same should be done for digital device screens in nurses' stations that display patient information.

- Refer to and follow HIPAA rules to ensure privacy of all patient information (American Health Insurance, 1996; Dubbs, 2003).

- Provide acoustical privacy in examination and treatment rooms by installing walls instead of curtains (Barlas et al., 2001; Malcolm, 2001; Olsen and Sabin, 2003). One approach is to construct walls from the floor to the underside of the structural slab, fully insulate them with sound-attenuating material, cover both sides of the studs with drywall, and then caulk all perimeter joints. In addition, install sound-attenuating material around pipes or duct work to reduce noise (Conway et al., 1977).

* Provide separate, private recovery or consultation rooms for patients to discuss medical history and diagnoses with staff or to recover physically and emotionally from difficult procedures (Altman, 1977; Dubbs, 2003; Malcolm, 2001).

* Although many treatments (such as dialysis) may be best carried out in an open ward, also provide a private room for medical examinations and consultations (Dubbs, 2003; Ringoir, 1980).

Optimizing Comfort

Since patients often spend a long time (on average, 45 minutes) in treatment rooms as they wait for a physician or other caregiver, it is important to consider their comfort during the inevitable wait (Reuter, 1974; Zilm, Brimhall, and Ryan, 1978). The treatment room should be a comfortable, relaxing place. A calming atmosphere is especially important for patients undergoing procedures that use potentially frightening technology, such as a linear accelerator, heart catheter, or MRI machine. (See Research Box 6.1.)

RESEARCH BOX 6.1 PATIENT CONTROL OF DESIGN FEATURES IN HEMODIALYSIS UNITS

There is growing evidence that the ability to control one's environment can reduce stress (Steptoe and Appels, 1989).

In one study, questionnaires were administered to patients at 16 hemodialysis units in the greater Houston area. The surveys asked about perceptions of control in relation to four design features in the treatment environment: acoustics/noise, lighting, temperature, and privacy. In most of the study facilities, patients had little or no ability to control the bright fluorescent lighting, irregular noise levels, or uncomfortably cool temperatures, and they had limited privacy. This lack of control and privacy constituted a stressful treatment environment for patients already experiencing considerable physiological and emotional stress related to their illness (Bame et al., 1991).

Despite these design features, a high proportion of patients reported satisfaction; however, their level of satisfaction with the design features in their treatment environments did not correspond with their reports of experiences involving facility design. For example, 61 percent of the patients reported that they usually or always were too cold, and yet 64 percent expressed satisfaction with the temperature of the treatment room. Sixty percent of the patients reported that they wanted more privacy during dialysis, and yet 72 percent reported that they were satisfied with the degree of privacy in the treatment room.

The researchers explained this seemingly contradictory finding in several ways. On the one hand, patients may not realize that their comfort and preferences should directly affect their satisfaction with the treatment environment. Patients probably adapt to the environment

(continued)

RESEARCH BOX 6.1 (*Continued*)

because they don't expect that the treatment environment will be designed to accommodate their needs. They typically take on a passive patient role, with expectations corresponding to their past health-facility experiences. On the other hand, this patient population simply may not be conscious of their environment. They may be so preoccupied with their illnesses or feel so overwhelmed by the demands of their treatment and of managing everyday life that they focus inward. They may regard the treatment environment as a low priority in relation to their other concerns. Furthermore, patients may not consider their treatment environment because they have never experienced a health facility designed to accommodate their needs. Thus, they have neither the frame of reference for what a "good" design could be nor expectations that their facility should be any different. Nevertheless, even though patients in this study were not critical of their facility's design, they clearly indicated that they preferred greater control of temperature, noise, and privacy within their treatment environment.

Design decision-makers should consider all features and details when creating comfortable diagnostic and treatment spaces. For instance, incandescent table lamps may produce a more comforting ambience than overhead fluorescent lights (Hayward and Gates, 1981). And, a setting that appears cold and institutional may reduce a patient's willingness to talk about intimate details with a physician. (See Research Box 6.2.)

RESEARCH BOX 6.2 DESIGNING FOR SELF-DISCLOSURE

Healthcare staff members often need detailed information from patients in order to diagnose an illness or determine proper treatment. The degree to which patients feel comfortable talking about personal issues may influence their ability to reveal this information (Chaikin, Derlega, and Miller, 1976).

Realizing that there may also be environmental factors involved, researchers at Old Dominion University in Norfolk, Virginia, examined the effect of room environment on self-disclosure (Langan, Wagner, and Buchanan, 1979). The study compared participant behavior within an architecturally "hard" room to that in an architecturally "soft" room. The "hard" room was relatively bare, with cinderblock walls, a brown tile floor, and simple furniture. The "soft" room added a rug, pictures on the wall, indirect lighting, magazines, some upholstered furniture, and a variety of odds and ends.

Participants in the study, psychology students, were interviewed by a counselor and asked to talk about themselves. The researchers examined videos of the sessions to determine the amount of self-disclosure. Results showed that those interviewed in the "soft" room were significantly more willing to discuss revealing details than those interviewed in the "hard" room.

The following design suggestions will help make treatment rooms comfortable for patients and visitors:

- When possible, provide two comfortable chairs in each examination or treatment room.

- If the protocol requires that patients are positioned for treatment while in the dark, provide a dim nightlight so they do not become disoriented (Conway et al., 1977).

- Minimize patient contact with medical equipment (Langan et al., 1979; Zubatkin, 1980).

- Use carpeting, wall coverings, wood paneling, or murals to soften the décor (Radiation unit improves, 1980).

- Select artwork likely to be perceived as calming by patients and visitors (prints, kites, mobiles, and so on) (Swartz, 1989). (See also chapter 7.)

- Consider providing patient-controlled music within the treatment room (Schweiger, 1991; Swartz, 1989).

- Prepare patients for the treatment by explaining what will be done.

For many patients, it is not pleasant to sit on an examining table wearing nothing but a patient gown. Examination and treatment rooms often seem designed more for the medical procedures that take place in them than for the patients who undergo those procedures. For example, some medical equipment (such as cardiac monitors) is sensitive to temperature and humidity fluctuations; others generate a great deal of heat. Consequently, treatment-room temperatures adjusted for equipment may be perceived by patients as too warm or too cool.

Attention to the following details can make a big difference:

- Attend to patients' thermal comfort in rooms that require particularly warm or cool temperatures (Altman, 1977; Ringoir, 1980).

- Because patients wearing hospital gowns may become chilled at a temperature comfortable for fully clothed staff, keep examination and treatment rooms warmer than staff areas (Altman, 1977; Ringoir, 1980).

- Consider using operating tables and mattresses that can be warmed (Bourke and Sadeghi, 2003).

- Where examination or treatment procedures are likely to be stressful, provide indirect, soft lighting. Avoid situations in which patients must stare into lights during treatment. If possible, provide a dimmer control (Langan et al., 1979).

- Help patients avoid being chilled by contact with metal medical instruments and equipment such as examination table stirrups. If possible, provide warmers for metal instruments.

Considering Lighting

It is important to provide optimum lighting in diagnostic and treatment areas as well as in inpatient rooms and other areas of the health facility. Some patients and visitors have particular lighting sensitivities and others have preferences about types of lighting.

Human beings thrive on natural light. As researchers explain, the combination of sun and sky (radiation), with its rhythmic changes in level, provides people with the basis for visual information to see brightness and react efficiently to the environment; it provides levels of light and light modulation necessary for controlling levels of melatonin, a hormone important in the regulation of biorhythms; and it provides the amount and balance of ultraviolet light needed for skeletal formation and maintenance (Brainard, 1995; Thorington, 1985). Exposure to bright light has been associated with improvements in alertness, mood, sleep quality, and a number of health outcomes. (See chapter 7.)

Healthcare providers have an interest in optimizing lighting in order to promote patient recovery and provide working conditions that allow staff to function effectively. For instance, evidence suggests that bright-light exposure could help night-shift workers maintain alertness and reduce errors by resetting or adapting their internal clocks (Brainard, 1995).

Lighting needs to provide proper intensity and color rendition without causing unnecessary glare or other uncomfortable effects (Fong, 2003; Fong and Nichelson, 2006; Souhrada, 1989). Lighting decisions should consider not only the properties of light sources but also the reflective properties of wallcoverings, flooring, and furnishings (Brainard, 1995; Fong and Nichelson, 2006).

Although incandescent bulbs are the most frequently used source of artificial illumination, and LEDs are becoming more popular, cool-white fluorescent lamps in fixtures with plastic diffusers have been frequently employed in health facilities. (See Research Box 6.3.)

RESEARCH BOX 6.3 IS FLUORESCENT LIGHTING HEALTHY?

Some people have adverse reactions to working under fluorescent lighting. Common complaints include eyestrain, fatigue, jumpiness, irritability, headaches, interference with hearing aids, and (for some people) skin lesions. One solution is to turn off the fluorescents and use an incandescent lamp or two when daylight is not available.

Standard cool-white fluorescent lighting is widely used in businesses, hospitals, and factories throughout the world, often in the absence of windows. Research has focused on chronic health effects. For instance, there is a body of evidence suggesting that frequent, extended exposure to standard fluorescent lighting at work and home increases the risk of melanoma, at least among males (Beral et al., 1982; Elwood, 1986; Elwood, Williamson, and Stapleton, 1986; English et al., 1985; Maxwell and Elwood, 1986; Pasternack, Dubin, and Moseson, 1983; Walter et al., 1992). The results are mixed, but four studies that assessed respondents' degrees of exposure to fluorescent lighting using direct interviews, rather than mailed questionnaires or phone interviews, found a significant association of fluorescent lighting with skin disorders (Walter et al., 1992).

Some researchers claim that standard cool-white fluorescents increase hyperactivity among schoolchildren (Mayron, 1978; Mayron, Ott, and Mayron, 1974). There have been reports from public-health officials suggesting that malfunctioning fluorescents may leak toxic chemicals and lead to outbreaks of illness—from eye irritation to nausea—among people nearby (Harris, 1985; Tavris, Field, and Brumback, 1984).

The exact cause of the broad array of symptoms noted by users and researchers remains largely a matter of continuing research, speculation, and debate. One claim is that the rapid flickering from fluorescent lamps at certain wavelengths is responsible for eyestrain and headaches. One proposed solution is for people in the vicinity of fluorescents to wear tinted eyeglasses (Wilkins and Wilkinson, 1991).

A parallel argument concerning melanoma is that standard fluorescents have a much greater energy flux in the 290- to 295-nanometer ultraviolet B (UVB) range than does solar energy. However, research shows that emission of UVA and UVB from these lamps is minimal and that emission is typically blocked by plastic fixture covers (Griffiths and Fairney, 1988; Ott, 1985).

Another researcher suggests that many of the reported abnormal biological effects are the result of radio-frequency and/or X-ray emissions similar to those given off by digital devices. He proposes controlling the emissions with a grounded wire-grid shielding, instead of a plastic diffuser (De Flora et al., 1990; Ott, 1973).

Known for their ability to light a large area inexpensively, standard cool-white fluorescents have the disadvantage of severely reducing the color spectrum by putting most of their energy into the yellow-green portion. One commonly perceived effect of this is to create an unnatural color rendition of human skin. Another is that, true to the name, such lamps emphasize a color combination people commonly perceive as cold. A third disadvantage is the inability of such lamps to supply the type and levels of ultraviolet radiation needed by humans for producing D hormones (vitamin D) (Davies, 1985; Thorington, 1985). Low light levels are also a problem. In order to conserve energy, fluorescent lamps are often used at illumination levels commensurate with twilight. However, the body is not able to properly regulate melatonin production at such light levels. Nor does the static nature of fluorescent lighting provide the natural time cues that humans expect and need during the day.

When patient and staff areas are illuminated by standard fluorescent lighting, rather than by natural light, the risk of sensory deprivation increases. As research about lighting and windows has demonstrated (see chapter 7), lighting conditions in some healthcare facilities may lead to sensory deprivation, depression, and reduced feelings of well-being among patients and staff.

The demand for artificial illumination that more closely resembles ordinary daylight has brought several alternatives to the market. Full-spectrum fluorescent lighting is one such alternative; however, these lights are considerably more expensive and less energy-efficient than other artificial lights. And most lighting researchers agree that full-spectrum lighting does not provide health benefits associated with natural lighting, despite claims by its proponents (Full-Spectrum Lighting, 2005; Joseph, 2006).

Not all daylight or deluxe bulbs offer equal illumination qualities. When choosing lighting, decision-makers should consider two particular aspects of lamp color: Color Rendering Index (CRI) and color temperature. Lighting researchers recommend choosing one lamp color in all spaces, to maintain a consistent quality of light. In order to provide neutral lighting that brings out the true colors of objects (good color rendering), a CRI in the mid-80,000s and color temperature between 3,000 and 3,500 degrees Kelvin are recommended (Fong and Nichelson, 2006).

Designers should consider the following guidelines when choosing lighting for examination and treatment rooms:

- Integrate daylight with indirect artificial lighting to create a soothing effect for patients (Fong, 2003; Fong and Nichelson, 2006).

- Install one lamp color in all patient areas, including patient access corridors, to allow health professionals to make consistent assessments of skin color (Fong, 2003; Fong and Nichelson, 2006).

- Use lighting levels high enough to provide good visibility, but not so high that they produce glare and cause patient discomfort (Fong, 2003; Fong and Nichelson, 2006).

- Consider installing fixed light sources with dimming switches or switches for multiple light levels (Fong, 2003; Fong and Nichelson, 2006).

- Install wall-mounted or ceiling-suspended indirect lighting fixtures to illuminate all areas of an exam room (Fong, 2003).

- Use supplemental lighting that is fixed or portable, depending on the tasks performed in the room (Fong, 2003; Fong and Nichelson, 2006).

- Choose examination lighting that provides effective lighting over a circular area no larger than 2 feet (~0.6 meters) in diameter (Fong, 2003).

Reducing Noise

Noise in healthcare facilities can be a source of stress for many patients and visitors (Hurst, 1966). Some sounds are so loud or noticeable as to be disturbing: sounds of pain that increase other patients' own anxieties, sounds of laughter that seem inappropriate to the setting, and sounds of conversations that can compromise privacy. The effects of pain and medication can heighten patients' negative reactions to sound. Patients and visitors typically have little or no control over noise, an often-inescapable feature of the physical environment.

Noise may lead to increased heart rates. Startle effects from sudden loud sounds may produce inaccurate blood-pressure measurements (Bakalar, 2008; Cmiel et al., 2004; Haslam, 1970; Storlie, 1976). However, it is difficult to determine the extent of negative physiological and psychological changes specifically attributed to noise, rather than to pain and general discomfort.

One study found that the layout of a treatment facility was more effective at reducing noise than were sound-absorbing tiles and walls. (See Research Box 6.4.) More recent studies indicate that sound-absorbing ceiling tiles can significantly reduce noise and corresponding sleep arousals (Berg, 2001; Joseph and Ulrich, 2007). In addition to insulating rooms and using sound-absorbing tiles, efforts to reduce noise in hospitals include increasing staff sensitivity, providing separate staff lounge areas, installing hydraulic door closers and rubber pads on door frames, reducing the volume of nearby phones and medical equipment, and using padded charts and chart racks (Cmiel et al., 2004; Duffy and Florell, 1990; Grumet, 1993; Hansell, 1984; Mazer, 2005; Williams, 1989; Williams and Murphy, 1991).

RESEARCH BOX 6.4 ACOUSTIC DESIGN AND NOISE IN HEMODIALYSIS UNITS

Noisy environments increase stress and decrease work performance. Higher levels of noise interfere with patients' abilities to relax or sleep, distract staff's attention from monitoring patients' conditions, and hamper communication among patients and staff, particularly for older patients with hearing limitations.

A study of 55 hemodialysis facilities in Texas revealed that noise exceeded recommended levels (Bame, 1992). Noise was measured at a sample of patient stations at each facility. General-purpose sound meters measured sound levels according to the decibel A scale. All facilities included in the study had mean noise levels over standards set for comparable hospital environments (27 to 47 decibels on the A scale) (Beranek, Blazier, and Figwer, 1971; Egan, 1972; Sound Research Laboratories Limited, 1976). Only one facility fell within an acceptable noise range for large or open office environments (42 to 52 decibels). Seven percent of the facilities were "noisy" (52 to 55 decibels on the A scale). Typical of conditions in lobbies, corridors, laboratory work spaces, and secretarial areas, 79 percent of the facilities had "very noisy" conditions (55 to 65 decibels on the A scale), comparable to conditions expected at industrial shops, garages, and machinery rooms (Egan, 1972). Fourteen percent of the facilities averaged even higher noise levels, at more than 65 decibels.

Acoustic design features, including acoustic ceiling tiles, textured wall coverings, wall cabinets, and shelves, did not effectively reduce the high noise levels. However, noise levels did vary significantly according to acoustic-screening characteristics present in different treatment-room layouts.

Five layout classifications were developed according to the arrangement of patient stations: parallel, pinwheel, bay, U-shaped, and peripheral. Parallel layouts had two, three, four, or six rows of patient treatment stations. Pinwheel arrangements had four patients around a floor-to-ceiling column built to accommodate plumbing and electricity access. Bays were small groupings of three to six treatment stations separated by partition counters. A U-shaped layout had patient stations around three walls, with a nursing station along the fourth wall. Peripheral layouts had patient stations all around the outside walls of the treatment room.

(continued)

RESEARCH BOX 6.4 (*Continued*)

The concentration of sounds reverberating within a bay of treatment stations contributed to a significantly higher noise level. Conversely, a layout of treatment stations arranged as a pinwheel was significantly quieter, reflecting sound more randomly because of the geometry of treatment stations configured at right angles. Treatment stations arranged either in parallel rows or around the walls (U-shaped and peripheral layouts) had noisy environments, louder than the pinwheel layout but quieter than the bay arrangement. Thus, the different treatment room layouts directly affected their noise levels.

Listening to Music

Listening to music may be beneficial for patients undergoing minor medical procedures. These patients may experience anxiety as a result of symptoms of the underlying disease, uncertainty of diagnosis, and fear of the unknown (Colt, Powers, and Shanks, 1999). (For a discussion of the special therapeutic effects of music for people with dementia, see chapter 9.)

Music interventions can reduce patient anxiety and improve well-being. Early studies suggested that music could be used as an "audioanalgesic" to help patients relax during minor medical and dental procedures. Dental studies have posited several factors that may contribute to this effect: the auditory stimuli of the music may suppress pain neurologically; music may mask the sound of the dental drill, which is often a source of conditioned anxiety; the music may have a conditioned relaxing effect; or music may serve as a simple distraction (Schweiger, 1991).

Results of more recent studies on the effect of music during invasive procedures do not all lead to the same conclusion. Two literature reviews reported mixed evidence of the effects on patient anxiety of listening to music during medical procedures (Evans, 2002; Kemper and Danhauer, 2005). Some studies reported a reduction in anxiety for patients exposed to music during outpatient bronchoscopy, sigmoidoscopy, cesarean delivery, and minor surgery with local anaesthesia (Chang and Chen, 2005; Dubois, Bartter, and Pratter, 1995; Mok and Wong, 2003; Palakanis et al., 1994). A review of 29 studies found that music reduced anxiety for patients receiving normal care, but not for patients undergoing invasive procedures (e.g., bronchoscopy, cataract surgery, and urological procedures) (Evans, 2002). (See Research Box 6.5.)

RESEARCH BOX 6.5 CAN MUSIC AFFECT PATIENT ANXIETY AND COMFORT?

The effect of music on patient anxiety during invasive medical procedures is difficult to determine, given contradictory results across studies. A number of methodological factors may contribute to these differences: (1) chosen measure of anxiety; (2) study design; (3) music selection; (4) use of anti-anxiety medication or sedatives; (5) medical procedures; and (6) researcher bias. Two studies of bronchoscopy reveal ambiguous findings regarding the effects of music.

One study examined the effect of music on anxiety levels in patients undergoing flexible fiber-optic bronchoscopy (Colt et al., 1999). Sixty patients were randomly assigned either to a control group or a music group. Both groups wore headphones throughout the procedure, but one group heard recorded relaxation music, while the other group heard nothing (silence). The music consisted of piano improvisations at a tempo of 60 beats per minute.

All patients received localized anaesthesia and did not receive sedatives or anxioloytics (drugs for reducing anxiety symptoms). However, medication for comfort (IV midaxolam) was administered during the procedure, if requested by the patient.

Procedure-related anxiety was measured using the State-Trait Anxiety Inventory (STAI), a self-report measure of present (state) anxiety and general (trait) anxiety. Patients were asked to focus only on the period of the bronchoscopy while responding to the questions. Patients completed the STAI within one hour before and one hour after the bronchoscopy procedure.

Results revealed that relaxation music did not decrease procedure-related state anxiety. No statistically significant differences were found between pre-procedure and post-procedure anxiety. Similarly, there were no statistically or clinically significant differences between the music group and control (silence) group.

Conversely, another researcher found positive effects of music on patient comfort during a bronchoscopy (Dubois, Bartter, and Pratter, 1995). Forty-nine patients were randomly assigned to a music group or a control group. During the procedure, the music group used headphones and portable CD-players to listen to pop rock (a style of music from the 1970s and '80s). The control group underwent the procedure as usual, without music.

Physiological measures were monitored, including heart rate, blood pressure, and oxygen saturation before and during the bronchoscopy. The amount and type of sedation was also documented. Following the bronchoscopy, patients responded to written questions about their comfort during the procedure.

The study found that music was associated with greater comfort and less coughing than in the control group. Physiological measures and medications given during the procedure did not differ significantly between the groups.

In these two studies, the researchers used different types of music (piano improvisations vs. pop rock). The researchers also tested the effects of music using different measures (anxiety vs. physiological measures and patient comfort). Differences in study design make it difficult to generalize across studies.

The music interventions investigated in many studies refer to patients listening to music using headphones. However, some music-therapy approaches involve more than simply listening to music and can have different levels of participation by patients and music therapists. For example, in Music-Based Imagery (MBI), the patient describes images of relaxing and safe experiences to a music therapist, who creates music and lyrics for the images and incorporates cues for rhythmic deep breathing. The patient is instructed to hold the images in mind and focus on breathing. Another approach, Musical Alternative Engagement (MAE), is more participatory in that the patient hums, sings, or otherwise physically responds to cues in the music.

Two studies explored the effect of Music-Based Imagery and Musical Alternative Engagement on pulse, pain, anxiety, and tension of burn patients during dressing changes and wound debridement (Fratianne et al., 2001; Prensner et al., 2001). They found MBI and MAE significantly reduced self-reported pain early in the debridement process; however, these techniques seemed less effective during the most painful aspects of the procedure.

Some adverse effects of music have been identified. Although rare, "music epilepsy" is a condition where a music stimulus can trigger a seizure. Music can also bother people with a low tolerance for noise, such as those with brain damage (Brown and Theorell, 2005). Therefore, patient history and medical conditions are important considerations in determining whether music could be beneficial. Most adverse effects of music can be prevented through individualized music selection and presentation methods, as well as by providing patients with the choice of whether or not to listen to music (Brown and Theorell, 2005).

Experiencing Positive Distractions

Patients tend to fear being diagnosed with a serious disease and/or needing painful treatment. Waiting with nothing to do gives them time to dwell on those fears and other worries. Anxiety may be alleviated, at least in part, when examination and treatment areas provide positive distractions—things for patients to focus their attention on during their time in the health facility (Reizenstein, Grant, and Vaitkus, 1981 [unpub.]).

Consider these guidelines:

- When patients undergo lengthy treatment procedures (such as dialysis or nuclear medicine scans) and visual privacy is not a concern, avoid separating patients and their companions. Allowing patients to watch the activities occurring around them may provide distraction (Simple, efficient departmental design, 1977).

- Where examination or treatment procedures are apt to be lengthy, consider providing television, radio, music, digital devices, and current magazines. Provide patients with choices about programming (Ringoir, 1980).

- Give patients something to focus their attention on. If possible, provide windows into the hallway or the outdoors or hang artwork on walls and ceilings (Oberlander, 1979; Radiation unit improves, 1980; Sandberg, 1987; Zubatkin, 1980).

- Provide a patient-to-staff communication system in examination rooms.

- During particularly stressful procedures, such as radiation therapy or MRI, enable patients to communicate with technicians or companions.

- During lengthy procedures, provide patients with the option of viewing monitors that show the progress of their treatment. This reassures some patients and helps them feel part of the overall process (Zubatkin, 1980).

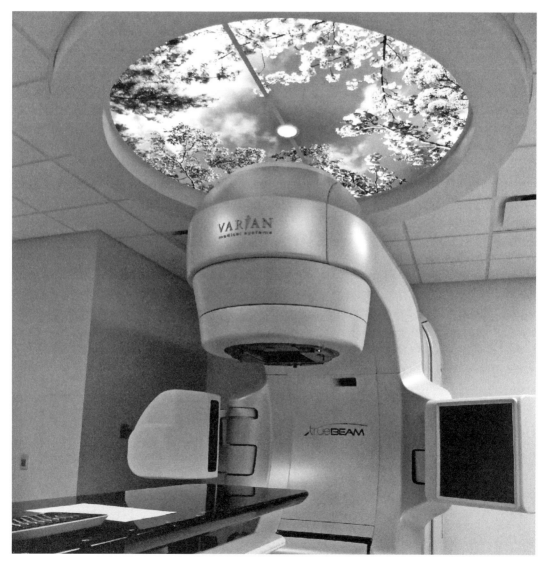

This radiation therapy treatment room features a ceiling view of colorful, internally lit trees, providing positive distraction for patients.

Photo credit: Courtesy of St. Joseph Mercy Chelsea

- Consider providing other types of distraction. Although not necessarily appropriate for every patient, aromatherapy, for instance, may be welcomed by people who find "hospital smells" unpleasant.

Virtual reality (VR) technology can be employed not only as a source of entertainment but also as a powerful distraction for patients undergoing medical procedures (Ma, Jain, and Anderson, 2014; Perhakaran et al., 2016). Virtual reality allows users to interact with a digitally-simulated environment using a head-mounted display, helmet, or other device. Programs engage multiple senses to enhance the patient's feeling of being immersed in the simulated environment. For instance, some headsets produce visual images accompanied with related sounds (Steptoe and Appels, 1989). Other devices can detect the patient's head, hand, and foot movements and change the view accordingly (Bame et al., 1991). A variety of virtual environments are available, including walks through a forest, deep-sea diving adventures, and museum tours (Brodeur, 2015; Kipping et al., 2012; Ma et al., 2014; Steptoe and Appels, 1989).

Some treatment centers have explored the use of virtual reality as a technique for distracting patients during medical procedures (Gold, Kant, and Kim, 2005; Kipping et al., 2012; Loyola University Health System, 2008; Wright, Hoffman, and Sweet, 2005). Audiovisual VR used by patients undergoing chemotherapy treatments has been associated with reductions in symptoms of distress and fatigue immediately following the treatment, with patients estimating the time spent in treatment as significantly less than the actual time spent (Steptoe and Appels, 1989). Burn patients using virtual reality during physical therapy report less pain and less time spent thinking about pain, as well as requiring less analgesic medication (Bame et al., 1991; Collins, 2014; Kipping et al., 2012; Loyola University Health System, 2008). Researchers theorize that VR distracts patients from processing pain signals, thereby reducing their perception of pain (Bame et al., 1991), and suggest that better acute pain control may lower the risk of patients developing chronic or persistent pain at a later date (Collins, 2014). VR technologies are also being developed to address anxiety, stress, and post-traumatic stress disorder (Brodeur, 2015; Ma et al., 2014; Perhakaran et al., 2016).

Using Digital Devices

Patients and visitors need to be able to use cell phones and other digital devices so they can make arrangements and keep up with life outside the facility. Available electrical outlets will help patients and visitors keep their devices charged and they will likely use and appreciate Wi-Fi.

Using Restrooms and Water Fountains

Restrooms and water fountains need to be available to patients and visitors near each stop in the journey (waiting, dressing, gowned-waiting, and treatment). Gowned patients should not have to walk through public areas to get a drink of water, nor should visitors need to enter a treatment area to use a restroom (Altman, 1977; Burgun, 1976; Conway et al., 1977).

Facilitating Contact between Patients and Staff

The healthcare experience may leave patients feeling vulnerable and forgotten if they are left alone to wait for what seems like a long time. In order to feel secure, patients need to know that if anything goes wrong, they will be able to get help. Visible and easily reachable call buttons or cords need to be available in restrooms, examination rooms, dressing rooms, and other closed rooms (Langan et al., 1979). It is also important for staff to have visual access to diagnostic and treatment waiting areas (Kebart, 1974).

Accommodating Companions

Patients often bring along friends or relatives to provide support and distraction. For patients unable to dress themselves, companions are a great help. When patients are emotionally distraught, companions can act as intermediaries between patients and the staff delivering care. Although most companions sit and wait for patients in an outer waiting area, companions who accompany patients throughout the diagnostic and treatment experience need to be accommodated in the following ways:

- Provide at least one dressing room large enough to accommodate two people.
- Provide chairs in the gowned-waiting area for companions.
- Provide comfortable chairs in examination and treatment rooms for the patient and a companion.
- Provide access to restrooms, a water fountain, and vending machines for companions remaining in a waiting area.

Summary

- Patients visit healthcare facilities for many reasons, from routine physical examinations to life-threatening crises. Their physical conditions will differ widely, as will their emotional states. They may be very familiar or totally unfamiliar with the facility and treatment processes, which may range from pain-free to painful and from stress-free to frightening. They may come alone or with one or more companions. At every stage, patients require both design and policies that humanize the experience; preserve their sense of control and dignity; and mitigate the myriad annoyances and difficulties associated with medical diagnosis and treatment.
- In removing some or all clothing, the individual begins to take on the role of patient. A healthcare facility demonstrates respect for a patient's comfort, privacy, and dignity

by providing patient gowns that cover the body. Facilities should also make available comfortable, changing rooms with doors and equipped with privacy curtains, ample space and seating, provision for communication with staff, and safe storage for belongings. Transition and waiting areas should be out of public view and near restrooms and water fountains.

o   Design features of examination and treatment rooms should ensure patients' visual and acoustical privacy. Lighting should provide optimum conditions for medical examination and treatment, patient orientation and comfort, and effective staff functioning. Noise should be minimized by thoughtful architectural layouts, use of insulation and sound-absorbing features, and other design and behavioral considerations. Facilities should attend to patients' thermal comfort, offer them positive distractions while waiting, and consider the therapeutic benefits of offering individual music devices.

o   Patients and visitors will want to use and charge their digital devices while they wait. They need access to restrooms and water fountains. To feel secure, they must know that staff have visual access to diagnostic and treatment areas and that visible and reachable call buttons or cords are available in closed rooms. Companions can provide valuable support and comfort to patients; their needs for space, seating, and amenities should also be met.

DISCUSSION QUESTIONS

1. What are some physical and emotional needs of patients when they visit examination, diagnostic, and treatment areas?

2. How can the design of hospital gowns and dressing areas address patients' needs for visual privacy and comfort?

3. What is the importance of acoustical privacy in waiting and treatment areas?

4. What factors are involved in providing optimal lighting in diagnostic and treatment areas?

5. Why is it desirable to reduce noise in diagnostic and treatment areas, and what policies and design decisions contribute to this outcome?

6. What factors should be considered regarding music in diagnostic and treatment areas?

7. What design features contribute to patient comfort in treatment areas?

8. What positive distractions can relieve patient anxiety during waiting and treatment?

9. What provisions should be made for companions accompanying patients to diagnostic and treatment areas?

Design Review Questions

Accommodating Patients' Needs in Diagnostic and Treatment Areas

☐ Will new patients be offered information before they undergo medical procedures?

☐ Will destinations be arranged in a way that allows patients to proceed from space to space without walking long distances? (Conway et al., 1977; Green, 1976; Kebart, 1974; Simple, efficient departmental design, 1977)

☐ Will patient routes and destinations be clearly marked?

☐ Will examination and treatment rooms be clearly identified so patients leaving the area can find their way back?

Undressing and Dressing

☐ Will dressing rooms have lockable doors? (Ringoir, 1980)

☐ Will dressing room doors indicate when the room is occupied? (Conway et al., 1977)

☐ Will curtains or doors on dressing cubicles provide visual privacy?

☐ Will restrooms and water fountains be located close to gowned-waiting areas and out of public view? (Lindheim, 1971; Ringoir, 1980)

☐ Will patients be out of public view as they travel between dressing areas, gowned-waiting areas, and examination or treatment rooms?

☐ Will at least one dressing room or cubicle be large enough to accommodate a wheelchair user and a companion? (Lindheim, 1971)

☐ Will comfortable chairs be provided in dressing areas? (Burgun, 1976; Lindheim, 1971)

☐ If dressing areas are also used as waiting spaces, will ample space and numbers of chairs be provided so patients can wait comfortably?

☐ Will a stool or other piece of furniture be provided to help patients tie their shoes if they have difficulty bending over? (Burgun, 1976; Lindheim, 1971)

☐ Will the dressing area be kept slightly warmer than the rest of the facility? (Burgun, 1976; Lindheim, 1971)

☐ Will there be a mirror in the dressing area that can be seen by wheelchair users, short people, and tall people?

☐ Will dressing area be carpeted?

Design That Cares: Planning Health Facilities for Patients and Visitors, third edition, by Janet R. Carpman and Myron A. Grant. ©2016 by Jossey-Bass.

☐ Will easily accessible hooks and shelves be provided in dressing areas for storing clothing and personal items?

☐ Will dressing areas be well lit?

☐ While in dressing areas, will patients be provided with some way to communicate with staff? (Lindheim, 1971)

☐ If patients cannot securely lock their belongings in the dressing area, will a locker or bag be provided? (Reizenstein et al., 1981 [unpub.]; Reizenstein and Grant, 1981 [unpub.])

☐ If lockers are provided, will they be secure? (Reizenstein et al., 1981 [unpub.]; Reizenstein and Grant, 1981 [unpub.])

Waiting While Wearing a Hospital Gown

☐ Will separate gowned-waiting areas be provided for men and women? Will the facility provide a modest hospital gown or a robe? (Reizenstein et al., 1981 [unpub.]; Reizenstein and Grant, 1981[unpub.])

☐ Will a sufficient number of seats be available for patients and several companions in the gowned-waiting area?

Maintaining Privacy

☐ Will examination and treatment rooms be designed so patients cannot be seen by passersby when the doors are open? (Burgun, 1976)

☐ Will privacy curtains be provided in examination and treatment rooms and will staff be encouraged to use them?

☐ Will the layout of furnishings in examination and treatment rooms be designed with consideration of patients' visual and acoustical privacy?

☐ If closed-circuit television monitors are used, will they be kept out of the view of passersby? (Conway et al., 1977)

☐ Will HIPAA rules be followed to ensure patient privacy? (American Health Insurance, 1996; Dubbs, 2003)

☐ Will examination and treatment rooms provide acoustical privacy? (Conway et al., 1977)

☐ Will sound-attenuating materials be used to insulate pipes and duct work in examination and treatment rooms? (Conway et al., 1977)

☐ Will private consultation and recovery rooms be available? (Altman, 1977)

☐ When treatment such as renal dialysis is carried out in an open ward, will a private examination room also be available? (Ringoir, 1980)

Optimizing Comfort

☐ Will two comfortable chairs be available in each examination or treatment room?

☐ Will a nightlight or low lighting be provided for patients being treated in darkened rooms? (Conway et al., 1977)

☐ Will patient contact with medical equipment be minimized? (Langan et al., 1979; Zubatkin, 1980)

☐ Will the décor of the treatment room reflect a warm, comforting ambiance? (Radiation unit improves, 1980)

☐ Will artwork be selected for its calming properties?

☐ Will there be patient-controlled music within the examination room, in order to mask outside noise and promote relaxation? (Schweiger, 1991; Swartz, 1989)

☐ Will patients be informed about the nature of their examination or treatment?

☐ Will examination, treatment, and gowned-waiting areas be kept warm enough for patients wearing hospital gowns? (Altman, 1977; Ringoir, 1980)

☐ Can operating tables and mattresses be warmed? (Bourke and Sadeghi, 2003)

☐ Will lighting in procedure areas be designed so it does not shine in patients' eyes? (Langan et al., 1979)

☐ Where examination or treatment procedures are likely to be stressful, will soft, indirect lighting be provided? (Langan et al., 1979)

☐ Will patients be protected from contact with cold medical instruments and equipment?

Considering Lighting

☐ Will artificial lighting be used to closely resemble daylight?

☐ Will lighting provide proper intensity and color rendition without causing glare? (Fong, 2003; Fong and Nichelson, 2006; Souhrada, 1989)

☐ Will the reflective properties of wallcoverings, flooring, and furnishings be considered? (Brainard, 1995; Fong and Nichelson, 2006)

☐ Will a single lamp color be chosen for patient areas in order to provide consistency for medical personnel assessing skin color? (Fong, 2003; Fong and Nichelson, 2006)

☐ Will daylight be integrated with indirect artificial lighting to create a soothing effect for patients? (Fong, 2003; Fong and Nichelson, 2006)

☐ Will lighting levels be high enough to provide good visibility, but not so high as to cause glare and patient discomfort? (Fong, 2003; Fong and Nichelson, 2006)

☐ Will fixed light sources be considered, with dimming switches or switches for multiple light levels? (Fong, 2003)

☐ Will wall-mounted or ceiling-suspended indirect-light fixtures be installed to illuminate all areas of the exam room? (Fong, 2003)

☐ Will fixed or portable supplemental lighting be considered? (Fong, 2003; Fong and Nichelson, 2006)

☐ Will examination lighting fixtures provide effective lighting over a circular area no larger than 2 feet (~0.6 meters) in diameter? (Fong, 2003)

Reducing Noise

☐ Will staff be periodically reminded and encouraged to reduce ambient noise?

☐ Will patient areas provide acoustical privacy?

☐ Will noise reduction be considered in the layout of the treatment facility?

☐ Will sound-absorbing ceiling tiles be considered?

☐ Will additional steps be taken to reduce noise, including insulating rooms, installing hydraulic door closers and rubber pads on door frames, lowering the volume of phones and medical equipment, and using padded charts and chart racks? (Cmiel et al., 2004; Duffy and Florell, 1990; Grumet, 1993; Hansell, 1984; Mazer, 2005; Williams, 1989; Williams and Murphy, 1991)

Listening to Music

☐ Will patients be given the choice to listen to music during treatment and medical procedures?

☐ Will a variety of music selections be available to patients?

☐ Will cultural preferences be considered when staff develop patient playlists?

☐ Before patients are offered music, will their medical conditions be assessed to determine any potential adverse effects?

☐ Will other types of music-therapy approaches be considered beyond simply listening to music?

Design That Cares: Planning Health Facilities for Patients and Visitors, third edition, by Janet R. Carpman and Myron A. Grant. ©2016 by Jossey-Bass.

Experiencing Positive Distractions

☐ When examination or treatment procedures are likely to be lengthy, will companions be able to stay with patients? (Simple, efficient departmental design, 1977)

☐ When examination or treatment procedures are likely to be lengthy, will television, radio, music, digital devices, and current magazines be available? (Ringoir, 1980)

☐ When visual privacy is not needed, will windows allow views to the outdoors or to the hallway? (Oberlander, 1979; Radiation unit improves, 1980; Zubatkin, 1980)

☐ Will examination and treatment rooms contain artwork on the walls and/or ceilings? (Oberlander, 1979; Radiation unit improves, 1980; Zubatkin, 1980)

☐ While patients are in an examination or treatment room, will there be a way for them to communicate with staff?

☐ During lengthy procedures, will patients be able to view monitors showing the progress of their treatment? (Zubatkin, 1980)

☐ Will other sorts of positive distractions be considered, such as aromatherapy?

☐ Will virtual-reality technology be considered as a source of entertainment and positive distraction? (Bame et al., 1991; Brodeur, 2015; Collins, 2014; Gold et al., 2005; Kipping et al., 2012; Loyola University Health System, 2008; Ma et al., 2014; Perhakaran et al., 2016; Steptoe and Appels, 1989; Wright et al., 2005)

Using Digital Devices

☐ Will electrical outlets be numerous and convenient so patients and visitors can charge their digital devices? Will Wi-Fi be available?

Using Restrooms and Water Fountains

☐ Will restrooms and drinking fountains be available and conveniently located? (Altman, 1977; Burgun, 1976; Conway et al., 1977)

☐ Will restrooms and drinking fountains be located so that gowned patients do not have to enter public areas and companions do not have to enter treatment areas to use them? (Altman, 1977; Burgun, 1976; Conway et al., 1977)

Facilitating Contact between Patients and Staff

☐ Will waiting areas be under the visual supervision of staff? (Kebart, 1974)

☐ Will call buttons be visible and reachable in patient toilets, as well as in examination, treatment, and dressing rooms? (Langan et al., 1979)

Accommodating Companions

☐ Will at least one dressing area be large enough to accommodate a patient and a companion?

☐ Will chairs for companions be provided in gowned-waiting areas?

☐ Will comfortable chairs for patients and companions be provided in examination and treatment rooms?

☐ If companions are not allowed in treatment rooms, will comfortable waiting areas be provided for them?

☐ Will there be access to restrooms, drinking fountains, and vending machines for companions in waiting areas?

Design That Cares: Planning Health Facilities for Patients and Visitors, third edition, by Janet R. Carpman and Myron A. Grant. ©2016 by Jossey-Bass.

References

Altman, W. CAT scanning and patient inconvenience. *New England Journal of Medicine* 297(4):226–27, July 28, 1977.

American Health Insurance Portability and Accountability Act of 1996, 45 CFR Part 160 and Part 164: HIPAA Privacy Rule and Compliance. www.hipaa-101.com/hipaa-privacy.htm.

Bakalar, N. Sleeping through noise, but still feeling its effects. *New York Times*, March 4, 2008, p. D6.

Bame, S. I. Dialysis treatment room design. Research report. College of Architecture, Texas A & M University, College Station, 1992.

Bame, S. I., Bettenhausen, K., Eltinge, J., Hill, R., Morgan, R., Ulrich, R., et al. Aesthetic and control dimensions of health facility design: The case of hemodialysis units. *Proceedings from the Third Annual National Conference on Health Facility Planning, Design, and Construction,* 144–57. Chicago: American Hospital Association, 1991.

Barlas, D., Sama, A. E., Ward, M. F., and Lesser, M. L. Comparison of the auditory and visual privacy of Emergency Department treatment areas with curtains versus those with solid walls. *Annals of Emergency Medicine* 38(2):135–39, August 2001.

Beral, V., Evans, S., Shaw, H., and Milton, G. Malignant melanoma and exposure to fluorescent lighting at work. *Lancet* 2(8293):290–93, August 7, 1982.

Beranek, L. L., Blazier, W. E., and Figwer, J. J. Preferred noise criterion (PNC) curves and their application to rooms. *Journal of the Acoustical Society of America* 50:1223–28, 1971.

Berg, S. Impact of reduced reverberation time on sound-induced arousals during sleep. *Sleep* 24(3): 289–92, 2001.

Bourke, D. L., and Sadeghi, M. A warm bed. *Anesthesia and Analgesia* 96(4):1238, April 2003.

Brainard, G. The future is now: Implications of the effect of light on hormones, brain, and behavior. *Journal of Healthcare Design* 7:49–56, 1995.

Brodeur, M. A. Finding actual tranquility in virtual reality. *Boston Globe,* April 0, 2015. www.bostonglobe .com/arts/2015/04/04/large/bqWlhjYw5y7EyzzHPDEaWL/story.html.

Brown, S., and Theorell, T. The social uses of background music for personal enhancement. In S. Brown and U. Volgsten, editors. *Music and Manipulation: On the Social Uses and Social Control of Music,* 126–60. New York: Berghahn Books, 2005.

Burgun, J. A. Construction considerations for ambulatory care facilities. *Hospitals* 50(3):79–84, February 1, 1976.

Chaikin, A., Derlega, V., and Miller, S. Effects of room environment on self-disclosure in a counseling analogue. *Journal of Counseling Psychology* 23(5):479–81, September 1976.

Chang, S., and Chen, C. Effects of music therapy on women's physiologic measures, anxiety, and satisfaction during cesarean delivery. *Research in Nursing and Health* 28(6):453–61, December 2005.

Cmiel, C. A., Karr, D. M., Gasser, D. M., Oliphant, L. M., and Neveau, A. J. Noise control: A nursing team's approach to sleep promotion: Respecting the silence creates a healthier environment for your patients. *American Journal of Nursing* 104(2):40–48, February 2004.

Collins, S. A virtual refuge from real pain. WebMD Health News. WebMD Special Report. 2014. www .webmd.com/news/breaking-news/brain-training/20141211/pain-virtual-reality.

Colt, H., Powers, A., and Shanks, T. Effect of music on state anxiety scores in patients undergoing fiber-optic bronchoscopy. *Chest* 116(3):819–24, September 1999.

Conway, D. J., Zeisel, J., et al. Radiation therapy centers: Social and behavioral issues for design. Unpublished research report, Engineering Design Branch, National Institutes of Health, Bethesda, MD, July 1977.

Davies, D. M. Calcium metabolism in healthy men deprived of sunlight. In R. J. Wurtman, J. J. Baum, and J. T. Potts Jr., editors. *The Medical and Biological Effects of Light*, 21–27. New York: New York Academy of Sciences, 1985.

De Flora, S., Camoirano, A., Izzotti, A., and Bennicelli, C. Potent genotoxicity of halogen lamps, compared to fluorescent light and sunlight. *Carcinogenesis* 11(12):2171–77, December 1990.

Dubbs, D. Privacy please! *Health Facilities Management* 16(8):20–24, August 2003.

Dubois, J. M., Bartter, T., and Pratter, M. R. Music improves patient comfort level during outpatient bronchoscopy. *Chest* 108(1):129–30, 1995.

Duffy, T. M., and Florell, J. M. Intensive care units. In Proceedings from the Second Symposium on Health Care Interior Design. *Journal of Health Care Design* 2:167–79, 1990.

Egan, M. D. *Concepts in Architectural Acoustics.* New York: McGraw-Hill, 1972.

Elwood, J. M. Could melanoma be caused by fluorescent light? A review of relevant epidemiology. In R. P. Gallagher, editor. *Epidemiology of Malignant Melanoma.* Berlin: Springer, 1986.

Elwood, J. M., Williamson, C., and Stapleton, P. J. Malignant melanoma in relation to moles, pigmentation, and exposure to fluorescent and other lighting sources. *British Journal of Cancer* 53(1):65–74, January 1986.

English, D. R., Rouse, I. L., Xu, Z., Watt, J. D., Holman, C. D., Heenan, P. J., and Armstrong, B. K. Cutaneous malignant melanoma and fluorescent lighting. *Journal of the National Cancer Institute* 74(6):1191–97, June 1985.

Evans, D. The effectiveness of music as an intervention for hospital patients: A systematic review. *Journal of Advanced Nursing* 37(1):8, January 2002.

Fong, D. B. Illuminating thoughts: Devising lighting strategies for clinical spaces. *Health Facilities Management*, 24–29, July 2003.

Fong, D. B., and Nichelson, K. Evidence-based lighting design. *Healthcare Design* 6(5):50–53, September 2006.

Fratianne, R. B., Prensner, J. D., Huston, M. J., Super, D. M., Yowler, C. J., and Standley, J. The effect of music-based imagery and musical alternate engagement on the burn debridement process. *Journal of Burn Care and Rehabilitation* 22(1):47–53, January–February 2001.

Full-spectrum lighting: Nothing but the truth. *Buildings*, November. 2005. www.buildings.com/articles/detail.aspx?contentID=2797.

Gold, J. I., Kant, A. J., and Kim, S. H. Virtual anesthesia: The use of virtual reality for pain distraction during acute medical interventions. In *Seminars in Anesthesia, Perioperative Medicine and Pain* 24(4):203–10. Philadelphia: WB Saunders, December 2005.

Green, A. Changes in care call for design flexibility. *Hospitals* 50(3):67–69, February 1, 1976.

Griffiths, A. P., and Fairney, A. Fluorescent lights, ultraviolet lamps, and cutaneous melanoma [letter]. *British Medical Journal* 297(6649):647–50, September 10, 1988.

Grumet, G. W. Pandemonium in the modern hospital. *New England Journal of Medicine* 328(6):433–37, February 11, 1993.

Hansell, H. The behavioral effects of noise on man: The patient with "intensive care unit psychosis." *Heart and Lung* 13(1):59–65, January 1984.

Harris, M. G. PCB exposure from fluorescent lights [letter]. *American Journal of Public Health* 75(8):892, August 1985.

Haslam, P. Noise in hospitals: Its effect on the patient. *Nursing Clinics of North America* 5(4):715–24, December 1970.

Hayward, D. G., and Gates, L. B. Lighting affects the social character of a space. Working paper, Environmental Institute, University of Massachusetts, Amherst, 1981.

Hurst, T. W. Is noise important in hospital? *International Journal of Nursing Studies* 3:125–35, 1966.

Joseph, A. The impact of light on outcomes in healthcare settings. *Center for Health Design.* Issue paper No. 2, 1–12, August 2006.

Joseph, A., and Ulrich, R. Sound control for improved outcomes in healthcare settings. *Center for Health Design.* Issue paper No. 4:1–15, January 2007.

Kebart, R. C. Innovative designs for a diagnostic radiology department. *Radiologic Technology* 45(4): 260–66, January–February 1974.

Keenan, L., and Goldman, E. Positive imaging: Design as marketing tool in diagnosis centers. *Administrative Radiology* 8(2):36–41, February 1989.

Kemper, K. J., and Danhauer, S. C. Music as therapy. *Southern Medical Journal* 98(3):282–88, March 2005.

Kipping, B., Rodger, S., Miller, K., and Kimble, R. M. Virtual reality for acute pain reduction in adolescents undergoing burn wound care: A prospective randomized controlled trial. *Burns* 38(5):650–57, 2012.

Langan, J., Wagner, H., and Buchanan, J. Design concepts of a nuclear medicine department. *Journal of Nuclear Medicine* 20(10):1093–94, October 1979.

Lindheim, R. *Uncoupling the Radiology System.* Chicago: Hospital Research and Educational Trust, 1971.

Loyola University Health System. Virtual-reality video game to help burn patients play their way to pain relief. *ScienceDaily.* March 22, 2008. www.sciencedaily.com/releases/2008/03/080319152744.htm.

Ma, M., Jain, L. C., and Anderson, P., eds. *Virtual, Augmented Reality and Serious Games for Healthcare 1,* Vol. 1. Berlin: Springer, 2014.

Malcolm, H. A. Does privacy matter? Former patients discuss their perceptions of privacy in shared hospital rooms. *International Journal for Healthcare Professionals* 12(2):156–66, March 2001.

Maxwell, K. J., and Elwood, J. M. Could melanoma be caused by fluorescent light? A review of relevant physics. In R. P. Gallagher, editor. *Epidemiology of Malignant Melanoma*, 137–43. Berlin: Springer, 1986.

Mayron, L. Hyperactivity from fluorescent lighting—fact or fancy: A commentary on the report by O'Leary, Rosenbaum, and Hughes. *Journal of Abnormal Child Psychology* 6(3):291–94, September 1978.

Mayron, L. W., Ott, J., Nations, R., and Mayron, E. L. Light, radiation and academic behavior. *Academic Therapy* 10(1):33–47, Fall 1974.

Mazer, S. E. Speech privacy: Beyond architectural solutions. Paper presented at Noise Conference. Minneapolis, MN, October 17–19, 2005.

Mok, E., and Wong, K. Effects of music on patient anxiety. *Association of Perioperative Registered Nurses Journal* 77(2):401–4, 406, 409–10, February 2003.

Oberlander, R. Beauty in a hospital aids the cure. *Hospitals* 53(6):74–75, March 16, 1979.

Olsen, J. C., and Sabin, B. R. Emergency Department patient perceptions of privacy and confidentiality. *Journal of Emergency Medicine* 25(3):329–33, October 2003.

Ott, J. N. Color and light: Their effects on plants, animals and people. *International Journal of Biosocial Research* 7(special issue):1–33, 1985.

Ott, J. N. *Heat and Light.* Old Greenwich, CT: Devin-Adair, 1973.

Palakanis, K. C., DeNobile, J. W., Sweeney, W. B., and Blankenship, C. L. Effect of music therapy on state anxiety in patients undergoing flexible sigmoidoscopy. *Diseases of the Colon and Rectum* 37(5): 478–81, May 1994.

Pasternack, B. S., Dubin, N., and Moseson, M. Malignant melanoma and exposure to fluorescent lighting at work [letter]. *Lancet* 1(8326, pt. 1):704, March 26, 1983.

Perhakaran, G., Yusof, A. M., Rusli, M. E., Yusoff, M.Z.M., Mahalil, I., and Zainuddin, A.R.R. A study of meditation effectiveness for virtual reality based stress therapy using EEG measurement and questionnaire approaches. In *Innovation in Medicine and Healthcare 2015*, 365–73. New York: Springer Nature, 2016.

Prensner, J. D., Yowler, C. J., Smith, L. F., Steele, A. L., and Fratianne, R. B. Music therapy for assistance with pain and anxiety management in burn treatment. *Journal of Burn Care Rehabilitation* 22(1): 83–88, January–February 2001.

Radiation unit improves patient access and comfort. *Hospitals* 53(18):57–58, September 16, 1980.

Reizenstein, J. E., and Grant, M. A. Patient activities and schematic design preferences. Unpublished research report No. 2, Patient and Visitor Participation Project, Office of Hospital Planning, Research and Development, University of Michigan, Ann Arbor, 1981a.

_____. Patient and visitor issues: Currently unmet needs and suggested solutions. Unpublished report No. 4a, Patient and Visitor Participation Project, Office of Hospital Planning, Research and Development, University of Michigan, Ann Arbor, 1981b.

Reizenstein, J. E., Grant, M. A., and Vaitkus, M. A. Visitor activities and schematic design preferences. Unpublished research report No. 4, Patient and Visitor Participation Project, Office of Hospital Planning, Research and Development, University of Michigan, Ann Arbor, 1981.

Ringoir, S. Design and function of a hospital artificial kidney centre. *International Journal of Artificial Organs* 3(3):134–35, May 1980.

Rueter, L. Providing room to care. *Hospitals* 48(4):62–65, February 16, 1974.

Sandberg, D. Ceiling art in the surgical holding area: A twofold treasure [letter]. *Perioperative Nursing Quarterly* 3(1):53–54, 1987.

Schweiger, A. B. The healing sound of music. *Ann Arbor News*, December 16, 1991, p. D1.

Simple, efficient departmental design suits function, growth of nuclear medicine. *Hospitals* 51(10): 30–32, May 16, 1977.

Souhrada, L. Lighting decisions affect image, morale, efficiency. *Health Facilities Management* 2(5): 19–27, May 1989.

Sound Research Laboratories Limited. *Practical Building Acoustics,* pp. 38–39, 125–26, 165–66. Suffolk, UK: SRL, 1976.

Steptoe, A., and Appels, A., eds. *Stress, Personal Control, and Health.* Chichester, UK: John Wiley, 1989.

Storlie, F. J. Does urban noise represent a hazard to health? Dissertation submitted to Portland State University, Portland, OR, 1976. [Available from ProQuest, 789 E. Eisenhower Parkway, Ann Arbor, MI 48108.]

Swartz, J. The doctor's office: Poor design may cost you patients. *Canadian Medical Association Journal* 140:320–21, February 1989.

Tavris, D. R., Field, L., and Brumback, C. L. Outbreak of illness due to volatilized asphalt coming from a malfunctioning fluorescent lighting fixture. *American Journal of Public Health* 74(6):614–15, June 1984.

Thorington, L. Spectral, irradiance, and temporal aspects of natural and artificial light. In R. J. Wurtman, J. J. Baum, and J. T. Potts Jr., editors. *The Medical and Biological Effects of Light,* 29–54. New York: New York Academy of Sciences, 1985. [Published as vol. 453 of *Annals of the New York Academy of Sciences.*]

Walter, S. D., Marrett, L. D., Shannon, H. S., From, L., and Hertzman, C. The association of cutaneous malignant melanoma and fluorescent light exposure. *American Journal of Epidemiology* 135(7): 749–62, April 1, 1992.

Wilkins, A. J., and Wilkinson, P. A tint to reduce eye-strain from fluorescent lighting? Preliminary observations. *Ophthalmic and Physiological Optics* 11(2):172–75, April 1991.

Williams, M., and Murphy, J. Noise in critical care units: A quality assurance approach. *Journal of Nursing Care Quality* 6(1):53–59, 1991.

Williams, M. A. Physical environment of the intensive care unit and elderly patients. *Critical Care Nursing Quarterly* 12(1):52–60, 1989.

Wright, J. L., Hoffman, H. G., and Sweet, R. M. Virtual reality as an adjunctive pain control during transurethral microwave thermotherapy. *Urology* 66(6):1320-e1, 2005.

Zilm, F., Brimhall, D., and Ryan, D. Ambulatory care survey paves way to the future. *Hospitals* 52(11): 79–83, June 1, 1978.

Zubatkin, A. Psychological impact of medical equipment on patients. *Journal of Clinical Engineering* 5(3):250–55, July–September 1980.

CHAPTER 7

INPATIENT ROOMS AND BATHS

At home, at work, and in the community, people enjoy a variety of settings during the course of a day. But hospital inpatients spend the majority of their time in one room. It becomes their bedroom, living room, dining room, and physician's office. This chapter discusses how acute care inpatient rooms can be designed to meet the needs of patients and visitors for control over social contact, physical comfort, and ease of communication among themselves and with healthcare staff. (See also chapter 9.)

This chapter also covers the inpatient bathroom, a space that needs to be designed with special care because patients may be weak from surgery or medications and may have difficulty using conventional bathroom facilities. We discuss safety features, accessibility, ease of use, and space for staff to assist patients. The chapter also looks at inpatient and family lounges, which offer patients and visitors a change of scene and places where small groups can gather. Finally, we consider intensive care units (ICUs) and some design features that can make these typically intimidating, high-tech environments more humane, such as providing for patient privacy, reducing emotional stress and sensory overload, attending to patients' preferences regarding lighting and temperature, and providing for family members' needs.

LEARNING OBJECTIVES
- Become familiar with ways in which the design of acute care inpatient rooms and bathrooms can accommodate patients' needs.
- Understand the purpose and design features of patient lounges.
- Know how design can help accommodate family and visitors in and around inpatient rooms.
- Become aware of design features that can make intensive care units less intimidating and more humane for patients and visitors.

Acute Care Inpatient Rooms

Size and Layout

The optimal size of private or semiprivate acute care patient rooms is frequently debated by medical and nursing staff, hospital planners, and designers. In addition, room size is often subject to federal and/or state regulations.

Government regulations are usually framed only in minimum square footages. As a result, planners may think these regulations need to be supplemented by performance criteria based on the requirements of patients, visitors, and staff, and by a systematic process for projecting space needs (Hayward et al., 1985).

Unfortunately, as with so many hospital design features, there has been little systematic analysis of how rooms of different sizes function in different hospitals. As Research Box 7.1 shows, the hospital planning team at the University of Michigan Medical Center looked into the question of patient room size by evaluating full-scale mock-up rooms.

Acuity-Adaptable Patient Rooms

A number of hospitals have explored universal or acuity-adaptable room design (Chaudhury, Mahmood, and Valente, 2005; Gallant and Lanning, 2001; Joseph, 2006b;

RESEARCH BOX 7.1 USING FULL-SCALE MOCK-UPS AS A DESIGN TOOL

Designing an optimally-sized patient room and bath has implications for patient health and facility costs. A patient's life may depend on the ability of staff to perform emergency procedures in these spaces. Patient room designs may be repeated hundreds of times in a given healthcare facility.

Because there can be a significant difference between the amount of space estimated to accommodate equipment and procedures and the actual amount needed, it may be cost-effective to construct full-scale mock-ups, simulate and test a range of room-use scenarios with hospital staff and standardized patients (people trained to portray patients in healthcare simulations), analyze the results, and modify the design accordingly. Researchers and designers at the University of Michigan Medical Center did just that (King, Marans, and Solomon, 1982).

Full-scale mock-ups of a private room and bath, a semiprivate room and bath, and an ICU room were constructed in order to evaluate each room's design under a variety of common healthcare delivery situations. Twenty-seven scenarios (such as moving a patient from the bed; using the sink, toilet, and shower; and providing emergency treatment) were simulated.

Given the initial design of these spaces, the researchers found that, on the whole, the rooms were too small and that fixed equipment and furniture were inefficiently placed. Analyses of the scenarios showed a variety of problems, including difficulty encountered when maneuvering a stretcher around a staff sink, too little room for staff performing emergency procedures at the head and foot of the patient bed, and the need to move room furniture, including the other patient's bed, when transferring a patient to and from bed. Problems were also found pertaining to patients' and visitors' needs. Room designs were modified in accordance with these findings.

Kwan, 2011; Scalise et al., 2004; Spear, 1997). These single-patient rooms are designed to accommodate patients needing care involving varying levels of acuity during their hospital stay, so they don't need to be transferred to different rooms. One study of a cardiac unit with an acuity-adaptable room design reported a 90 percent decrease in patient transfers, 70 percent fewer medication errors, a 75 percent decrease in patient falls (because of better staff observation), and an increase in patient satisfaction compared to previously designed units; some other hospitals experienced similar benefits (Maze, 2009; Scalise et al., 2004).

Such outcomes, however, have proved difficult to sustain (Kwan, 2011). In addition, not all staff members are attracted to the acuity-adaptable room model, since it eliminates specialized nursing roles (such as acute care versus critical care nurses) to which they are accustomed, and tends to increase rounding times, since patients are not "cohorted" together (Gallant and Lanning, 2001; Maze, 2009; Scalise et al., 2004). Acuity-adaptable rooms also need to be larger than traditional patient rooms, typically in the range of 280–300 net square feet (~26–28 net square meters), with a longer headwall and more clearance to provide sufficient clinical space for special equipment and procedures (Cahnman, 2010; Gallant and Lanning, 2001).

Nevertheless, healthcare facilities still seek ways to bridge acuity levels and eliminate patient transfers (Cahnman, 2010). Variations on the original concept continue to emerge under such names as *flex-up, flex-down, universal room*, and *single-stay unit* (Kwan, 2011).

Other considerations for inpatient rooms are related to room organization. There is a trend toward designing identical, "same-handed" rooms rather than traditional "mirror-image" ones with a shared headwall between every two rooms. Same-handed design can reduce noise transmission between patient rooms (Patient room design, 2011). When patient headwalls are placed back to back, the holes in the headwalls that accommodate electrical and gas lines, switches, and other equipment allow noise to pass from one room to the other. Proponents also argue that a same-handed layout permits total standardization and, by lessening the cognitive burden on caregivers, leads to greater efficiency and patient safety. Little empirical research has been carried out, however, and results remain inconclusive (Patient room design, 2011; Stouffer, 2010).

Space for Families and Visitors

Dedicated space in the patient room for family and visitors has become a standard feature of healthcare-facility design; families and friends are now recognized as allies for the quality and safety of patient care. (See Research Box 7.2.) Evidence-based design supports organizing the patient room layout in three zones: staff, patient, and family, with the family zone usually placed farthest from the room door (Bunker-Hellmich, 2010; Cahnman, 2010; Changing the Concept, 2014; Patient Rooms, 2014; Taylor, 2009).

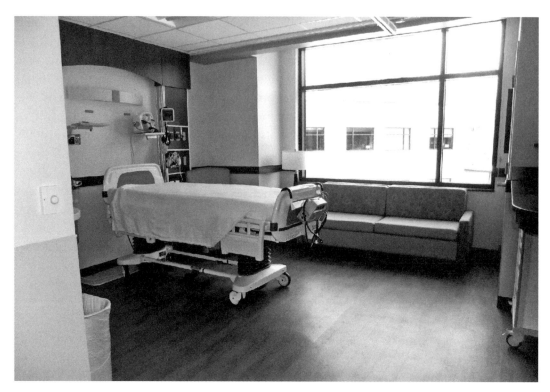

This inpatient room features an outdoor view, a convertible couch for visitors, and a shelf for personal items.

Photo credit: Courtesy of St. Joseph Mercy Chelsea

RESEARCH BOX 7.2   DOES PROGRESSIVE CARE MAKE A DIFFERENCE?

In order to improve the quality of care, some researchers and medical facilities have proposed transforming the traditional, institutional-style hospital atmosphere of inpatient units into a more homelike "progressive care" environment.

The goal of such self-care or progressive care units is to make the hospital setting less alienating for short-term and ambulatory patients. One proposed way of accomplishing this is to provide patients more options for socializing, and another is to improve the quality of basic amenities such as food service, lounges, and dining rooms. Progressive care encourages self-care, independence in decision-making, and greater control by patients over their social and physical environments. Proponents of progressive care believe that convalescing patients recover more quickly and stay in better spirits when they are in a less institutional setting, separated from very ill patients.

One researcher compared the effectiveness of a progressive care unit with a traditional one at a large Catholic hospital in the eastern United States (Olsen, 1984). The progressive care unit was designed to provide both day-bed service for patients in need of medical observation or stabilization and hospital-bed service for surgical and cardiac patients. This study compared 30 similar, non-cardiac, surgical patients in each of two units, irrespective of length of stay.

The layout of the progressive care unit was a "racetrack-shaped" corridor, with all rooms—six triples, a double, and a single—having their own baths and furniture typical of hospital rooms. The halls were decorated and well lit, as were the patient lounge and dining room, which were located on opposite ends of the wing. The dining area contained four imitation-butcher-block tables with kitchen chairs, and a pantry with a well-stocked refrigerator was located nearby. These facilities were available for use by ambulatory patients who had their physicians' permission to eat regular meals.

The traditional care unit had a capacity of eighteen, with four doubles and ten single rooms. The units had identical exposures, but the traditional unit lacked a formal lounge, dining room, pantry, or day-bed section. The author describes its layout as T-shaped and its ambience as dreary.

In order to understand patients' experiences and behaviors in the two units, the researcher interviewed them on the unit and mailed each a questionnaire after discharge. In addition, patient behavior was mapped on the basis of observations made every fifteen minutes for six hours in the afternoons and evenings. Patients were matched by diagnosis between the two units.

The author reports that relative to patients on the traditional unit, the progressive care patients rated their environment as significantly more pleasant and cheerful. Overall, these patients felt less confined and considered their unit as less institutional and more stimulating. These findings stayed stable despite the unexpected conversion during the study of three rooms in the hospital unit to cardiac care.

At the same time, there was no difference between the two units in how depressed or upset patients felt at being exposed to sicker patients. Contrary to the researcher's expectations, patients rated nursing care similarly on both units, thus eliminating it as a confounding factor.

In terms of behavior, although the progressive care surgical patients were an average of ten years older than those in the traditional unit (56.6 years old, as compared to 46.4), they moved around and socialized more and exhibited less passivity. Progressive care day-bed patients also socialized more than traditional care patients and spent more time out of their rooms. In all, progressive care surgical patients said they felt more as if they were in a friendly hotel than in a hospital.

According to the Centers for Disease Control and Prevention, one of every 20 patients admitted to a hospital acquires an infection there (The Hospital Room of the Future, 2013). Since infection is spread more frequently by contact than by airborne transmission, it is now evidence-based practice and a frequent code requirement to provide a visible handwashing sink at the entrance of each patient room (Cahnman, 2010; Facility Guidelines Institute, 2014).

The sink should be easily accessible by both staff and visitors and placed far enough from the patient bed to eliminate the danger of splash contact. Motion detectors and electronic timers can encourage compliance and proper use. Locating the sink strategically within the patient's line of sight enables patients to play a role in monitoring staff handwashing, thus reinforcing both hygienic procedures and a sense of empowerment (Cullinan and Wolf, 2010).

Locating the Patient Bathroom

A key consideration for room layout is placement of the patient bathroom: on the hallway wall ("inboard"), on the window wall ("outboard"), or on a wall between patient rooms ("midboard" or "nested") (Maze, 2009; Scalise et al., 2004). An inboard location has several advantages: it results in the largest family zone, more window area and thus more daylight, greater visual privacy from the corridor, and more insulation from corridor noise. An inboard bath has several disadvantages, including a smaller staff area, making it difficult to fit in the handwashing sink, digital device for charting, and workspace. An inboard bath also makes it difficult to fit in the pass-through patient server for supplies and medications that is a key component in infection control (Horwitz-Bennett, 2014). Researchers note that the growing complexity and equipment needs of the staff zone may result in pushing the patient bed into the family zone (Bunker-Hellmich, 2010). The vestibule area can be a "pinch point" for maneuvering the bed in and out of the room; and the room door and bathroom door can interfere with each other (McCullough, 2010). Most problematic is that an inboard bath layout limits staff's ability to observe patients from the corridor and makes it difficult to monitor patients from decentralized caregiver stations, although some experts maintain that patient checks should be made at bedside, not from the corridor (Maze, 2009). Some of these disadvantages can be mitigated by placing the bathroom on the footwall side of the room, by designing the room door with glazing, and by pulling back a corner of the bathroom to improve sight lines (Maze, 2009).

An outboard patient bathroom allows maximum patient visibility from the corridor or nurses' station, allows for a larger staff zone, and is better suited for patient transfer (Horwitz-Bennett, 2014). Although this layout restricts the size of the family zone, the zone is a more clearly defined nook, and patients and caregivers have an unobstructed travel path (Horwitz-Bennett, 2014).

A nested configuration, with the patient bathrooms of two adjacent rooms placed on the shared interior wall, provides larger family space, good views to the outdoors, and good patient visibility (Maze, 2009). This layout, however, makes a same-handed design impossible. Also, by contributing to the length of the building, it increases staff travel distances.

A further design consideration for the placement of the inpatient bathroom is whether to locate it on the headwall or the footwall of the patient room. A footwall location offers the most flexibility, allowing maximum headwall space, good patient views to the outside, and a visually clear path to the bathroom, as well as unobstructed room for a bassinet or visitor chair on the outboard side of the patient bed (Horwitz-Bennett, 2014). It also provides for better staff visibility of the patient from the corridor or nurses' station.

A headwall placement of the inpatient bath results in a shorter path between the patient bed and the bathroom and allows for a handrail for patient support along the headwall. Studies have found that most patient falls take place on the way to the bathroom (Horwitz-Bennett, 2014). Systematic research is needed to determine whether a shorter path and a handrail reduce patient falls, because these may also encourage patients to attempt the trip without needed assistance (Bunker-Hellmich, 2010; McCullough, 2010).

Some research has shown that the location of the bathroom is less important than having a well-lit, clear path and nonslip floors (McCullough, 2010). One response to the problem of patient falls is to install a ceiling-mounted lift system between the bed and the toilet to assist in moving and turning patients and mitigate the risk of injury to patients and staff (Bunker-Hellmich, 2010).

Unfortunately, no single patient room configuration is optimal for all patient and staff needs. Suitable room configuration must always take into account the specific context (Pati et al., 2009).

Guidelines for Patient Room Size and Layout

Facilities are likely to have differing requirements for patient room size. A hospital may have been built many years ago and remain constrained by the original construction. Others may be limited by cost or building codes, and still others may feel the need to provide more than the average amount of space. In acknowledging this variety of needs and approaches, we offer a few performance criteria for room size and layout, rather than recommending specific dimensions. Facilities can follow the criteria that best suit their needs and develop a workable room size through a participatory design process (Hayward et al., 1985). (See chapter 11.)

To determine optimum size and layout of acute care rooms that satisfy the needs of patients and visitors:

- Consider using full-scale mock-ups to systematically analyze proposed designs for acute care and ICU patient rooms.

- Consider the design requirements of particular patient units when deciding among room layouts for inboard, outboard, or nested bathrooms, and headwall or footwall placement (Pati et al., 2009).

- Consider placing the doorway in line with the foot of the bed, rather than in line with the head of the bed.

- Provide ample circulation space so medical emergency teams and equipment can easily gain access to the patient.

- Size, arrange, and furnish rooms to maximize patient mobility, rehabilitation, weight-bearing exercise, and ambulation potential (Facility Guidelines Institute, 2014).

- Provide an easily accessible handwashing sink at the entrance to each patient room (Cahnman, 2010; Facility Guidelines Institute, 2014).

- Provide space for a wardrobe, bedside stand, overbed table, and patient chair, in addition to the bed.

- Provide a family zone with at least one visitor chair.

- Provide circulation area around the beds so visitors can place their chairs on either side of the patient's bed.

- Provide a well-lit, clear path between the patient bed and the bathroom (McCullough, 2010).

- Consider installing a ceiling-mounted lift system between the bed and bathroom.

- Provide space and an unobstructed circulation area to ensure access for wheelchairs, rolling IV poles, and walkers.

- Provide space in private rooms to accommodate cots or beds for overnight visitors. (See chapter 10.)

Number of Occupants

No longer are the multiple-bed, open wards inspired by Florence Nightingale the norm for patients in US hospitals. Today, patients want more privacy and noise control. Many hospitals provide only private rooms. Others provide both private and semiprivate rooms in addition to small suites of three or four patient beds.

As a result of research on the health effects of single- versus multiple-occupancy rooms, guidelines on hospital design now recommend single-patient rooms for all new hospital construction and remodeling (Facility Guidelines Institute, 2014). Research studies reveal a number of advantages of single-patient rooms (Chaudhury et al., 2005; Detsky and Etchells, 2008). The spread of infections has been shown to be lower in single-patient rooms (Ben-Abraham et al., 2002; Chaudhury et al., 2005; Detsky and Etchells, 2008; Ulrich et al., 2004; Van Enk, 2006; Zimring et al., 2006). Single-patient rooms have also been associated with decreases in patient transfers, lengths of stay, noise levels, and sleep disturbances (Chaudhury et al., 2005; Detsky and Etchells, 2008). Patient satisfaction and privacy are greater in single-patient rooms (Chaudhury et al., 2005; Detsky and Etchells, 2008; Janssen et al., 2000).

Despite the increasing use of private rooms, not all patients expect or desire the privacy these rooms offer. Several studies show that some patients prefer multi-patient rooms over single-patient rooms (Chaudhury et al., 2005; Detsky and Etchells, 2008; Jolley, 2005; Miller et al., 1998; Pease, 2002). One study found that if cost were no object, 45 percent would choose a private room, 48 percent would choose a semi-private room, and 7 percent would prefer a multiple-bed room (Reizenstein and Grant, 1981 [unpub. No. 2]). The fact that approximately half the patients in this study said they would choose a semi-private room, even if cost were no object, may surprise some designers and planners, because privacy seems to be such a rare and desirable commodity in hospitals. However, it seems many people are willing to trade privacy for company. Many patients enjoy having someone close by to talk with during their hospital stays.

In addition, some patients fear what would happen if they had a medical emergency. They feel more secure knowing there is someone nearby who could call for help, rather than feeling dependent on a call button or the chance a nurse might happen by when needed. For example, in two surveys conducted by Austrian student nurses, about 40 percent of respondents expressed fear of not being able to receive help at the right moment. Those expressing such fears were older and disproportionately female. Not surprisingly, the desire for privacy was inversely associated with the severity of illness: nearly two-thirds said they would want a single room after a tonsillectomy, but only 38.5 percent would want a single room after a stroke (Spork, 1990).

For patients hospitalized for extended periods of time, such as rehabilitation patients, multiple-bed suites may provide valuable social contact. One creative response to this issue is the so-called "super suite," consisting of a semi-private room with two bathrooms, one per patient, and a pocket wall that can be opened or closed depending on privacy needs (It's the Right Thing to Do, 2014).

Control Over Social Contact

The relationship of various elements within the patient room (the bed, views from the window, the doorway, and the bathroom) affects the patient's ability to control social contact, including visual and acoustical privacy and interactions with other patients, visitors, and staff. In determining the optimal arrangements of elements, it is important to consider patients' preferences because these may differ from the preferences of healthcare staff.

Visual Privacy

One area of potential conflict between patient and staff preferences is the ease with which patients can see into and be seen from the hallway. Although patients may like having a view into the hallway, they do not necessarily want people looking in on them. For patients, a door or interior window (between the room and the hallway) can provide a visual link between their rather confined rooms and the busy corridor.

While looking out, they may feel more a part of the rest of the hospital and enjoy the opportunity to people-watch, provided that they can manipulate the interior window covering. If curtains are used for this purpose, they should be made of specially treated fabric to mitigate the problem of transmitting infection (Cahnman, 2010). One privacy option uses electrically charged glass that can be made opaque at the flick of a switch (Reiling, Hughes, and Murphy, 2008). A further advantage is that e-glass, like integral blinds, reduces the cleanable surface of these windows (Cahnman, 2010). For staff, the door and interior window can provide easy visual monitoring of the patient.

The same concern applies to exterior windows. Patient room windows on the ground floor with views to gardens and other public spaces can compromise patient privacy if certain precautions are not taken. Designers should consider tinted windows or private porch areas

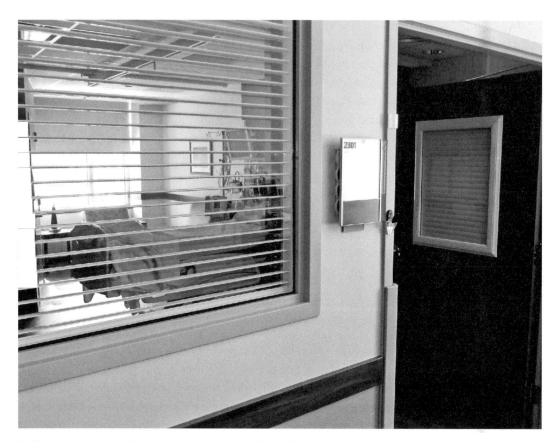

The blinds in this patient room interior window are manipulated from inside, allowing patients and visitors to control views in both directions.

Photo credit: Courtesy of St. Joseph Mercy Chelsea

outside these patient rooms to preserve patient privacy and prevent people outside from look-ing into patient rooms (Sherman et al., 2005).

While patients' desires for visual privacy are understandable, the primary concern of a healthcare facility must be patient health and safety. Arguments can be made for designing all nursing units, not merely the ICU, for maximum patient visibility, with outboard bathrooms and glass interior walls and with privacy provisions, such as blinds or curtains deployable at the discretion of clinical staff (Hardy, 2006). Some rooms have even been designed with the headwall canted toward the corridor for better patient visibility (Cullinan and Wolf, 2010). In these, as in all other design decisions, the clinical context must be considered and solutions arrived at in consultation with healthcare-facility staff.

Patients have expressed their opinions about the arrangements of beds within a semi-private room. Whether beds are placed next to each other (side by side) or facing each other (toe to toe), issues of choice and territory arise. In one study, patients preferred the side-by-side arrangement and did not like the idea of patients facing each other. Some patients said that

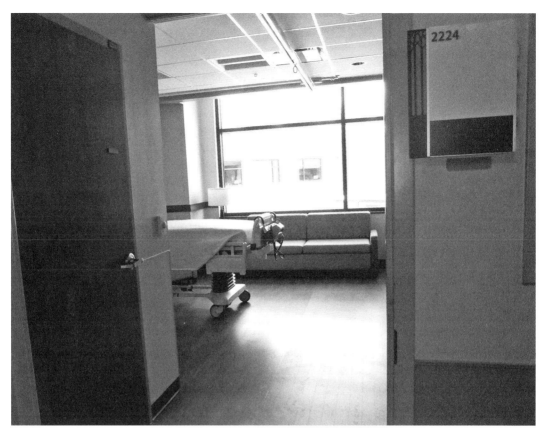

The layout of this room, with the toilet on the left, means that the patient's head cannot be seen from the doorway. This protects patient privacy, but the tradeoff is that staff will need to step into the room in order to observe.

Photo credit: Courtesy of St. Joseph Mercy Chelsea

they would not want someone "staring" at them all the time. Others pointed out that one patient's light might shine in the other's eyes (Reizenstein and Grant, 1981 [unpub. No. 1]). However, they also recognized a major disadvantage of the side-by-side arrangement: one patient would tend to claim the window as his or her territory, and the other patient would tend to claim the door area (Reizenstein and Grant, 1981 [unpub. No. 1]). The toe-to-toe arrangement provides more equitable territories.

Some approaches to the design of semi-private patient rooms combine the best features of side-by-side and toe-to-toe arrangements in trapezoid- or diamond-shaped rooms, where beds are positioned at 90 degrees to one another. In these designs, both patients have equal access to the door and window (Barker, 1985; Prototype hospital room, 1985).

Privacy curtains, used by almost all patients during the course of their hospitalizations, also reflect concern about unwanted exposure. As one study found, cubicle curtains are pulled for a variety of reasons, including blocking out light and shielding patients from view when using a bedpan, being examined or treated, dressing or undressing, sleeping, receiving a bed bath, or talking with visitors (Reizenstein and Grant, 1981 [unpub. No. 23]). Although few patients in this study thought cubicle curtains provided much visual or acoustical privacy, being able to manipulate the curtains was very important to them.

One way of returning some degree of control to hospitalized patients, who otherwise relinquish much of their usual autonomy, is to enable them to regulate visual access to and from their beds. A cubicle curtain is one way to provide this control, but many non-ambulatory patients (such as rehabilitation patients and orthopedic patients in traction) have to depend on hospital staff to open and close the curtain. A motorized curtain with a remote can allow non-ambulatory patients to control their visual privacy without leaving the bed. Motorized curtains can also be operated by staff. Although motorized curtains tend to be costly, some require little maintenance.

In designing an inpatient room to maximize patient control over visual privacy, consider these guidelines:

- If windows are located between patient rooms and hallways, ensure that patients have bedside remotes that control the interior blinds or shades (Reizenstein and Grant, 1981 [unpub. No. 1]).

- For ground-level rooms with views to a courtyard or other exterior space, consider providing tinted exterior windows or private porch areas outside patient rooms in order to prevent outsiders from seeing into patient rooms (Reizenstein and Grant, 1981 [unpub. No. 1]; Sherman et al., 2005).

- In a side-by-side, semi-private room, be attentive to patient complaints regarding the limited outside view for the bed closer to the hallway (Reizenstein and Grant, 1981 [unpub. No. 1]).

- In a toe-to-toe semi-private room, enable patients to control their views of each other, and make sure that the bed light of one patient does not shine in the eyes of the other (Reizenstein and Grant, 1981 [unpub. No. 1]).

- Consider providing motorized cubicle curtains with remote controls, in areas other than ICUs where patients are most likely to be non-ambulatory and hospitalized for extended periods of time (Reizenstein and Grant, 1981 [unpub. No. 1]).

In addition to considerations for room layout, it is important to protect the privacy of a patient's medical information. Medical charts and digital displays in nurses' stations and on mobile charting carts should be positioned so passersby cannot view them (Dubbs, 2003). Screensavers or programs that time-out quickly can be installed on digital devices to prevent others from viewing private medical information (Dubbs, 2003).

Acoustical Privacy

Acoustical privacy—the ability of a patient and family to talk together without being overheard or without having to listen to other conversations—is often at a premium in patient rooms. Acoustical privacy is naturally more difficult to achieve in semi-private rooms or suites than in private rooms. Although patients and visitors can attempt to keep their voices low or discuss private matters only when the other patient is out of the room, a lack of acoustical privacy can be stressful. It is often difficult for patients and visitors to choose another setting for private conversations within a healthcare facility, because lobbies, lounges, waiting areas, and cafeterias are likely to be crowded. Fear of being overheard has even led some patients to withhold personal information or history from health practitioners (Barlas et al., 2001; Malcolm, 2005).

Sound travels between a patient's room and surrounding spaces, including other patient rooms, hallways, and waiting areas. Consequently, private information may be inadvertently overheard. Sound-attenuating materials between patient rooms (such as wall insulation) and within rooms (such as carpeting and other sound-absorbing surfaces) can help alleviate this problem. Patients can also be asked to keep their doors closed when privacy is at issue and staff can be asked to avoid conversations directly outside patient rooms.

Consider these design guidelines for achieving acoustical privacy within patient rooms:

- Consider providing walls instead of curtains between patients in semi-private rooms in order to promote acoustical privacy (Barlas et al., 2001; Malcolm, 2005; Olsen and Sabin, 2003).

- If care staff need visual access to patients, consider transparent sound barriers as a substitute for walls in order to provide acoustical privacy (Mazer, 2005).

- Use sound-attenuating materials in patient room walls (Leibrock, 1990).

- Consider the use of fire-retardant, easily washable wall fabric to muffle sounds and protect walls from wheelchair abrasion (Hiatt, 1991; Leibrock, 1990).

- Provide a private room or setting where patients, visitors, and practitioners can hold confidential conversations (Dubbs, 2003; Malcolm, 2005).

- Locate only quiet functions near patient rooms.

- Acoustically contain nurse and physician work areas on patient floors.

Color

Color is a useful design device for making inpatient rooms feel less institutional and more homelike, and has been frequently discussed in the hospital design literature. Beliefs about color effects tend to spread quickly, despite a lack of grounding in empirical evidence. Although many authors agree that "hospital white" and "hospital green" should be avoided, arguments have been made for both the use of "cool" colors (green and blue) and "warm" colors (red, pink, coral, and orange) with little apparent agreement or solid research to support either position (Birren, 1979; Chaney, 1973; Edwards, 1979; Rabin, 1981). Several researchers have conducted studies to explore how color is used in the hospital environment and how it affects patients. (See Research Boxes 7.3 and 7.4.)

RESEARCH BOX 7.3 DO PATIENT ROOM WALL COLORS AFFECT RECOVERY?

Some colors have been said to have healing properties (Edge, 2003; Marberry and Zagon, 1995; Moore, 2000). For instance, the color orange has been called a universal healer (Edge, 2003). In 2003, a researcher at the University of Florida studied whether color has positive effects on healing and whether some colors are more effective than others in promoting healing.

The pilot study involved 39 cardiac patients, including 10 surgery patients and 29 patients under observation. Ages ranged from 26 to 89. The patients were randomly assigned to double-occupancy rooms that varied in the color of the wall at the foot of the patient's bed. The wall colors were beige, mid-tone purple, green, or orange. On the last day of their hospital stay, the patients' anxiety levels, lengths of stay, and medication requests were measured.

Findings suggest that color did not have an effect on patient recovery. There were no significant relationships between wall color and anxiety level, length of stay, or pain medication requests. The researcher reported that the lack of statistically significant effects could be due to small sample size.

Interviews with patients and staff indicated that most participants believed color should be incorporated into patient rooms in hospitals. Certain patients who appeared to be from a lower socioeconomic background than the other participants, however, said they felt comfortable being in the beige room because the color helped reinforce the feeling of being in a hospital receiving medical care (Edge, 2003).

RESEARCH BOX 7.4 WHAT IS THE EVIDENCE REGARDING EFFECTS OF COLOR ON HUMAN BEHAVIOR?

One group of researchers conducted a review of the literature on color in healthcare in an attempt to determine which color effects on human health and behavior, if any, are evidence-based (Tofle et al., 2004; Young, 2007). They reviewed more than 3,000 references related to theories of color and focused on those applicable to healthcare settings. The study concluded that many claims regarding human responses to color lack solid empirical evidence. There is too little evidence to suggest that specific colors *cause* certain healthcare outcomes or behaviors. In addition, although some studies show a correlation between color and mood, there is no evidence that specific colors are linked to or cause any particular emotion. In terms of people's perceptions of space (for example, spaciousness or confinement), studies suggest that the brightness or darkness (value) of a color, rather than a specific hue, and the level of contrast between objects and their background make a difference in mood or emotion. It is generally agreed that spaciousness can be enhanced with lighter walls and lower contrast (Tofle et al., 2004).

The literature review compared design guidelines for color in healthcare settings across eight sources and found many contradictions, particularly related to specific colors. Claims regarding the healing powers of certain colors were unsubstantiated and seemed to reflect the designers' individual beliefs. In several cases, the same color was recommended by some authors and discouraged by others. For example, some designers noted that yellow can promote optimism and improve mood, while others said yellow can be unsettling and can create sickly-looking skin tones (Tofle et al., 2004). Some said deeper colors offer stability, while others claimed dark colors can contribute to depression. Finally, some designers encouraged the use of a full spectrum of color to enliven the space rather than restricting colors to beige, white, and gray (Malkin, 2006; Marberry and Zagon, 1995; Zagon, 1993). However, positive aspects of white also were noted (Edge, 2003; Tofle et al., 2004).

Results of the analysis indicated conflicting recommendations by designers, making the choice of colors for a given space difficult to determine (Tofle et al., 2004). As a result of their findings, the authors of the literature review advise against creating universal guidelines for color in healthcare settings, given the lack of strong evidence on which to base them.

The literature review of color in healthcare environments described in Research Box 7.4 is fairly consistent with a previous literature review of color research intended to inform the design of NASA space station interiors. The NASA literature review summarized the empirical evidence about human responses to color and how, if at all, color influences people's perceptions of a setting or their behaviors in that setting (Beach et al., 1988). The researchers report that so much has been written about color that the distinction between facts and myths has become blurry. One such myth concerns use of "easy eye green" (Bernardo, 1983):

Hospitals replaced the color white on both walls and clothing with the color green, in order to minimize the afterimages experienced by operating room staff. It was incorrectly inferred that a color used in hospitals to aid visual tasks would also benefit other work environments. It was not so much the hue component of this color but its relative lightness that was important in the surgical suite. Another hue with the same degree of lightness might have worked just as well if not better (Beach et al., 1988, p. 2).

The NASA researchers' conclusions from their analysis of more than 200 color-related studies include the following points:

- The common claim that red is expansive and green is constrictive and tranquilizing is not supported by research evidence, nor are claims that red impairs and green and blue enhance fine motor coordination, motor performance, or judgment abilities (Beach et al., 1988).

- "Physiological arousal responses to color are of a short duration and a transitory nature" (Beach et al., 1988, p. 24).

- Red (and other colors) may have signal and symbolic properties under certain circumstances, but the effects of increased production and alertness are at most of short duration, and the basic association is a learned one (Beach et al., 1988).

- A positive reaction to color is a mixture of social and emotional context and general fashion as well as a specific response to the interaction among light source, background color, and object color. The contrast of objects with background color is the most important factor (Beach et al., 1988).

- Generally, blue is preferred most and yellow-red least, but many other factors may come into play (Beach et al., 1988).

- Preference for color is alterable by changing purity and brightness, illumination, background, imagined color combinations, and considering cultural and other factors (Beach et al., 1988).

- Brighter colors are typically judged "lighter" in weight. Higher purity (chroma) and lower brightness (value) is the key to a "weight" impression, with hue (color) adding little (Beach et al., 1988).

- "Warm colors advance and cool ones recede" is overly simplistic, at best (Beach et al., 1988).

- Wall brightness affects perceived room size and distance estimation. Lightly colored space appears larger—about 15 percent larger with white—but blue may recede, depending on its purity (white is not a favorite color, but appears more open and less complex) (Beach et al., 1988).

- Light distribution is much more important than color for spaciousness effects. Bright lighting at a room's periphery gives a greater sense of spaciousness and is mostly produced by the "wall washing" of the light rather than the sheer amount of light (Beach et al., 1988).

- "Abrupt lines of contrast can be used to perceptually widen walls or lower ceilings, as long as the viewer's perspective is taken into account. But decoratively striping a wall area at eye level only introduces a strong sense of 'constriction' into a space due to the advancement produced by this element relative to its background" (Beach et al., 1988, p. 80).

- The most successful wall colors for living rooms are warm in hue, high in brightness, and lower in purity (saturation) (Beach et al., 1988).

- "The ability of a product's color to harmonize well with other products' colors is critical to its acceptance," as well as whether it reflects the "character" of the product, including its image and function, irrespective of people's general preference for the color (Beach et al., 1988, p. 84; Minato, 1977).

- For building exteriors, people like yellow-red more than blue, and they like various shades from yellow to beige, or those that look like natural wood (Beach et al., 1988).

- Perceived appropriateness of colors varies with the function and style of an interior, including its decoration, and with education and sociocultural norms (taste). Characteristic appearance preferences for each style are unique to that style. For example, people have "prototypes" or "ideas" as to what a style of room should look like and, therefore, what colors are appropriate (Beach et al., 1988).

♦ Personal control over some aspects of one's setting overrides expected behavioral color effects chosen by outside means (Beach et al., 1988).

♦ Architects learn styles and color, but non-architects need extrinsic contexts for evaluation, which leads to conflicts. Designers should not generally accept people's preferences as is or impose their own, which are based on contradictory and often erroneous principles (Beach et al., 1988).

Given a lack of strong evidence on which to base them, guidelines for specific colors in healthcare settings are not provided here. Still, the problem remains of choosing the "best" colors, and in a time of high healthcare costs, color is sometimes the most readily available tool for change. Based on findings from the literature, researchers recommend that designers choose colors based on the intended use of the space and the role of color within the space (Tofle et al., 2004). Other factors to consider include geographic location, user characteristics (for example, age and culture), lighting sources, and size and shape of the room (Tofle et al., 2004). Many researchers discourage designers from relying solely on personal preferences for color decisions because preferences vary greatly among individuals (Beach et al., 1988; Tofle et al., 2004; Young, 2007).

Lighting

Light plays a critical role in sleep/wake cycles, alertness, and energy levels through its effects on melatonin production and the body's circadian rhythm (biological events that occur at regular intervals) (Brainard, 1995; Joseph, 2006a). (See chapter 6.) Several studies indicate that exposure to sunlight and artificial bright light can affect health outcomes. Numerous studies have shown that bright light is effective in reducing depression among patients with bipolar disorder or seasonal affective disorder (Benedetti, 2001; Beauchemin and Hays, 1996; Joseph, 2006a; Ulrich et al., 2006). Exposure to natural sunlight has also been associated with reduced agitation in dementia patients (Ulrich et al., 2006).

Studies have documented shorter hospital stays for patients in sunny rooms. This effect was found for patients with depression as well as for cardiac patients in the ICU (Beauchemin and Hays, 1996, 1998; Benedetti, 2001). (See Research Box 7.15 later in the chapter.) Other researchers have reported reduced pain for surgery patients (Walch et al., 2005). (See Research Box 7.5.)

RESEARCH BOX 7.5 DOES EXPOSURE TO SUNLIGHT REDUCE REQUESTS FOR PAIN MEDICATIONS?

Research indicates that exposure to natural light can increase concentrations of serotonin in the central nervous system. Serotonin plays a vital role in regulating body temperature, mood,

(continued)

RESEARCH BOX 7.5 (*Continued*)

appetite, sleep, and metabolism. It can also block pain pathways in the central nervous system. This suggests that exposure to natural sunlight may reduce pain through its effects on serotonin concentrations (Walch et al., 2005).

A research group was interested in testing whether post-surgical patients in sunny rooms required less pain medication than patients in dim rooms. The sample consisted of 89 patients who had undergone elective spinal surgeries. After discharge from the post-anaesthesia care unit, patients were assigned to sunny rooms on the east side of the building or dim rooms on the west side, based on room availability. Pain medication was administered to patients as needed.

Researchers used three measures of morning and afternoon sunlight intensity: directly from the window, reflecting off the patient, and reflecting off interior surfaces. They found that patients in sunny rooms received an average of 46 percent more natural sunlight per day than did patients in dim rooms.

Baseline data indicated that patients did not differ in terms of demographics, initial pain scores upon leaving the PACU, or optimism ratings (as a personality trait).

Findings revealed that patients in the dim rooms received 28 percent more pain medication per hour during the length of their stay than did patients in sunny rooms. A significant difference in pain medication use between the two groups was found on the first post-operative day. Pain medication costs for patients in sunny rooms were on average 21 percent lower than similar costs for patients in dim rooms.

With regard to psychological variables, patients in sunny rooms reported significantly less perceived stress upon discharge than did patients in dim rooms. There were no significant differences between groups on measures of depression or mood.

Daylight and indirect artificial lighting in patient rooms can contribute to a soothing environment. However, direct sun can be too bright and produce glare. Therefore, windows should have blinds, shades, or drapes, ideally a double set for both sheer and opaque coverage (Fong, 2003; Fong and Nichelson, 2006; Patient Rooms, 2014). The reflective properties of wall coverings, flooring, and furnishings should also be considered in order to reduce glare (Brainard, 1995; Fong and Nichelson, 2006).

Lighting can contribute to comfort, ambience, and task accomplishment in the patient room. Various activities require specific lighting features. For instance, an examination by medical staff requires the patient's body or part of the body to be well illuminated by a light source that minimizes shadows and is as close to natural light as possible. (One alternative is to provide a large, diffuse field of light that illuminates the whole bed.) Nursing staff need a general room light so patients can be visually monitored from the hall or from just inside the room. Low-level lighting for nighttime monitoring is often required by code. Housekeeping staff require lighting that is bright enough to expose hidden areas that need cleaning.

Patients' and visitors' lighting-related concerns involve ambience and non-medical functions. They need low lighting for watching television or talking quietly, task lighting over the bed for reading or writing, medium-level lighting for more animated conversation with a number of visitors, and a dim nightlight for late visits to the bathroom. Because their lighting needs are varied, it makes sense to design a flexible system that offers several different light sources, each adjustable by multiple switching or dimmers. This system should include controls at the patient's bedside (Fong and Nichelson, 2006).

Lighting can make a room look larger or smaller; can emphasize certain features of the room, such as setting off an alcove or highlighting a particular part of the décor; and can make sick patients look healthy or healthy ones look sick.

The following considerations are important to planning and designing a lighting system (see also chapter 6):

- Provide general room lighting, adjustable by multiple switching and/or rheostats. Make sure illumination levels can be adjusted for the time of day, the amount of sunshine in the room, the task being attempted, and the patient's vision (Beck and Meyer, 1982; Fong, 2003; Fong and Nichelson, 2006; Hayward, 1974).

- Consider the reflective properties of wall coverings, floors, and furnishings in order to reduce glare (Brainard, 1995; Fong and Nichelson, 2006).

- Place lighting controls within easy reach of both staff and patients (Fong and Nichelson, 2006).

- Provide a reading light above or close to the patient's bed.

- Select lighting fixtures that allow the patient to adjust the light upward and downward (Beck and Meyer, 1982; Fong and Nichelson, 2006; Fong, 2003; Lam, 1977; Rosenfeld, 1971).

- Provide nighttime lighting that illuminates the path between the patient's bed and the bathroom.

- Avoid examination or general room lighting that may cast unflattering shadows or give an unnatural tone to the patient's skin (Benya, 1989; Fong, 2003; Torrice, 1989).

- Install a single lamp color in all patient areas to enable staff to give a consistent diagnosis when assessing skin color (Fong, 2003; Fong and Nichelson, 2006).

- Provide examination and general room lighting that has color characteristics as close as possible to natural daylight. Lighting sources with a Color Rendering Index in the mid-80,000s and color temperature between 3,000 and 3,500 degrees Kelvin are recommended for neutral lighting with good color rendering (Fong and Nichelson, 2006).

- Provide some indirect lighting in patient rooms so patients and visitors do not need to contend with lights that are too bright (Beck and Meyer, 1982; Benya, 1989; Boyce, 1981;

Rosenfeld, 1971). This could include lights with dimmers, recessed downlights, or wall-washers (Fong and Nichelson, 2006).

- Consider using a mix of fluorescent and incandescent lighting (Benya, 1989; Boyce, 1981).

Style in Healthcare Settings

With a view to relieving stress and enhancing the patient's physical and psychological comfort, healthcare-facility designers have increasingly sought to avoid the impersonal, cold-feeling, stereotypically "institutional" look of health facilities of the past and replace it with a more comforting, warm-feeling, contemporary "residential" environment. Design elements such as fashionable colors, varied textures and patterns, soft lighting, and products that use or mimic natural materials such as wood, marble, and travertine have been deployed (Cullinan and Wolf, 2010; Horwitz-Bennett, 2014). The aim, as expressed by one hospital administrator, is to change the patient room "from a clinical environment to a personal bedroom away from home" (Frellick, 2014). With a high-end aesthetic and amenities such as decorative sconces and towel warmers, design can even approach a hospitality-like ambiance (Horwitz-Bennett, 2014).

This aesthetic, however, may run counter to the demands of medical technology and infection control and become difficult, as well as costly, to achieve. Materials and finishes must be durable enough to withstand rigorous cleaning. Surfaces should be as seamless as possible, without joints and corners that can harbor bacteria. Strategies must be developed to avoid positioning medical equipment so that it leads to an "overwhelming amount of visual noise and institutional clutter," in constant view of the patient and family (Battisto and Allison, 2014). It's also important that responses to so-called homelike and hospitality-oriented design features will vary according to the experience, background, socioeconomic status, and culture of the health facility's patients and visitors.

Some design decision-makers are adopting a different, "21st-century" approach to the healthcare environment. Instead of striving to make health facilities appear "homelike," they employ smooth, curved surfaces and space-age materials "to be true," in the words of one designer, "to what a hospital is," to shape a healing environment by means of simplicity, sleek lines, a neutral color palette, and the latest technology (Cullinan and Wolf, 2010; Ferenc, 2014). Proposed models employ backlit displays and touchscreens on almost every surface for access to medical information. Sensors are embedded in walls and furniture to reduce the need for manual record-keeping, for greater efficiency and fewer medical errors (Flaherty, 2013).

Selection of design criteria will necessarily vary from facility to facility. Choices will depend not only on the philosophy of a given healthcare facility, but also on the particular character and requirements of individual units within a facility and on its patient population.

Inpatient Room Furnishings

Not only do patients have little variety in the settings they encounter during hospitalization, within their rooms, there are few alternative places to sit or lie down during the course of a day.

Patient beds and chairs are the most frequently used design features, and their designs greatly affect patient comfort.

Patient Beds

Patients who spend long periods of time in bed must conduct a variety of activities without getting up. They must be able to adjust the bed and move the overbed table in order to eat; manipulate the bed so they can sleep comfortably; and adjust it so they can read, talk, or find a comfortable position for watching television. To facilitate these tasks, the bed's controls must be easy to understand and manipulate. Even so, it may be helpful for staff members to point out and demonstrate to new patients how to work the various buttons and switches in their rooms.

The following guidelines may help in designing and selecting patient bed controls:

- Provide standing assists such as bedrails (Facility Guidelines Institute, 2014; Carpman and Grant, 1984 [unpub. No. 25]; Soloman and Gaudette, 1984).

- Provide controls for the bed, nurse call, light, and television that are easily understood and operable by patients who are lying flat or sitting upright. Controls need to be lighted for nighttime use (Carpman and Grant, 1984 [unpub. No. 25]; Soloman and Gaudette, 1984).

- Provide controls that patients can operate with either hand, because one hand may be injured or immobilized and because patients may be left- or right-handed (Carpman and Grant, 1984 [unpub. No. 25]; Soloman and Gaudette, 1984).

- If controls are to be used by patients who have difficulty with hand manipulation, provide pressure-sensitive control buttons (Carpman and Grant, 1984 [unpub. No. 25]; Soloman and Gaudette, 1984).

- Place the inpatient telephone where it can be easily reached and manipulated with either hand (Carpman and Grant, 1984 [unpub. No. 25]; Soloman and Gaudette, 1984).

Patient Chairs

Patient chairs are often used as an alternative place for reading, eating, and watching television. A visitor may sit in a chair for hours, talking with or just keeping the patient company. Because patient chairs are so heavily used, one might expect them to be designed as carefully as patient beds, with special attention given to comfort and physical support. Unfortunately, it is rare to find patient chairs that satisfy all important comfort-related criteria. Yet patient chairs must meet the requirements of patients who vary in size, weight, and physical condition; for example, there will likely be a need for chairs that accommodate obese patients. Furthermore, it is important to consider staff and management's requirements for patient chairs, including ease of movement, cleaning, and maintenance, along with cost and appearance.

Consider the following guidelines:

- Select patient chairs that will be comfortable for long periods of time (Carpman and Grant, 1984 [unpub. No. 25]; Soloman and Gaudette, 1984).

- Select patient chairs that provide back and lumbar support, are easy to get into and out of, have sturdy and comfortable arms, and can be moved easily (Carpman and Grant, 1984 [unpub. No. 25]; Soloman and Gaudette, 1984).

- Provide patient chairs with standing assists such as extended armrests (Carpman and Grant, 1984 [unpub. No. 25]; Facility Guidelines Institute, 2014; Soloman and Gaudette, 1984).

- Select chairs that enable patients to elevate their feet (Carpman and Grant, 1984 [unpub. No. 25]; Facility Guidelines Institute, 2014; Lowry, 1989; Soloman and Gaudette, 1984).

- Avoid trip hazards, such as separate footstools or ottomans (Carpman and Grant, 1984 [unpub. No. 25]; Facility Guidelines Institute, 2014; Lowry, 1989; Soloman and Gaudette, 1984).

- Select chair-covering materials that are comfortable and easy to clean (Baier, 1989; Carpman and Grant, 1984 [unpub. No. 25]; Lowry, 1989; Soloman and Gaudette, 1984).

- Because the size, weight, and physical condition of patients vary, consider purchasing chairs that can be easily adjusted to satisfy numerous support and configuration demands (Carpman and Grant, 1984 [unpub. No. 25]; Soloman and Gaudette, 1984).

- Select chairs with legs that do not extend laterally or forward beyond the chair seat (Carpman and Grant, 1984 [unpub. No. 25]; Facility Guidelines Institute, 2014; Soloman and Gaudette, 1984).

- Make chairs available that are wide enough to accommodate obese patients (Carpman and Grant, 1984 [unpub. No. 25]; Soloman and Gaudette, 1984).

Storage for Belongings

When people stay in a hotel, hospital, or other unfamiliar and relatively impersonal place for a period of time, they often bring along a few personal possessions to make the strange environment more homelike. Even though almost all basic needs will be met regarding food, clothing, communication, and even positive distractions, patients tend to bring a number of possessions anyway. In an effort to cheer up patients, visitors may bring even more things.

Not surprisingly, clothing is the most common type of belonging brought to the hospital (Reizenstein, Vaitkus, and Grant, 1982). Most patients bring shoes, socks, shirts, pants, bathrobes, slippers, and underwear. In areas that have cold winters, they also bring a coat or jacket, boots, gloves, and often a scarf, hat, or sweater. Although clothing storage is more of a problem in winter, storage is needed year-round for basic items. There are also individual differences: hospitals may need to accommodate patients who bring ten pairs of underwear and pajamas as well as those who bring two, or they will need to limit what can be brought.

Hospital patients also bring toiletries. The variety of toiletries brought and the size of different patients' collections may vary enormously. At the very least, there should be space available for patients to store a comb, brush, toothbrush, toothpaste, shaving equipment, shampoo, deodorant, cologne or aftershave lotion, makeup, and lotion.

Space is needed for reading materials, writing supplies, and digital devices, if these are allowed. Visitors often bring flowers, greeting cards, knickknacks, books, and food, hoping to contribute to their patient's well-being by brightening up the environment. It is important that space be available for these as well.

Regardless of who brought the items, if there is too little space for storage, items will get in the way of healthcare staff. In addition to the patient wardrobe, the overbed table and bedside stand provide needed space. Storage areas need to be easy to access. Drawers and doors should require little effort to push and pull.

In designing and selecting storage areas, consider the following guidelines:

Overbed Tables

* Provide overbed tables that people with limited dexterity can easily adjust to various heights.

* Make sure overbed tables are stable and cannot be easily tipped over.

* Provide storage space inside overbed tables, with easy access from both sides.

* Provide an adjustable mirror in overbed tables that can be easily used from either side.

* Make sure the drawer and mirror are easily manipulated by people with limited dexterity.

* Select an overbed table that can be easily used as a writing surface while the patient is seated in a chair.

* Make sure staff are trained to show patients and visitors how to use overbed tables (Carpman and Grant, 1984 [unpub. No. 25]; Soloman and Gaudette, 1984).

Bedside Stands

* Select bedside stands that can be easily moved so bedridden patients can reach the top surface and drawers.

* Select bedside stands with drawers that can be easily opened by people with limited dexterity (Carpman and Grant, 1984 [unpub. No. 25]; King et al., 1982; Soloman and Gaudette, 1984).

Wardrobes

* Design or select wardrobes with sufficient capacity to store winter outerwear, shoes or boots, some clothing, underwear, a suitcase, and other small possessions.

* Provide a small lockable drawer within the wardrobe.

* Select opening and closing hardware that can be easily used by people with limited dexterity (Carpman and Grant, 1984 [unpub. No. 25]; King et al., 1982; Reizenstein and Grant, 1982; Soloman and Gaudette, 1984)

* Place the clothes rod at a height that can be reached by wheelchair users or make the clothes rod adjustable.

* Position the wardrobe within the room so it does not impede circulation or other room functions.

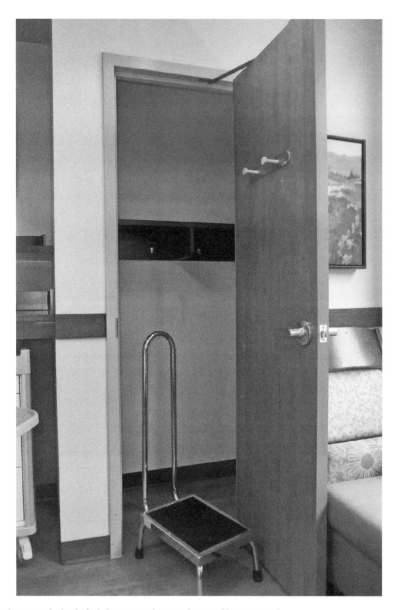

This patient room closet provides hooks for belongings and storage for items like a step stool.
Photo credit: Courtesy of St. Joseph Mercy Chelsea

- Place a few hooks inside the wardrobe for bathrobes and other clothing (Carpman and Grant, 1984 [unpub. No. 25]; King et al., 1982; Reizenstein and Grant, 1982; Soloman and Gaudette, 1984)

Other Storage

- Provide a tackboard so that patients can display cards and mementos.

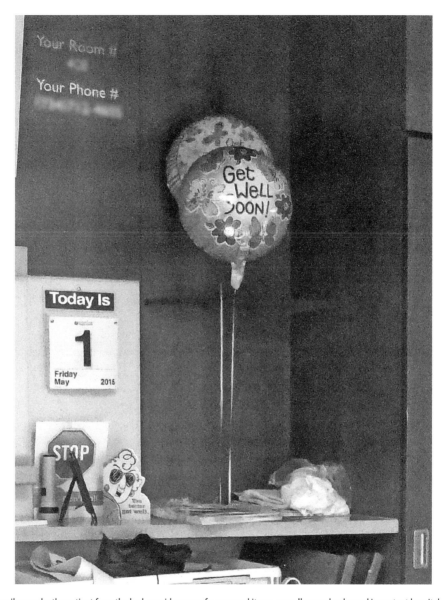

This area, easily seen by the patient from the bed, provides space for personal items, as well as a calendar and important hospital information.

Photo credit: Courtesy of St. Joseph Mercy Ann Arbor

- Provide a shelf for displaying flowers and other personal items. Make sure this shelf is sufficiently wide and has enough vertical clearance to accommodate large flower arrangements. It needs to be positioned so it will not be bumped and should have no sharp corners.

- Provide hooks for visitors' coats behind the door or in some other unobtrusive location (Carpman and Grant, 1984 [unpub. No. 25]; King et al., 1982; Reizenstein et al., 1982; Soloman and Gaudette, 1984).

Televisions

In the hospital, television helps patients pass the time, acts as "company," and helps provide positive distraction. Some hospitals are expanding their television services to include on-demand patient information programs and interactive features (Robert Wood Johnson University Hospital, 2008). For many patients, it matters less what programs are watched than that television is available. Television also serves a social function; it provides an activity that patients can share with family and friends (Carpman and Grant, 1984 [unpub. No. 11]).

Several types of televisions are often used: large, wall-mounted flat screen or ceiling-suspended models and small, personal-size models, usually suspended on arms. There are advantages and disadvantages associated with each.

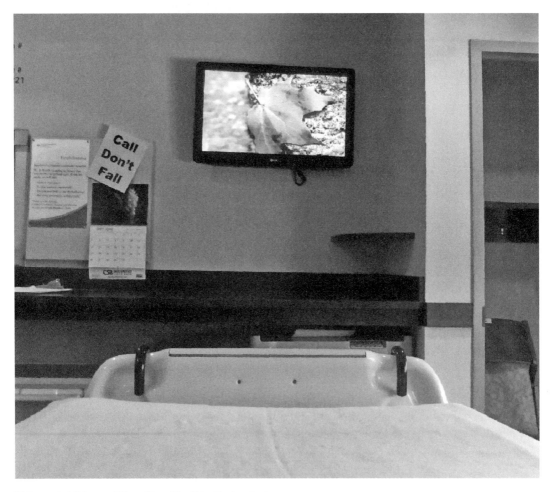

Wall-mounted, flat-screen TVs provide positive distraction in patient rooms.

Photo credit: Courtesy of St. Joseph Mercy Chelsea

A study at the University of Michigan compared preferences of patients and nurses for wall-mounted televisions and arm-suspended televisions (Carpman and Grant, 1984 [unpub. No. 11]). Patients were split on their stated preferences (40 percent preferred the wall television, 37 percent preferred the arm television) and a large proportion (23 percent) could not decide which was preferable. However, nurses strongly preferred the larger wall-mounted television because it did not get in their way as much as the small television did.

The large television had other advantages: it accommodated viewing by groups (a patient and several visitors) and was easier to see. However, some patients found the large television less preferable because it was difficult to watch in a comfortable position. Some patients also reported that the other patient's privacy curtain could be pulled in front of the large television, blocking their own view.

Those who preferred the small arm-mounted television liked its closeness to the patient's face, its relative quiet, its ease of adjustment, and the fact that privacy curtains could not block it. Some patients said its screen was too small to see easily; others said it sometimes got in their way.

Television sound needs to be controlled so it does not bother other patients. One way of minimizing TV sound is to provide personal audio devices such as pillow speakers or earphones.

Another important issue is that of television sharing. Different preferences for television programs, viewing times, and volume make many patients unwilling to share a television with another patient. Consequently, to avoid potential problems, it is advisable to provide one television per patient.

Increasingly, digital devices are being incorporated into inpatient room design. Television and internet access can be integrated into a flat-screen monitor or media wall providing TV and movie channels, connection to classroom or work through webcams, medical education programming, music services, and medical information and images relayed by clinicians from staff computers (Cahnman, 2010; Patient Rooms, 2014). Access can be by means of handheld controls or even from a digital tablet mounted in the overbed table (Ferenc, 2014).

Clocks

With the activities and demands of their everyday lives temporarily suspended, time passes slowly for many inpatients. Most patients want to know the time in order to keep track of schedules for medical procedures, medications, visiting hours, television programs, and the like (Baier, 1989). Because patients are often discouraged from bringing digital devices or watches, clocks need to be provided within the patient room. Consider the following design guidelines:

- Place a clock in each patient room so it is visible from the bed and yet not directly in the patient's line of sight.

- If analog rather than digital clocks are used, select clocks with numbers and hour-, minute-, and second hands that are legible from the bed.

Artwork

Patients appreciate having pleasant and interesting things to look at. Most like to look outside, watch television, and see their get-well cards. Many patients also enjoy having some artwork in their rooms. Although patients have a degree of control over other views (they can close the shades or turn off the television) and have some variety in what they see (views change with the weather and time of day, television channels can be flipped, bulletin board displays can be altered), artwork usually remains static. If patients happen to like the piece of art in their room, there may be no complaint. But if they do not, it may add to the stress they are already experiencing (Baron and Greene, 1984).

Because artwork displayed in the patient room has the potential for being a source of pleasure and even for being somewhat therapeutic, it is important to select art that patients like to look at (D'Alessio, 1986; Nanda, Eisen, and Baladandayuthapani, 2008; Ulrich and Gilpin, 2003). But, can subjective preferences be generalized? Are there certain characteristics of artwork that are widely appealing to hospitalized patients? Several studies on patients' relative preferences for different types of artwork suggest that patients prefer artwork depicting natural subjects and settings, and that representational styles are preferred over abstractions (Carpman and Grant, 1984 [unpub. No. 32]; Nanda et al., 2008). The study described in Research Box 7.6 also found that patients' preferences differed from the preferences of people with art or design backgrounds (Nanda et al., 2008).

RESEARCH BOX 7.6 WHAT TYPES OF ARTWORK DO PATIENTS PREFER?

In an effort to better understand patients' and designers' preferences for artwork in hospitals, a group of researchers compared the preferences of patients at St. Luke's Episcopal Hospital (Houston) to those of undergraduate students in interior design and architecture programs (Nanda et al., 2008). Preferences were based on ratings of how the artwork made the respondents feel (for example, better, worse, no impact) and whether they would select the artwork for their room. Sixty-seven hospital patients, 75 interior design students, and 50 architecture students were surveyed. Patients' ages ranged from 33 to 65.

Artwork chosen for the study included both representational and abstract images. Concerns about the quality of abstract artwork used in previous preference studies led to the selection of best-sellers from three popular online art vendors. Abstract images included contemporary abstract art with graphic forms, stylized nature images, and classic works by Vincent van Gogh and Gustav Klimt. Representational images were chosen in accordance with guidelines for artwork in healthcare settings based on both theory and previous empirical studies (Ulrich and Gilpin, 2003). These pieces of art portrayed realistic images with nature content, including landscapes, waterscapes, flowers, animals in natural surroundings, and humans in natural surroundings. The abstract and representational images were similar in composition, content, and quality.

Findings revealed that patients ranked all realistic images with nature content significantly higher than the best-selling abstract images both for the way the image made them feel and the desire to select the image for their room. The strong preference for realism-based nature settings by patients provides support for previous guidelines concerning art in hospital settings.

All respondents gave high ratings to images with nature settings and lush foliage, indicating a universal appeal for these types of images.

Differences were found between the preferences of patients and design students. Design students rated abstract art significantly higher than did patients, and patients rated realistic nature art significantly higher than did design students. Differences also emerged in the strength of the relationship between respondents' emotional responses to the art (how it made them feel) and choice of art for their rooms. Patients' selections for their rooms were closely linked to how the art made them feel, whereas this link was not strong for the design students. The researchers emphasize that it is important for designers to understand the difference between their personal preferences and the preferences of patients (Nanda et al., 2008).

In another study exploring patients' preferences for artwork, realistic images of nature settings ranked consistently high across age groups (Carpman and Grant, 1984 [unpub. No. 32]). However, evidence from other studies suggests that preferences may differ between adolescents and adults. The study described in Research Box 7.6 indicated higher preferences for realistic nature settings by patients ages 33–65 than by undergraduate design students. Similar differences between adolescents and adult populations have been noted in other preference studies of nature settings (Kaplan and Kaplan, 1989, 1995). These studies showed that teenagers' preferences were consistently lower for more natural settings than those of other age groups (Balling and Falk, 1982; Medina, 1983). In a different type of study, exploring preferences for features of a hospital room, adolescents rated paintings of trees and grass as the least-preferred amenity, below televisions, music, and telephones (Blumberg and Devlin, 2006). Because of these potential differences, researchers and designers should further explore how adolescents' preferences differ from those of other age groups across all types of health-facility design issues.

Some hospitals operate their inpatient artwork program on the principle that patients should be able to choose the art they look at (Nanda, Hathorn, and Neumann, 2007). These hospitals operate an "art cart" containing a collection of framed art reproductions. Volunteers or staff members periodically take the art cart to inpatients, who then make their own selections. This way, long-term patients do not have to look at a piece of art they do not care for and can also enjoy some variety. A study of an art cart program at St. Luke's Episcopal Hospital in Houston found that the majority of patients valued having the choice of artwork in their room (Nanda, 2006; Nanda et al., 2007). Most patients welcomed a change in the artwork; however, not everyone wanted change. Occasionally patients became attached to the artwork in their rooms. Providing a choice gave the patients a sense of control over their surroundings (Nanda, 2006).

In selecting artwork for inpatient rooms, consider the following guidelines:

- Adopt an art cart program so patients are given choices about the artwork in their rooms (Carpman and Grant, 1984 [unpub. No. 32]; Nanda, 2006; Nanda et al., 2007).

- Locate the artwork-hanging mechanism so the artwork can be seen from the patient's bed (Carpman and Grant, 1984 [unpub. No. 32]; Nanda, 2006).

- Include artwork with natural subjects and settings such as water scenes and landscapes (Carpman and Grant, 1984 [unpub. No. 32]; Nanda et al., 2008; Ulrich and Gilpin, 2003).

- Include more pieces of representational art than of abstract art (Collins, 1975; Miller and Goldman, 1984; Nanda et al., 2008).

- Include more photographs and paintings than posters with text.

- Include images that are texturally complex (Carpman and Grant, 1984 [unpub. No. 32]).

- Consider mobiles as an artwork alternative (Carpman and Grant, 1984 [unpub. No. 32]).

- Avoid images of urban scenes, portraits, muted or dark colors, and poster art with text (Carpman and Grant, 1984 [unpub. No. 32]).

- Consider differences in designers' versus patients' preferences for artwork (Nanda et al., 2008).

In addition to traditional forms of artwork that hang on the wall, some hospitals are exploring the use of virtual skylights and virtual windows that display nature settings using backlit panels in ceilings and walls (Corcoran, 2007). This approach may be particularly useful in basements and interior rooms where access to the outdoors is not possible, as well as in areas where patients wait on gurneys or undergo treatment while looking at the ceiling.

An Outside View

Views to the outdoors are particularly important to patients. Looking out the window gives them something to do, helps orient them to the time of day, season, and weather, and—depending on the nature of the view—provides a source of pleasure (Alexander, 1973; Collins, 1975; Keep, 1977). Having a pleasant, natural view can also be therapeutic (Heerwagen, 1990; Ulrich, 1984). (See chapter 8.) The importance of an outside view was illustrated in a study that gave patients a hypothetical choice between an interior window (in a room with an outboard bathroom) and a large exterior window with an outside view (in a room with an inboard bathroom). The latter arrangement was less private for patients because they might be seen walking to and from the bathroom by people in the hallway. It also did not permit a view to hallway activity. Still, it was preferred by the vast majority of patients (more than 71 percent). The availability of a generous outside view outweighed both the desire to have a view into the hallway and the greater visual privacy offered by the other arrangement (Reizenstein and Grant, 1981 [unpub. No. 1]).

Regarding views to the outside, the American Society for Healthcare Engineering recommends in its 2014 *Guidelines for Design and Construction of Hospitals and Outpatient Facilities* that "a window in each patient room, the views from it, and the diurnal cycle of natural light afforded by it are important for the psychological well-being of all patients . . . each patient room shall be provided with natural light by means of a window to the outside" (Facility Guidelines Institute, 2014). But providing just any window is not sufficient. How the window is designed, the type of view, and whether the window can be covered are also important considerations. (See Research Box 7.7.) For example:

- Provide windows that are as large as possible.

- Place window sills between ~20 and 30 inches (~50.8–76.2 centimeters) high to allow patients in beds and wheelchairs to see outside (Cooper Marcus and Barnes, 1999).

- Position windows so bedridden patients can see both sky and ground (Cooper Marcus and Barnes, 1999; Verderber and Reuman, 1987).

- Consider angling the bed so the patient can easily see out of the window (Patient Rooms, 2014; Zeit, 2013).

- Provide windows to enable patients to see out, but that minimize the potential for others to see in (Cooper Marcus and Barnes, 1999). Preserve patient privacy by using tinted windows or private porch areas (Sherman et al., 2005).

- If possible, provide views of activity going on at street level (Verderber and Reuman, 1987).

- Make sure visual access to windows is unobstructed by furniture, vents, or oversized sills (Verderber and Reuman, 1987).

- Provide window coverings that can be easily manipulated by patients and visitors. Enable patients to manipulate shades from the bed (Cullinan and Wolf, 2010).

- Provide window coverings that enable the room to be completely darkened at night: ideally, provide both sheer and opaque shades for two levels of light control (Patient Rooms, 2014).

- Select windows that avoid undue heat gain.

RESEARCH BOX 7.7 WINDOWS AND WELL-BEING ON A PHYSICAL MEDICINE AND REHABILITATION UNIT

Windows bring the outside in. Some research suggests that a lack of windows in hospitals (and offices) negatively affects the mental and physical health of patients and staff. Sensory deprivation in treatment units, psychological depression, and a diminished sense of well-being are commonly reported symptoms of people in windowless rooms.

In a study of Physical Medicine and Rehabilitation (PM&R) in six Chicago-area hospitals, one researcher analyzed elements that contribute to satisfactory "person–window transactions"

(continued)

RESEARCH BOX 7.7 (*Continued*)

(Verderber, 1986). He looked at preferences expressed by patients and staff with regard to a series of color photographs of patient units, therapeutic treatment areas, and staff offices, and the degree of patient and staff satisfaction with windows in their own units, as well as the extent to which each group reported engaging in behavior associated with the presence or absence of windows.

The 125 patients and 125 staff in the study expressed the strongest preference for photographs showing views of outside scenes of cityscapes and street life. The next strongest preference was for "substitutes" (plants) and representations of nature (pictures, calendars). Conditions without windows were preferred very little. Between patients and staff, the former preferred cityscapes, and the latter favored views of street life.

Both sets of respondents indicated that rooms with large windows looking out on a concrete building 25 feet (~7.6 meters) away, or small, poorly placed windows with monotonous views were the functional equivalent of rooms without windows.

Neither PM&R patients nor staff were very satisfied with the views from their windows, and views from treatment areas were generally considered the worst. Patients were also moderately dissatisfied with their inability to maintain personal control over the operation of windows, screens, and curtains. Other characteristics of rooms with ineffective windows included window sills too high from the floor, windows too distant from the viewer, and views obscured by walls, screens, and furnishings.

In a further study, the researcher and a colleague hypothesized that patients are more adversely affected than staff by windowless or practically windowless conditions and that patients lacking the choice of window usage have lower health status than those having such a choice (Verderber and Reuman, 1987).

To test this hypothesis, the researchers interviewed staff and observed daytime patterns of room use within each PM&R unit for seven days. Staff completed questionnaires evaluating patients' health status and well-being, as well as their own occupational outlook and level of job satisfaction. The authors were able to identify several conditions under which patients' lack of access to windows apparently slowed the pace of recovery or actually led to diminished health.

For instance, patients with good vision and healthy gait who were able to get to windows experienced a sense of greater well-being. However, patients with the following conditions, who were stationed in windowless areas, experienced a decrease in health status: low vision, confined to bed or using a wheelchair at a distance from windows, limited upper body usage, or experiencing a chronic disability or illness.

Among the staff, those working in windowless areas or distant from windows reported feeling a diminished sense of well-being. Staff able to frequently use window screens and curtains and those part-time staff working where window sills were moderate in height experienced a greater sense of well-being than did other staff members.

The authors suggest that full-sized windows should be an integral part of therapeutic treatment areas and that the staff position patients, whether or not they are ambulatory, as close as possible to windows with interesting views and low sills. Giving patients maximum possible control to adjust window curtains and screens also helps counter the sense of helplessness that many patients feel.

Reducing Noise on Acute Care Units

Many studies indicate that noise levels in acute care units consistently exceed the recommended levels of noise in hospitals (Balogh et al., 1993; Cmiel et al., 2004; McLaughlin et al., 1996; Scalise, 2004; Ulrich et al., 2004). In addition to staff, patient, and visitor conversations, noise in patient rooms arises from staff activity, telephones, televisions, nurse-call systems, and medical equipment. Noise can negatively affect patient healing by increasing blood pressure and sleep disturbances (Bakalar, 2008; Cmiel et al., 2004; Haslam, 1970; Storlie, 1976).

When possible, patients who are hard of hearing should be placed in the patient rooms nearest to noisy areas, such as nurses' stations. Other noisy activity areas should be placed away from patient rooms. Nurse and physician work areas on patient floors should be acoustically contained. Options for reducing noise include installing sound-absorbing tiles, using hydraulic door closers and rubber pads on door frames, and employing padded charts and chart racks (Cmiel et al., 2004; Duffy and Florell, 1990; Grumet, 1993; Hansell, 1984; Mazer, 2005; Williams, 1989; Williams and Murphy, 1991). (See "Reducing Noise in ICUs" later in this chapter.)

Using Music Therapeutically

Although unwanted sounds can be disturbing to patients and visitors in a health facility, musical sounds considered beautiful or soothing by patients or visitors can have a positive effect. Music has long been believed to aid the healing process. But it was not until the early 1980s that researchers began systematically assessing the relationship between music and recovery (Standley, 1986). Since then, the number of related studies has grown considerably.

Seven literature reviews between 1995 and 2007 identified numerous studies testing the effects of music on patients' pain and anxiety in a variety of medical settings (Cardozo, 2004; Cepeda et al., 2006; Cooke, Chaboyer, and Hiratos, 2005; Evans, 2002; Henry, 1995; Joseph and Ulrich, 2007; Kemper and Danhauer, 2005). In some studies, mood and satisfaction were also evaluated. Many of these studies found beneficial effects of music on patients' pain and anxiety, leading to the conclusion that music can be a simple, low-cost way to improve patient well-being in a variety of medical settings. (For a discussion of the therapeutic effects of music for people with dementia, see chapter 9.)

In the studies reviewed, music intervention was conducted in the pre-operative stage, during treatment or surgery, in the post-operative stage, during post-anaesthesia care, or in intensive care. Two literature reviews focus solely on patients in ICUs (Cardozo, 2004; Henry, 1995). The types of medical procedures or conditions represented in the studies also vary. They include mechanical ventilation, cardiac surgery, cancer surgery or treatment, sigmoidoscopy, cesarean delivery, childbirth, and burn treatment. Other studies have indicated positive effects of music on hospitalized infants (Chapman, 1975; Owens, 1979).

Effects of Music on Anxiety and Mood

Anxiety is typical among patients before, during, and after medical procedures and surgery. Fear, uncertainty, unfamiliarity, and discomfort can contribute to feelings of anxiety. Anxiety can affect patients psychologically and physically. Patients may experience feelings of apprehension, tension, nervousness, and worry. Anxiety also can lead to increases in heart rate, respiratory rate, blood pressure, and cortisol levels.

A review of more than 50 studies evaluating the effects of music indicates that it can reduce anxiety and improve mood (Kemper and Danhauer, 2005). This literature found that listening to preferred music was more effective than uninterrupted rest in reducing anxiety in mechanically ventilated patients in the ICU (Wong, Lopez-Nahas, and Molassiotis, 2001). Another group of researchers found music intervention during post-operative care following coronary bypass surgery to be associated with a significant improvement in mood compared to a group that received only rest (Barnason, Zimmerman, and Nieveen, 1995).

Effects of Music on Pain

A number of studies indicate that music also can help reduce pain (Chan et al., 2006; Locsin, 1981; Nilsson et al., 2003; Shertzer and Keck, 2001). However, some researchers have expressed methodological concerns regarding studies on music and pain. Their concerns include small sample sizes, nonrandom assignment, and lack of a control group (Kemper and Danhauer, 2005).

A more recent literature review, which also assessed methodological quality of the studies, provides supporting evidence of the relationship between music and pain reduction (Cepeda et al., 2006). This review included 51 studies that involved 1,876 subjects and evaluated pain during diagnostic procedures, pain following surgery, and chronic or labor pain. Exposure to music was associated with a reduction in pain intensity and analgesic requirements. Pain intensity was evaluated in 31 of the 51 studies. In pooling the results, the authors estimated that subjects exposed to music had an average 0.4 units (on a 0–10 scale) less pain than unexposed subjects. When patients were exposed to music, their needs for strong pain relievers (narcotics or opiates) were reduced, as reported in 13 of the 51 studies. Authors estimated that patients who listened to music required 18.8 percent less morphine two hours after surgery than patients not exposed to music. Similar results (15.4 percent less morphine) were found 24 hours after surgery. Requirements for opiates during painful procedures were also lower in the music group, but these results were not statistically significant.

Although reductions in pain intensity and the need for opiates were found for patients exposed to music, the magnitude of the benefit was small. Music has favorable but limited effects on pain. Thus, music should not be considered a primary method for pain management, but a combination of music and other pain-relief methods could prove valuable. Several other researchers caution against the use of music in place of medication and other pain management methods (Cardozo, 2004; Cepeda et al., 2006; Chlan, 2000; Henry, 1995). (See Research Box 7.8.)

Guided imagery, both alone and in combination with music, is another relaxation technique associated with a reduction in pain and anxiety in postsurgical patients (Halpin et al., 2002; Kshettry et al., 2006; Renzi, Peticca, and Pescatori, 2000; Tusek et al., 1996). For example, a study of colorectal surgery patients found that guided imagery significantly reduced postoperative anxiety, pain, and medication intake and increased patient satisfaction (Tusek et al., 1996). Similarly, a combination of music, imagery, and light massage was shown to reduce pain and tension during early recovery from open heart surgery (Kshettry et al., 2006).

RESEARCH BOX 7.8 DOES MUSIC REDUCE PAIN INTENSITY IN SURGICAL PATIENTS?

Swedish researchers were interested in the effect of music on post-operative recovery of day-surgery patients (Nilsson et al., 2003). Their study included 183 patients receiving varicose vein or hernia-repair surgery. Patients were assigned to one of three groups: music, music with therapeutic suggestions, and silence. Using an audiotape player and headphones, patients listened to their assigned tape from the time of arrival in the Post-Anaesthesia Care Unit (PACU) and for as long as the patient wanted to listen.

For the two intervention groups, the music group listened to soft classical music and the "music with therapy" group listened to relaxing music accompanied by encouraging suggestions recorded in a male voice by a person trained in hypnotherapy. Therapeutic suggestions related to feelings of relaxation, security, rapid healing, quick recovery, and absence of pain. The control group listened to a blank tape.

The researchers assessed a number of variables to measure patient recovery, including heart rate, oxygen saturation, pain intensity (reported by patients), morphine intake, psychological well-being (reported by patients), anxiety (using the State-Trait Anxiety Inventory), and presence of symptoms (for example, headache, urinary problems, nausea, fatigue).

Researchers found that pain intensity was significantly lower for the music and "music with therapy" groups than for the control group. The intervention groups also experienced higher

(continued)

RESEARCH BOX 7.8 (*Continued*)

oxygen saturation than the control group, although the difference was not clinically significant. There were no significant differences between groups for the other variables.

The study indicates that music can lessen post-operative pain in day-surgery patients. Music alone and music with therapy appeared to be equally effective in reducing pain.

These results were fairly consistent with a previous study of 24 female gynecological and obstetric patients (Locsin, 1981). Half of the patients listened to music for 15–30 minutes every other hour; the other half did not listen to music.

Based on results of an overt-pain-reaction rating scale devised by the researcher, the study groups exhibited several significant differences. Those who listened to music showed fewer overt facial expressions of pain, had lower blood pressure, and exhibited a relatively smaller increase in pulse rate during either the first or second 24-hour post-operative period, or both. The researcher notes that the lower blood pressure and pulse rate readings are indicators of less pain. At the same time, the groups showed no significant differences in respiratory rate, overt verbal physiological–autonomic response, or amount of pain-relieving medication administered, although the non-music group did have more analgesics dispensed to them.

As for the patients' subjective reactions to the music, two-thirds said that it lessened the pain and a third said that the music was an effective distraction. Most preferred instrumental music or a combination of vocal and instrumental music, and all respondents recommended that post-operative patients have music available to them.

Types of Music and Permission to Choose

Different types of music can lead to different physiological responses. Steady, slow, and repetitive low-pitched music has been thought to facilitate the relaxation response and quiet the mind, whereas fast, high-pitched music can heighten physiological responses and raise tension (Cardozo, 2004).

One researcher tested the effects of different types of music on mood, tension, and mental clarity (McCraty et al., 1998). One type of music analyzed was "designer music," music composed to improve the listeners' mental state and boost immunity through its effect on the autonomic nervous system. Respondents who listened to designer music, New Age, and classical showed a reduction in tension. Respondents who listened to New Age music also experienced an increase in relaxation. Designer music was associated with the greatest number of benefits, including significant increases in relaxation, mental clarity, and vigor, as well as decreases in hostility, fatigue, and sadness. "Grunge" music was associated with significant increases in hostility, sadness, tension, and fatigue.

The type of music analyzed varies across studies. Some patients were allowed to bring their own music, while others were provided with slow rhythm, classical, tranquil, or New Age music. In a study in which patients could choose from classical, country, jazz, popular, or show tunes, there was no correlation between type of music and decrease in stress or anxiety. However, some patients refused to participate because their preference was not available (Winter, Paskin, and Baker, 1994).

Respondents in several studies indicated the importance of having a choice of music (Cardozo, 2004; Cooke et al., 2005; Joseph and Ulrich, 2007). Although many authors advocate giving patients a choice of music, results of studies are mixed when assessing the effects of providing this choice on levels of anxiety and pain reduction. One systematic review of studies found similar effects on decreases in pain intensity regardless of whether the patient was permitted to select the music (Cepeda et al., 2006). Other studies found that providing the choice of music was a critical factor in lowering anxiety and promoting relaxation (Yung et al., 2002). Whether or not selecting their own music has a clinical effect, it does afford patients a degree of control over their healthcare experience.

Culture is an important consideration when staff provide music or determine the selection from which patients can choose. Studies on the effects of music on patients have been performed in many countries, including the United States, China, Australia, Taiwan, the United Kingdom, Denmark, and Sweden. In a study of the effects of music on anxiety in Chinese mechanically-ventilated patients, culture and language were principal factors in the choice of music (Wong et al., 2001).

Considerations Related to the Effects of Music

Because of the wide variety of methods used, types of interventions, medical procedures, and cultures represented in studies of music in healthcare settings, the general effect of music is not fully understood. Questions remain about how to administer music interventions, including when (for example, pre-operative, during, post-operative) and for which medical procedures music is most effective. Researchers recommend continuing the analysis of outcomes and effectiveness of music intervention (Henry, 1995).

In order to prevent unintended adverse consequences of music, it is important to consider the patient's medical condition. Although rare, negative effects of music are possible for people with "music epilepsy," in that seizures can be triggered by music (Brown and Theorell, 2005). Music can also bother people with hearing limitations and patients with brain damage who are very sensitive to noise (Brown and Theorell, 2005). Most adverse effects of music can be prevented through individualized music selection and by giving patients a choice about whether or not to listen to music (Brown and Theorell, 2005).

Medical and nursing staff need to be aware of additional cautions associated with music therapy. Staff should avoid types of music that can increase anxiety and should not play music too loud or for too long (Cardozo, 2004). Fifteen to ninety minutes of music is recommended; the time periods for music interventions in the studies fall within this range (Cardozo, 2004;

Cooke et al., 2005; Henry, 1995). Because of negative reactions to music played in a room without the patient's control (see "Music" section in chapter 5), it is preferable to provide individual, controllable listening devices with headphones. Accommodations (for example, sound quality, volume control) should be made for people with hearing limitations.

With these considerations in mind, music can be an inexpensive, safe, and effective way to improve the patient's experience. Evidence-based positive effects of music on anxiety, pain, and mood may encourage medical and nursing staff to offer music to their patients. Other recommended efforts include compiling a music library, assisting patients in making music choices, scheduling time for music interventions, and providing additional comfort techniques (Henry, 1995).

Inpatient Bathrooms

Bathrooms used by acute care inpatients require special attention to design, with safety issues as a particular concern. (See also chapter 9.) (See Research Box 7.9.)

RESEARCH BOX 7.9 MINIMIZING THE RISK OF PATIENT FALLS

Depending on their condition, patients may move about their rooms without supervision by medical staff, visitors, or fellow patients. With this freedom comes a risk of accidents and falls. In one retrospective study of "patient incident reports" in a 152-room acute care specialty hospital, researchers found that of 249 patient falls recorded during a 22-month period, 94 percent occurred within patient rooms (Morgan et al., 1985). Although the majority of these falls resulted in no apparent injury, three did cause injuries serious enough to prolong patients' hospital stays. Patients had the hardest time negotiating the area near their beds (41.0 percent) and in or near bathrooms (43.4 percent), with two-thirds of bathroom falls occurring by the toilet.

Those having the greatest difficulty were patients 65 or older, who accounted for a little more than half the falls. Older males fell more frequently: at almost twice the rate of older women, adjusted for length of stay. Among the women who fell, those 40 years or younger experienced the highest rate, although the reason for this is not clear.

In looking at the relationship between patient diagnosis and rate of falls, the authors found that patients who were admitted with "mental disorders" were more than twice as likely to have fallen as those with other diagnoses. Incomplete hospital records prevented the researchers from specifying further relationships among the diagnostic groups.

Of particular note was the distribution of falls by time of day. Although the researchers found that patient falls were evenly distributed (using three-hour time blocks), they suggest that this finding is in itself significant, because patients are less likely to be out of bed at night.

The results of this study—combined with a recognition that many, if not most, patient falls go unrecorded—emphasize the need for reducing the risk of avoidable accidents. To this end, the authors propose that hospitals modify rooms to minimize the distance between bed and bathroom and provide secure handholds. In addition, they recommend that designers consider the use of "forgiving" surfaces.

Patients using walkers, wheelchairs, or IV poles need easy access from the bathroom threshold to the sink, toilet, and shower (Heulat, 1991). The bathroom door swing should allow adequate clearance and not block the path to the toilet or sink. Because patients may become ill while inside the bathroom, the door must be openable from outside to allow staff to enter, as needed. Hinges and latch sets should allow doors to swing either inward or outward.

There needs to be enough space in the bathroom for staff to assist patients. The toilet room clearances recommended by the Americans with Disabilities Act are geared toward wheelchair users who are able to function under their own power and these clearances are often not ample enough to allow necessary staff assistance (Cahnman, 2010). An "open bathroom" concept has been proposed, with sliding doors that can be moved completely out of the way to recapture room space for caregivers and medical equipment. This bathroom is compact, flexible, and accommodates various needs, while containing costs (Ferenc, 2014).

For nighttime use, low light should be available in the bathroom. An illuminated switch may be helpful. The bathroom should be well ventilated, with a mechanical ventilation system that meets code or that provides a minimum of 10 air changes per hour (Facility Guidelines Institute, 2014). The bathroom should also be acoustically insulated from the surrounding spaces to help ensure privacy.

Sink Area

The sink area in a patient bathroom is used for washing, shaving, hair care, putting on makeup, and putting in contact lenses. To accommodate these grooming activities, patients need a sink, mirror, storage area, trash receptacle, electrical outlet, and towel rack.

Consider the following guidelines:

• To accommodate both ambulatory patients and wheelchair users, make sure the sink is at least 34½ inches (~87.6 centimeters) and no more than 36½ inches (~92.7 centimeters) high. (Check all applicable codes.) (Kira, 1977)

• Select sinks with smooth undersides that are free from obstructions (Popkin, 1980).

• Make sure exposed pipes are insulated in order to prevent burns and other injuries (Kira, 1977).

• Select a sink large enough to hold a small basin.

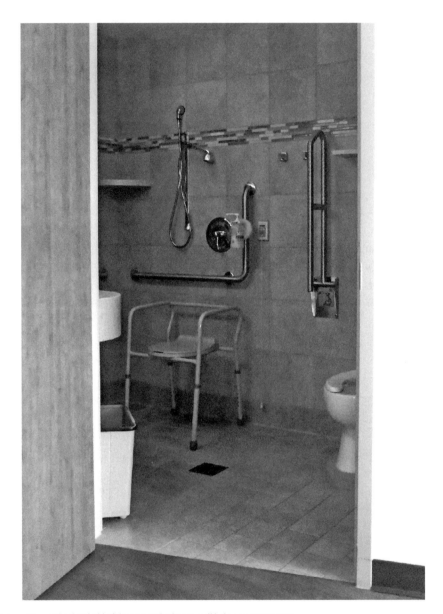

The smooth transition at the threshold of this patient bathroom will help prevent tripping.

Photo credit: Courtesy of St. Joseph Mercy Chelsea

- Select water control levers or knobs that can be reached and operated by patients with little strength or grasping ability (Baier, 1989).
- Make sure water control levers or knobs are labeled clearly.
- Select and position the mirror so that it can be seen by tall or ambulatory patients as well as by wheelchair users and short or seated patients.

- Provide electrical outlets in close, yet safe, proximity to the sink and mirror, so hair dryers and shavers can easily be used. Position these in compliance with codes and at a height that can be reached by wheelchair users or seated patients (Bergstrom, Cooper, and Simonsson, 1985).

- Provide storage shelves without sharp corners and large enough to hold patients' toiletries (Reizenstein et al., 1982).

- Place shelves within easy reach of a wheelchair user (King et al., 1982).

- Install towel racks strong enough to support a patient's weight.

- Install towel racks close to the sink and large enough to hold a washcloth and face towel for each patient.

Shower Area

For many patients, taking a bath or shower can be invigorating, relaxing, or even therapeutic. The shower can be a frightening place, however, for a patient newly ambulatory after a long stay in bed. Thus, safety is a key requirement in shower design. It is important to accommodate those who need staff assistance, as well as those who can shower independently or with a few aids.

Consider the following guidelines:

- Install nonslip flooring (Bergstrom et al., 1985; King et al., 1982; Kira, 1977).

- Provide a portable or foldable seat for those who cannot stand while showering (King et al., 1982; Kira, 1977).

- Provide a shower seat that is comfortable and non-slippery.

- Allow space in the shower area for two caregivers to assist a patient.

- Design the shower area so a patient can transfer from a wheelchair to a shower seat.

- Select and place grab bars that support a patient's weight as he or she stands, rises from a shower seat, or transfers from a wheelchair.

- Select shower controls and a shower head operable by patients with little strength or grasping ability.

- Select shower controls that can be easily read and understood by patients standing a few feet away.

- Make sure the shower controls and nozzle can be reached from both sitting and standing positions (Kira, 1977).

- Provide a hand-held shower head (King et al., 1982; Kira, 1977).

- Place the emergency call cord within easy reach of a seated or standing patient or one who has fallen (Bergstrom et al., 1985).

- Place the soap dish and space for shampoo within easy reach of a seated or standing patient.

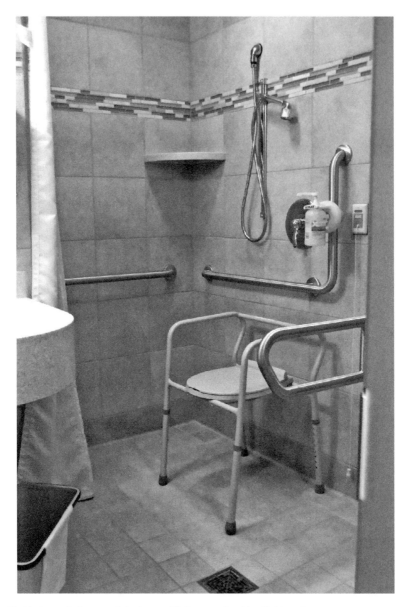

This accessible patient bathroom features a walk-in shower with shower seat and handheld nozzle.

Photo credit: Courtesy of St. Joseph Mercy Chelsea

- Provide hooks for clothing and towels close to the shower, but outside the spray area (Bergstrom et al., 1985; King et al., 1982).

Toilet Area

Key considerations when designing inpatient toilet areas are safety, ease of reaching for and manipulating the toilet paper dispenser and flushing lever, ease of sitting on and rising from the toilet, and the ability of the space to accommodate caregivers.

Consider these guidelines:

- Provide ample space in front of and directly alongside the toilet for two assistants to help the patient transfer from a wheelchair (Bergstrom et al., 1985; Kira, 1977).

- Design the area so that a patient can sit on the toilet while using the sink (Bergstrom et al., 1985).

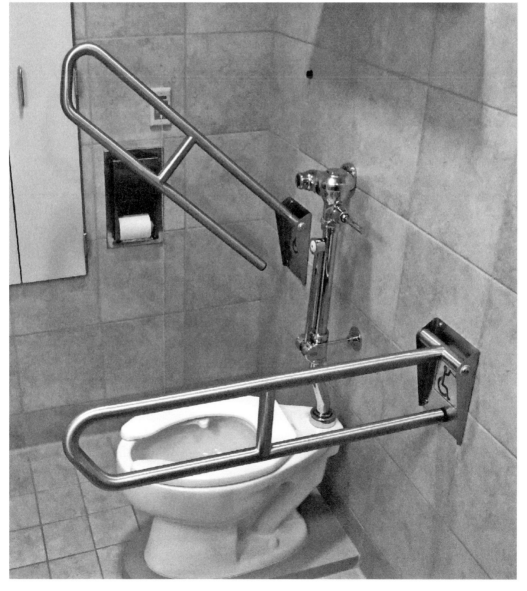

This inpatient toilet features adjustable handrails for both sides of the toilet. When not needed, they can be folded against the wall behind the toilet.

Photo credit: Courtesy of St. Joseph Mercy Chelsea

- Provide grab bars as support for patients sitting and rising (Baier, 1989; Bergstrom et al., 1985; King et al., 1982).

- Select toilets that are comfortable for older patients and high enough to facilitate easy wheelchair transfer.

- Position the toilet paper dispenser within easy reach of a person seated on the toilet (Bergstrom et al., 1985; King et al., 1982).

- Position the toilet flushing lever within easy reach of a person seated on the toilet (King et al., 1982; Kira, 1977).

- Select a toilet flushing lever that can be operated by patients with little strength or grasping ability (King et al., 1982; Kira, 1977).

- Locate an emergency call cord that can be easily reached from the toilet (Bergstrom et al., 1985).

- Provide a storage area that can be easily reached from the toilet (Bergstrom et al., 1985; Kira, 1977).

Inpatient Lounges

Many inpatients are encouraged to move around as part of the recovery process. They may be more likely to do so if they have appealing destinations to visit. A patient lounge can serve this purpose. The location of the lounge is critical. If it is centrally located, close enough to most patients' rooms, they will be more likely to make it a destination. A patient lounge at the far end of the hall or one shared with another unit may never be discovered or may seem too far away for a patient just beginning to walk again.

The size of the lounge is another important consideration. Although guidelines range from ~10 to 50 net square feet (~0.9–4.6 square meters) per bed, lounge size should be determined by the activities that will take place within it. If dining and special occasion parties will occur there, the room needs more space than if it will be used only for socializing and reading (Hamilton, 1983 [unpub. No. 1]; Kenny and Canter, 1978; Murtha, 1970).

In a study of patient lounges in three hospitals, researchers at the University of Saskatchewan documented lounge use and other design-related issues (Hamilton, 1983 [unpub. No. 1]). Through interviews with patients, visitors, and staff and by compiling a physical features checklist, researchers found that the patient lounges studied had common problems. They were too remotely located; too small, given the demand for use; too noisy, with noise spilling over into other patient areas; and arranged poorly, with activities such as television watching conflicting with visiting or game playing. Other problems included unattended children, uncomfortable furniture, and furniture that could not be easily rearranged.

Furnishings and entertainment options available within patient lounges may affect their use by patients. Lounges likely to attract patients will be furnished with comfortable, movable, and durable seating; contain plants and appealing artwork; provide outside views; and offer a variety of entertainment options, such as a television, music, pool table, table tennis, or a movie screen (Beckman, 1974; Bobrow and Thomas, 1976; Edwards, 1979; Hamilton, 1983 [unpub. No. 1]; Noble and Dixon, 1977; Olsen, Pershing, and Winkel, 1984; Reizenstein and Grant, 1981 [unpub. No. 6]). (See Research Box 7.10.)

RESEARCH BOX 7.10 CREATING UNUSUAL INPATIENT LOUNGES

Researchers at Bellevue Hospital in New York City joined forces with the 3M Company and Berkey K & L Custom Photographic Services to create and analyze some unique inpatient lounges (Olsen et al., 1984). They wanted to understand how the design of a lounge could play a role in enhancing patient morale. They hypothesized that well-designed lounges could draw patients out of their rooms, decreasing passivity and feelings of confinement. They also hypothesized that lounges might decrease boredom and provide an arena for social contact. The four identically-sized lounges in the study measured ~441 square feet (~41 square meters). Each room had two exterior walls with views of Manhattan or the East River. A 10-foot tall (~3.1-meter) partition wall located in the center of each room subdivided them into two distinct areas. Despite comfortable seating and commanding views, patients did not make much use of the lounges, finding them unattractive and unstimulating.

Two of the four lounges, located at opposite corners of a square floor for surgical patients, were selected for redesign using Scanmurals, which enlarged color photographs to floor-to-ceiling images. Audio systems in the redesigned lounges contained two-minute tapes of sounds related to the images.

One lounge became the "Harbor" lounge, with murals created from aerial photographs of New York Harbor, the East River, the Statue of Liberty, and the lower Manhattan skyline. Patients could push a button to hear sounds of sea gulls, lapping water, tugboats, and foghorns. The other lounge became the "Central Park" lounge, with photographs of the park's lake, a backdrop of the Manhattan skyline, a waterfall, a cluster of trees, and one of the park's ornamental bridges. This tape contained sounds of oars dipping into the lake, horses' hooves on cobblestones, vendors selling their wares, and a merry-go-round. Both lounges also contained park benches and large plants.

Observations of the use of all four lounges were made in the corridors and in the lounges both before and after the Scanmurals were installed. Patients were interviewed to learn what they thought of the lounges and how often they used them.

The analysis showed that the Scanmural lounges were successful for patients who visited them. Almost all patients reported liking the photomurals and sound systems, and most saw a positive relationship between the lounges and their own morale. The data indicated that the Scanmural lounges were perceived more positively than were the lounges without murals. However, observation data indicated that the effect of the Scanmural lounges on overall patient mobility was no greater than that of installing televisions in each lounge. One reason for this was that most patients who did not use the Scanmural lounges simply did not know about them.

(continued)

RESEARCH BOX 7.10 *(Continued)*

When asked about ways to make the Scanmural lounges more appealing to patients, both patients and staff suggested adding television, providing more comfortable seating, supplying games and magazines, and improving housekeeping. Staff suggested making music available with headphones.

This study makes two important points. First, attractive and interesting patient lounges will be enjoyed by patients, but only if they know the lounges exist. Innovative design must be accompanied by publicity. Second, lounges designed for a single purpose—in this case, experiencing special sights and sounds—may be less widely appealing than lounges designed to accommodate a number of different activities.

Additional considerations for patient lounges include:

- Because the patient lounge will be used by a number of people at a time, subareas within the room should be easily formed using furnishings or dividers (Hamilton, 1983 [unpub. No. 1]; Reizenstein and Grant, 1981 [unpub. No. 2]). In this way, small groups or individuals can comfortably participate in an activity without bothering others. Acoustic treatment is needed in lounges to keep lounge-related noises from disturbing other patients or staff.

- If patients can eat meals in the lounge, this will afford them companionship and an additional opportunity for a change of scene. If eating in the lounge is desired, tables need to be available. (Tables should be stored out of the way when not in use.) Because this is a patient-oriented space, staff need to be discouraged from using it themselves.

- People often want to inspect a social area before they enter it, to see what is going on and who is there. A glass panel in the lounge's door or wall will let patients preview lounge activity so that they can decide whether to participate (Howell et al., 1976).

- A separate, staffed inpatient lounge for teenagers is also desirable. Facilities can include digital devices, video games, equipment for listening to music, and perhaps an arcade-style basketball hoop. Storage should be provided for board games and arts and crafts supplies. A graffiti wall has been used successfully in one hospital (St. Louis Children's Hospital, 2014). Keep in mind that desirable design features for teens may vary over time.

Accommodating Visitors

Visitors may spend hours sitting with the patient, monitoring medical care, talking, reading, watching TV, or just being there to help if needed. They may adjust the patient's pillows, pull the privacy curtain, manipulate the lighting, get fresh water, assist the patient in using the bathroom, and represent the patient in communicating with staff. With increased recognition of the role played by the family in caregiving and the healing process, healthcare facility decision-makers see the importance of providing comfortable spaces and practical amenities for families and visitors. Design and policies that neglect visitors' needs can only worsen an already stressful situation.

Every patient room should contain a family zone. It should include at least one comfortable, movable chair that can be positioned within easy conversational distance of the bedridden patient, storage space for coats and personal belongings, and provisions for sharing mealtimes with the patient and staying overnight (Facility Guidelines Institute, 2014). In addition, visitors may want to use (and charge) digital devices in order to keep in touch with family, friends, and work colleagues.

Providing for Mealtimes

For most people, mealtimes are social times. Some patients find that eating even a thoughtfully prepared meal alone in bed can turn what is potentially a pleasant situation into a depressing one. To make mealtimes more enjoyable, many patients like company (Arneill and Frasca-Beaulieu, 2003). In addition to eating in the patient's room, visitors need a comfortable place to sit and a table to eat from. The surface should be large and stable enough for eating, writing, and supporting a digital device and be separate and distinct from surfaces used for clinical activities or the storage of medical supplies (Facility Guidelines Institute, 2014).

Providing a Place to Spend the Night

There are times when patients will want family members to stay overnight, especially on the night before surgery or when they are in pain. This is a particularly desirable option for patients in private rooms who do not want to be alone or who tend not to "bother" staff for what they need. A cot or pull-out sofa bed and a family shower and changing area should be available (Facility Guidelines Institute, 2014).

Having visitors spend the night in the inpatient room may not make sense for all patients, such as those in semi-private rooms or wards. Recognizing the importance of family support for patient well-being, however, healthcare facilities are developing policies to meet these needs (Changing the Concept, 2014). When patients in one University of Michigan study were asked whether they would like a family member or friend to be able to spend the night, more than 85 percent responded positively (Reizenstein and Grant, 1981 [unpub. No. 2]). (See chapter 10 for more details about overnight accommodations.)

Family Lounges

Family members and visitors will not be able to or want to spend all of their time in the patient's room. Family lounges, which can provide a needed change of scene, should be located near patient treatment areas. They should be furnished with comfortable chairs, tables, eating areas, beverage facilities, and perhaps a kitchenette. Restrooms should be located nearby. Where possible, a TV area should be physically or at least acoustically separated from quieter

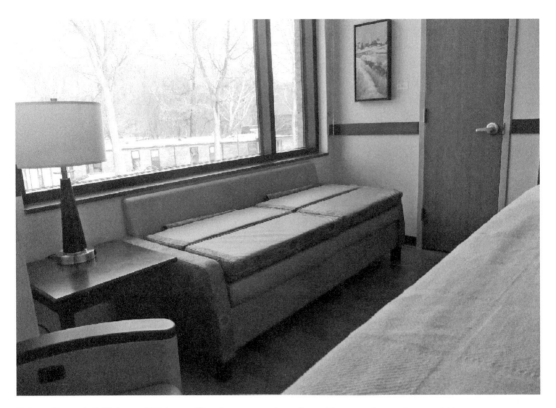

Cushions that can be folded out or folded up enable patient room couches to be used by companions staying overnight.
Photo credit: Courtesy of St. Joseph Mercy Chelsea

portions of the space. Laundry facilities are a desirable amenity, particularly near units such as pediatrics where families are likely to spend considerable time.

Family members and visitors will want to communicate with friends and other family about the patient's condition. They will also need to keep up with phone calls, text messages, emails, and work communications, and may wish to go online. Family lounges should provide shared devices with internet access and areas for using and charging personal digital devices.

Children visiting family and friends in a hospital have different design-related needs than adults do. Parents may have to bring their children with them, only to find that child-related needs have not been considered. These children, often bored or tired, may annoy other visitors in waiting areas, play in hallways where they get in the way of staff, or make noise that disturbs patients. When two parents or adults are present, they must often take turns watching the children and being with the patient, a situation that only increases stress (Reizenstein et al., 1981 [unpub. No. 4]). It is important that child-friendly spaces be included in family waiting areas. If possible, such areas should be somewhat separated from the quieter portions of the waiting areas, but easily visible to parents and other supervising adults. Toys, games, and video entertainment should be made available.

Attractive spaces should be provided for older children as well. Options include opening the teen patient lounge to siblings accompanying patients, or to siblings of patients in

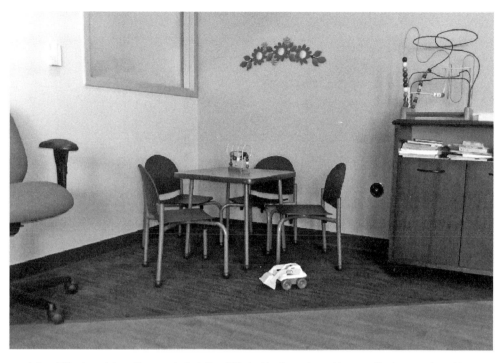

Accommodating children's needs in waiting areas by including child-sized furniture, along with toys and books, can make waiting more pleasant for both children and adults.

Photo credit: Courtesy of St. Joseph Mercy Chelsea

the neonatal intensive care unit, or other intensive care units (St. Louis Children's Hospital, 2014).

Intensive Care Units

For patients and family members, time spent in an ICU is likely to be one of the most physiologically and emotionally stressful periods of their lives. For many, ICUs represent a place where people die. Although this is obviously not always the case, the fears surrounding an ICU are pervasive and real. Design can act together with medical technology, healthcare staff, and hospital policies to create ICUs that are humane places for patients and their families.

Patients admitted to an ICU experience life-threatening illnesses or injuries that necessitate the use of specialized medical technologies. Even though their physical needs for immediate life support may be met by these technologies, studies show that ICU patients also need emotional support because they may feel helpless, confused, and afraid. Furthermore, their emotional stress can be magnified by other stressors associated with the ICU experience. Perhaps for the first time in their adult lives, all major decisions are being made for them. They lie in what seem like glass-enclosed fishbowls in which they are continually monitored by medical staff and noisy machines they do not understand.

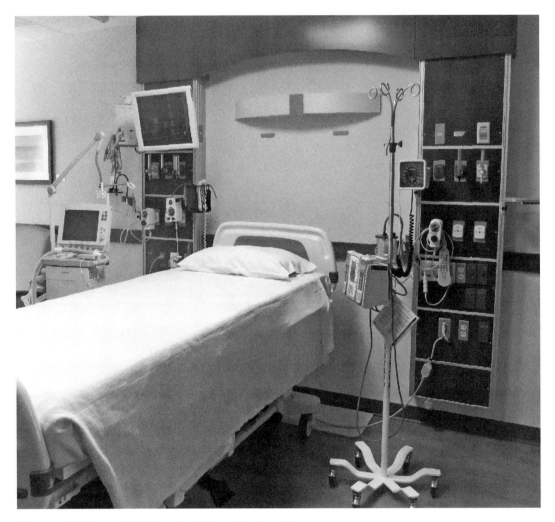

ICU rooms typically feature both built-in and portable medical equipment.
Photo credit: Courtesy of St. Joseph Mercy Chelsea

Providing Control Over Social Contact

Because ICU patients need high levels of vigilant medical care, these units are often designed for easy visual monitoring and quick access. This makes good medical sense, but if monitoring is not executed with care for the patient's psychological well-being, patients may feel robbed of their privacy. By following a few guidelines, however, increased privacy can be maintained without diminishing good medical care:

• To separate patients from one another and provide acoustical privacy, consider providing sliding glass doors (for visual monitoring) in private rooms and solid partitions or walls in semi-private rooms (Barlas et al., 2001; Hickler, 1969; Malcolm, 2005; Malin, 2011; Olsen and Sabin, 2003).

- Make sure that, upon request, patients can be visually shielded from outside view (Clipson and Wehrer, 1973).

- Provide acoustical privacy for patients so they can have confidential conversations with medical personnel and with their families (Barlas et al., 2001; Clipson and Wehrer, 1973; Dubbs, 2003; Malcolm, 2005).

- To ensure confidentiality and decrease anxiety, provide a space away from but close to the patient area for physicians to confer (Clipson and Wehrer, 1973).

- Provide acoustical and visual privacy for patients using the bedpan or commode, and make sure this equipment is stored out of sight (Clipson and Wehrer, 1973).

- Make sure digital displays in nurses' stations and medical records are not viewable by passersby (Dubbs, 2003).

Addressing Sensory Overload and Challenges of Maintaining Family Support

ICUs seem to be filled with tubes, wires, IV lines, bright lights, monitoring equipment, respirators, and other pieces of machinery. They are awash in activity. Patients may feel that they are being bombarded with noise, light, and pain. These patients, emotionally threatened by the very medical technology that is saving their lives, have traditionally been separated from family members for all but extremely short visits and thus deprived of much-needed human contact and emotional support. Policies and design decisions that enable and encourage the presence of loved ones in the ICU can help alleviate what can be, in the words of a distinguished physician who himself became a patient in a busy ICU, "a devastating psychological experience" (Relman, 2014).

Stresses created by equipment-related sensory overload and minimal social contact have been linked to "intensive care unit syndrome." This syndrome is characterized by hallucinations, delusions, psychotic episodes, and sleep disturbances that cannot be traced directly to the illness itself (Gowan, 1979; Keep, James, and Inman, 1980). Patients who experience ICU syndrome are likely to forget much of their stay in the ICU, misjudge their length of stay, and be disoriented about the time of day or day of the week (Laufman, 1981).

There is some evidence that the incidence of ICU syndrome can be reduced by careful attention to design details (Gowan, 1979; Keep et al., 1980). (See Research Box 7.11.) By providing a less-threatening environment (for example, limiting patient contact with medical equipment), increasing patient contact with others, providing windows and other orienting devices, and offering soothing music (see earlier section in this chapter), health facilities can limit the incidence of ICU syndrome (Wilson, 1972).

Consider the following design guidelines:

- Encourage visits by family members by providing ample space and comfortable bedside chairs (Clipson and Wehrer, 1973; Relman, 2014).

- Provide ways for patients and caregivers to keep each other within view (Clipson and Wehrer, 1973; Sturdavant, 1960).

- When patients are well enough to receive and make calls, provide a telephone within easy reach (Clipson and Wehrer, 1973).

- Provide a large clock and calendar in clear view, but not directly in front of each patient (Kornfeld, 1972; Task Force on Guidelines, 1988).

- Make sure each patient has a clear and comfortable view of the outside and that this view includes sky and ground (Beck and Meyer, 1982; Clipson and Wehrer, 1973; Gowan, 1979; Hickler, 1969; Keep, 1977; Keep et al., 1980; Popkin, 1980).

- Whenever possible, minimize patient contact with medical machinery, store unused equipment out of sight, reduce the cluttered appearance of tubes and wires, locate monitoring equipment out of the patient's direct line of sight, and explain the function of each monitor to the patient, as appropriate (Clipson and Wehrer, 1973; Duffy and Florell, 1990; Zubatkin, 1980).

- Allow patients to display personal possessions or cards by their bedsides and provide artwork and other interesting things to look at (Clipson and Wehrer, 1973).

- Avoid design details that can be visually confusing, such as abstract artwork or patterned curtains (Williams, 1991).

RESEARCH BOX 7.11   PROVIDING WINDOWS IN THE ICU PATIENT ROOM

A number of studies have examined effects of the presence and absence of windows on ICU patients.

One such study focused on patients who had stayed at least 48 hours in an ICU (Keep et al., 1980). Questionnaires examined patients' memories of their stay, asking about time orientation, memory of admission and discharge, incidence of hallucinations or delusions, problems with sleep, and amount of time spent there. Approximately 50 percent responded and indicated memory of their stay. Of those, almost two-thirds in an ICU with windows were able to make a good or fair estimation of their actual length of stay, but only 28 percent in a windowless unit were able to do so. Other questions resulted in similar findings on such issues as recall of admission to and discharge from the unit, orientation during their stay as to the time of day or day of week, and sleep and visual disturbances. Forty-eight percent of those in the windowless ICU reported having hallucinations or delusions, as opposed to 23 percent in the other unit.

In another study using hospital records instead of patients' recollections, an Arkansas physician measured the relative incidence of post-operative delirium in the ICUs of two general hospitals in the same town, one with windows to the outside and the other without (Wilson, 1972). The sample at each hospital comprised 50 consecutive post-operative ICU patients with similar background characteristics, types of surgical treatment, and post-operative clinical base measurements. Of the 50 patients in the windowless unit, 20 became delirious, but only 9 did so on the unit with windows to the outside. Symptomatically, these patients showed impairment of orientation, memory, intellectual function, and stability of judgment. Furthermore, although only 2 of 8 patients who had abnormally low hemoglobin or elevated blood urea nitrogen levels developed delirium in the unit with windows, 7 of 10 with comparable symptoms in the windowless ICU developed delirium.

Researchers at a hospital in Pennsylvania examined the effects of exposure to natural light on levels of analgesic medication. Patients recovering from elective spinal surgery were assigned to either "bright" or "dim" single-patient rooms of the unit in accordance with normal hospital protocol of room availability. Those patients housed in bright rooms (on average, 46 percent higher-intensity sunlight) reported less stress and marginally less perceived pain than patients in dim rooms, while taking 22 percent less analgesic medication per hour (Walch et al., 2005).

Although these results seem to provide a strong argument for inclusion of windows in ICUs, other research has produced more equivocal results. A study in two New Hampshire ICUs examined the effects of daylight and window views on patient pain levels and length of stay. ICU patients were randomly selected from cardiac surgery, pneumonia, and chronic obstructive pulmonary disease (COPD) admissions of one or more days. Findings supported the researchers' hypothesis that "increased light levels reduce pain perception and length of stay," but were not statistically significant. Findings suggested that "view was associated with reduced pain perception," but this also was not statistically significant (Shepley et al., 2012).

Another large study of 789 patients with subarachnoid hemorrhage who were treated in the neurological ICU at the Columbia University Medical Center (New York City) from August 1997 to April 2006 similarly found no differences in either short- or long-term functional outcomes, whether the patients received all of their care in a room with a window (57.7 percent) or one without (42.3 percent) (Wunsch et al., 2011).

Thus, there is a general consensus that further research is needed on the effects of windows in ICUs. However, some studies and anecdotal evidence supporting the potential importance of windows is such that numerous clinicians and specialty societies such as the Society of Critical Care Medicine recommend a window in every room (Fontaine, Briggs, and Pope-Smith, 2001; Guidelines/Practice Parameters, 1995).

Reducing Noise in ICUs

Common noises in the ICU include staff conversations, beeps and alarms, ringing telephones, and movement of equipment. Noise can make it difficult for patients to sleep and can lead to increased heart rates even while sleeping (Bakalar, 2008; Cmiel et al., 2004; Haslam, 1970; Storlie, 1976). Sleep deprivation in ICU patients has been found to contribute to impaired immune functioning, ventilation or breathing problems, and delirium (Cmiel et al., 2004; Parthasarathy and Tobin, 2004; Topf, Bookman, and Arand, 1996; Wallace et al., 1999). Adverse effects on the respiratory system may interfere with the weaning of patients from mechanical ventilation (Meyer et al., 1994). Noise may contribute to these negative health effects; however, it is difficult to determine the degree to which negative health effects are specifically due to noise.

Noise-related problems are further complicated by the fact that the effects of noise depend on its frequency and on the sensitivity of individual listeners. Sounds that annoy one patient may be stimulating or comforting to another (Hewitt, 2002; Redding, Hargest, and Minsky, 1976). For example, some patients reported finding comfort in hearing conversations and footsteps of the nurses (Hewitt, 2002). For some, the usual noises of conversations and traffic may help orient them and reduce confusion (Hewitt, 2002). In general, hospitals tend to be noisy places, with conditions not conducive to the restful, restorative atmosphere needed by most patients.

According to the US Environmental Protection Agency (EPA), recommended upper limits on continuous sound levels for hospitals are an average of 45 decibels or fewer over a 24-hour period (Public Health, Madison and Dane County, 2013; Topf, 1983). For sleeping conditions, the EPA and the World Health Organization (WHO) recommend 35 decibels (Balogh et al., 1993; Cmiel et al., 2004). An expert panel at the National Institutes of Health (NIH) Consensus Development Conference in 1990 reported that sounds at or above 85 decibels are potentially hazardous for hearing. Most permanent hearing loss is a result of exposures to sound levels over 85 decibels for eight hours a day over many years or a single exposure to abrupt sounds at high decibel levels (Noise and Hearing Loss, 1990).

Some examples of everyday noise levels are listed here to help put the EPA, WHO, and NIH standards in perspective (every 10-decibel increase is perceived by the human ear as being about twice as loud) (Cmiel et al., 2004; US Environmental Protection Agency, 1974):

- Rush hour traffic: 90 decibels
- Cafeteria at noon: 75 decibels
- Radio at full volume: 60 decibels
- Normal conversation: 60 decibels
- Whispering: 30 decibels

For comparison, the EPA-documented noise levels found within residences are as follows (US Environmental Protection Agency, 1974):

- Quiet suburban residence: 48–52 decibels
- Normal suburban residence: 53–57 decibels
- Urban residence: 58–62 decibels
- Noisy urban residence: 63–67 decibels
- Very noisy urban residence: 68–72 decibels

Several studies have reported noise levels in recovery rooms and acute care units to be consistently above 60 dB(A), surpassing EPA-recommended levels (Balogh et al., 1993; Cmiel et al., 2004; McLaughlin et al., 1996; Scalise, 2004; Ulrich et al., 2004). Peak sound levels ranged from 80 dB(A) to 113 dB(A)—reflecting sounds of bedside monitors, alarms, and phones during a staff shift change (Cmiel et al., 2004; Scalise, 2004). One study reported a night average of 45 dB(A), 10 dB higher than the EPA- and WHO-recommended 35 dB(A) (Cmiel et al., 2004). ICU equipment typically produces sounds of up to 75 decibels or more, and brief sounds lasting about one second may reach levels over 90 decibels at the patient's head (Balogh et al., 1993; Beck and Meyer, 1982; Martin, 1992). The frequent banging of metal bedpans and bed rails, floor-cleaning equipment used late in the evening, and alarms were among the most irritating noises (Balogh et al., 1993; Hurst, 1966; Storlie, 1976). (See Research Box 7.12.)

RESEARCH BOX 7.12 DOES LOUD NOISE WORSEN PAIN?

In a study of noise and its relationship to patient discomfort in a 10-bed post-surgical recovery room, one researcher hypothesized that more pain medications would be given during periods of high noise levels than during times of low noise levels (Minckley, 1968). To test this hypothesis, observations were made every half-hour from 8:30 a.m. to 6 p.m. during five randomly chosen workdays. Sound levels were recorded, as were their source and character, the numbers of patients and staff present, and the number of pain medications given. Patients were given additional pain medication in the recovery room only if their pain caused restlessness or they showed other signs of pain intolerance. In all, sound levels were documented 100 times and 544 pain medications were given.

Over twice the number of patients received pain medication when the sound level was high (60–70 decibels or higher) than when it was medium or low (40–60 decibels). When the sound level was in the lower range, increasing its duration did not lead to an increase in medication provided.

The sounds registering 60 decibels or greater included telephones ringing, children crying, and patients crying out, vomiting, snoring, and moaning. Of these, only snoring and ringing telephones elicited no verbal remarks from patients. In response to the other loud sounds, patients near the source complained. Typical comments were "How long do I have to lie here and listen to that?" or "Can't you do anything about him/ her?" The researcher also noted that the sound of staff laughter from across the room often brought expressions of irritation to patients' faces.

Higher sound levels tended to correspond to increased numbers of physicians in the recovery room rather than to increased numbers of nurses and patients. It is not clear whether physicians were less sensitive to potential patient discomfort or whether the physicians' presence generated increased medical activity and noise.

The researcher theorized that diminished control of their environment makes post-operative patients less able to tolerate loud sounds. Whether or not this is the central mechanism at work, it is apparent that increased noise decreases patient comfort.

Effects of Noise on Sleep

Several studies on patients' perception of sleep quality in the ICU indicated a reduction in sleep quality due to noise (Ulrich et al., 2004). Patients in one study reported that noise was perceived to be as disruptive to sleep as patient treatment and testing (Freedman, Kotzer, and Schwab, 1999). In another study, patients considered pain, tubes in the nose and mouth, and trouble sleeping because of noise to be the most important physical stressors in the ICU (Novaes et al., 1997).

A number of studies evaluate the effects of noise on sleep for patients in the ICU. Many of these studies found noise to be associated with sleep disruption (Freedman et al., 2001; Gabor et al., 2003; Reid, 2001; Topf et al., 1996; Topf and Davis, 1993; Topf and Thompson, 2001). In a study of mechanically ventilated patients, researchers found that noise was responsible for 20 percent of patient arousals and awakenings, while patient care activities accounted for 7 percent (Gabor et al., 2003). Another study found noise to be responsible for 11.5 percent of arousals and 17 percent of awakenings of mechanically ventilated patients (Freedman et al., 2001).

Although most researchers attribute sleep disruption to peak noise levels, other researchers found that the change in noise levels from baseline to peak was the main cause of sleep disruption. Providing "white noise" is one potential way to reduce the number of times a patient wakes up from changes in noise levels. White noise is a combination of sounds (at the same intensity at all frequencies) capable of masking conversations. Research suggests that white noise may be effective in reducing awakenings for patients by reducing the difference between background and peak noise (Stanchina et al., 2005).

However, the studies suggest that noise is not the only contributor to sleep disturbances. Patient discomfort, anxiety, and uncomfortable or unfamiliar beds also have been found to negatively affect sleep (Topf and Thompson, 2001). Several physiological factors associated with medical conditions, medications, and circadian rhythms can also disturb sleep (Reid, 2001). (See Research Box 7.13.)

RESEARCH BOX 7.13 DOES NOISE AFFECT THE QUALITY OF REM SLEEP?

Results from a study of healthy respondents exposed to typical sounds of a critical care unit (CCU) provide supporting evidence that noise can reduce REM (rapid eye movement) sleep (Topf and Davis, 1993). REM deprivation can lead to confusion, withdrawal, and poor recall of new material.

Seventy healthy subjects were randomly assigned to a noise condition or quiet condition. Subjects in the noise condition listened to an audiotape of sounds from a critical care unit during the night. The sounds emanated from equipment such as patient monitoring devices, ventilators, suction machines, chest tube drainage, and oscilloscopes, as well as from staff providing care. An alarm sounding at a level of 84 dB(A) was also recorded. Overall, the sound level averaged 56.3 dB(A), with a minimum of 50 dB(A) and a maximum of 86.8 dB(A).

REM sleep was measured using polysomnograph equipment for ten sleep variables. The variables included total REM sleep, number and duration of REM periods, density (number of eye movements per minute of REM period), and REM interval (time between REM cycles) for the first and second halves of the night.

The majority of REM sleep measures recorded indicated poorer REM sleep quality for subjects in the noise condition. Total REM activity and REM duration were significantly lower throughout the night for the noise group compared to the quiet group. It also took longer for the noise group to reach REM sleep, as indicated by longer REM intervals in the first half of the night. Thus, critical care unit noise can disrupt REM sleep in CCU patients.

Hospitals are dynamic environments filled with continual activity and noise, so it can be difficult to reduce noise levels. Nonetheless, researchers have made a number of recommendations for improvements. As a starting point, they suggest mounting a mix of periodic and continuous campaigns to increase staff sensitivity to loud talking and the need for extra caution in handling of supplies and equipment (Cmiel et al., 2004; Hansell, 1984; Haslam, 1970; Hilton, 1985; Kam, Dam, and Thompson, 1994; Whitfield, 1975; Williams and Murphy, 1991).

Other improvements include insulating hallways, diagnostic and treatment areas, nurses' stations, conference areas, and patients' rooms (Kam et al., 1994). A few studies have shown that installing sound-absorbing ceiling tiles can significantly reduce the amount of time a sound persists after the source has been removed (that is, reverberation time) (Berg, 2001; Joseph and Ulrich, 2007). One of these studies found a significant reduction in sleep arousals when effective sound-absorbing ceiling tiles were installed (Berg, 2001). In designing an ICU, designers should consider providing fully enclosed patient rooms, separating nurses' stations from patient rooms, or creating mini work stations, and directing all phone calls to a call center staffed by a trained medical receptionist in the waiting area (Joseph and Ulrich, 2007; Kam et al., 1994; Petterson, 2000). The creation of a dedicated service corridor has been shown to make an ICU significantly quieter, benefiting not only patients but also staff, who reported less stress and more job satisfaction (Wang et al., 2013).

Staff can also work with manufacturers and equipment technicians to reduce the sound levels generated by medical devices (Mazer, 2006). One researcher suggests that staff establish strict acoustical standards for all new equipment purchases, which might ultimately lead to changes in equipment design (Mazer, 2006). Telephones, monitors, and alarms could be designed to emit pleasant sounds at the lowest level consistent with good care (Hilton, 1985; Task Force on Guidelines, 1988). Another possibility is to replace overhead paging systems with cell phones or wireless communication devices carried by staff, although the effectiveness of this strategy is not yet fully understood (Joseph and Ulrich, 2007).

Other simple efforts such as padding the bottom of patient chart holders, medical carts, and receptacles of pneumatic tubing systems, lowering the volume on existing machines and phones, turning off unneeded machinery, and changing the hours of floor cleaning can have a considerable effect on noise reduction (Cmiel et al., 2004; Snyder-Halpern, 1985; Whitfield, 1975).

Music in ICUs

Under some conditions, music can mask noise and provide positive distraction for intensive care patients (see "Using Music Therapeutically" earlier in this chapter, for more details). When patients are well enough to want to listen to music, staff could provide personal music-listening devices with headphones and a library of music choices (Jenna, 1986; Williams, 1989).

Patient Comfort in ICUs

Intensive care patients are often in pain and may find it difficult to position themselves comfortably. They may also have a hard time sleeping. Consequently, it is important to pay attention to lighting levels, lighting quality, temperature, humidity, and the patient's ability to manipulate these systems from the bed. In addition, the design of patient furniture may facilitate both physical and psychological comfort.

Design guidelines for creating a more comfortable environment in ICUs include the following:

- If possible, provide windows in ICU patient rooms.
- Provide exposure to sunlight or other sources of bright light (see Research Box 7.5).
- Provide window shades, light dimmers, and double switching on grouped fluorescent fixtures so patients can adjust lighting to preferred levels (Clipson and Wehrer, 1973; Fong, 2003; Fong and Nichelson, 2006).
- Provide lenses and shades for light fixtures that produce non-glaring light (Clipson and Wehrer, 1973; Fong and Nichelson, 2006).
- Avoid situations in which lighting from the nurses' station disturbs patients trying to rest (Clipson and Wehrer, 1973; Duffy and Florell, 1990).
- Position nighttime lighting so nursing staff can monitor sleeping patients without disturbing their rest (Clipson and Wehrer, 1973).
- Keep ICU rooms at temperatures appropriate for the needs and preferences of critically ill patients (Clipson and Wehrer, 1973).
- Consider maintaining a relative humidity level of 50 percent in patient areas (Hickler, 1969).
- Place at least one comfortable, movable chair near the ICU patient's bed (Clipson and Wehrer, 1973; Ulrich, 1991).

RESEARCH BOX 7.14 HEALTH OUTCOMES FOR ICU PATIENTS IN SUNNY VERSUS SUNLESS ROOMS

After finding that depressed patients in sunny rooms had shorter hospital stays than depressed patients in sunless rooms, two researchers wondered whether ICU patients in sunny rooms had better health outcomes than patients in sunless rooms. An experiment in a cardiac ICU was conducted to test this hypothesis (Beauchemin and Hays, 1998).

The sample was limited to patients in the ICU who had suffered a first-time heart attack. Only patients staying in north-facing (dark) rooms or south-facing (sunny) rooms were included in the study. Age, gender, length of stay, room brightness, and patient outcome were recorded for 628 patients admitted to the ICU over a four-year period.

Researchers found that patients in sunny rooms had shorter hospital stays than patients in dark rooms. Women in particular showed a significant difference in the average length of stay: 2.3 days in the sunny rooms and 3.3 days in the darker rooms. Health trends indicate that women who have heart attacks tend to do less well than men (Beauchemin and Hays, 1998). However, in this study, the women treated in the sunny rooms did just as well as men.

Findings also revealed that deaths were consistently more frequent in the dark rooms, compared to the sunny rooms, in each of the four years studied. However, the researchers recommended further investigation of this relationship within a controlled experiment before making any conclusions.

As discussed earlier in this chapter, several studies indicate that exposure to sunlight can reduce depression, agitation, pain, and length of stay (Beauchemin and Hays, 1996, 1998; Benedetti, 2001; Ulrich et al., 2006; Walch et al., 2005). These studies provide strong support for providing windows in ICU patient rooms. If windows are not possible or do not provide enough natural lighting, other sources of bright light should be considered (see "Lighting" section earlier in this chapter). (See Research Box 7.14.)

Addressing ICU Visitors' Needs

Family members of ICU patients suffer great stress. They are worried about the welfare of their loved ones and about a questionable future. They often feel helpless as a result of being able to do little that will help their loved one. They may need to alter familiar patterns and roles, such as when adult children are faced with making decisions for their parents. (See Research Box 7.15.)

RESEARCH BOX 7.15 CARING FOR FAMILIES OF CRITICALLY ILL PATIENTS

When hospital staff pay attention to the needs of family and friends visiting critically ill patients, they help reduce anxiety for patients and families. Such care may engender positive feelings on the part of visitors toward the hospital and its staff (Molter, 1979).

To better understand ICU visitors' needs, one researcher questioned the relatives of 40 patients who had just moved to the general ward after at least three days in an ICU (Leske, 1986; Molter, 1979). The relatives were asked to evaluate each of 45 need statements and to indicate whether that need had been met and by whom. A follow-up interview ascertained demographics and information about whether relatives had other needs not covered in the inventory.

Results showed that although relatives' priorities differed, there was a consensus about their greatest needs. At least three of four respondents considered a combination of cognitive and emotional needs most important: to feel hope; to get good, timely, and understandable information from physicians and nurses about the patient's condition and progress; and to feel that the hospital staff cares about the patient and accepts the relatives' presence. At the next level of importance, many relatives ranked a variety of personal needs, such as having a restroom and telephone near the waiting area, comfortable furniture, a chaplain available to visit, and good food in the cafeteria.

Although the sample size was too small to determine statistically significant differences, the results suggested that younger visitors, 18–34 years old, felt more of a need for more detailed information about patient care and wayfinding than did visitors in other age categories. Whether this stemmed from having less experience in hospital settings or more education was not discussed. For lower socio-economic-status relatives, obtaining daily information from the physician, getting a chaplain's support, having a nearby telephone, and being allowed to visit at any hour were of greater importance than for other groups. But notably, none of these needs ranked among the top 10 overall.

Most of the time, relatives felt their needs were met, although often through their own resources, whether drawing on inner strength and religious beliefs or obtaining help from other hospital personnel not directly involved in patient care.

Only four of the important or very important needs were not met more than half the time. Of these, being able to talk to the physician daily and being informed by staff of a chaplain's services drew the most comments. Yet, paradoxically, although relatives appreciated the attention given them by staff, they did not necessarily expect it. Contrary to notions of offering "total patient care" that focuses on the needs of both patients and families, relatives in this study frequently saw healthcare as patient-centered and did not expect staff to be concerned about them (Craig, Cioni, and Morrison, 1986; Dyer, 1991; Leske, 1986; Molter, 1979).

Making relatives feel more involved in the treatment process requires a proactive program on the part of the staff, and several models toward that end have been proposed (Craig et al., 1986; Dyer, 1991; Simpson, 1991; Vogelsang, 1988). The common element is a coordinated program to meet relatives' most pressing needs for regular and accurate information, emotional support, and wayfinding ease.

Although ICU visitors want to help and comfort patients, they have traditionally been allowed only very short visits. And they must stay close by in case things take a turn for the worse. Their plight is one of frustration and worry. A dedicated ICU waiting area should be provided that offers comfort, privacy, and access to amenities. (For details on waiting area design, see chapter 5.) There should be good visual access between the waiting area and attending staff and direct access to information about the patient. Artwork, plants, and other items of visual interest should be provided, including, if possible, an outside view to nature. ICU waiting areas should include zones designed for sleeping, because companions of ICU patients often spend the night. Couches or fold-out beds will allow visitors to rest at least somewhat comfortably. Consultation and grieving rooms should be located adjacent to ICU waiting areas so that, particularly when a patient dies, family members can cope with their loss in private. (Consultation and grieving rooms are discussed in chapter 10.)

Hospital decision-makers should not dismiss the emotional needs of family members who perform important functions valuable to the patient's care and well-being. The nurturing and support that patients receive from their families are therapeutic and can help them regain health (Molter, 1979).

Once hospital decision-makers recognize the importance of families and visitors as an integral part of ICU patient care, time and resources can be devoted to their needs. For example, the concept of "intensive care for relatives" has been developed where trained personnel work directly with family members, helping them understand medical procedures, giving needed emotional support, and, when necessary, helping them begin a healthy grieving process (Hoover, 1979). A program of this type minimizes the potential conflict over policy issues between medical staff and family, allowing everyone to participate in patient care.

Summary

○ Acute care inpatient rooms should be designed to meet the needs of patients and visitors for privacy, physical comfort, and ease of communication among themselves and with healthcare staff. Private and semi-private rooms should be available. Acuity-adaptable room design should be considered. There should be space for medical equipment and patient furniture, including the bed, patient chair, bedside stand, overbed table, wardrobe, flower shelf, and tackboard, as well as at least one visitor chair and, in single-patient rooms, a cot or sofa bed for overnight stays. There should be ample and unobstructed circulation areas for medical emergency teams to easily gain access to the patient, for the patient to navigate using a wheelchair, IV pole, or walker, and for visitors to provide social contact and support.

o   Design of inpatient rooms should maximize patient control over visual and acoustical privacy. Noise should be reduced as much as possible. Rooms should have an outside view. Natural lighting should be integrated with adjustable artificial lighting; measures should be taken to reduce glare. Controls should be within easy reach of both staff and patients. One television per patient is desirable. The choice of artwork should align with patient preferences. The therapeutic use of music should be considered, with patients having choice of and control over any music made available.

o   The inpatient bathroom must be designed for accessibility, safety, and ease of use. Furnishings should be easily reached and operated by all patients, whether short, tall, or using a mobility device, or with little strength or grasping ability. Towel racks and grab bars should support a person's weight. Water control levers or knobs should be labeled clearly. Sharp corners should be avoided; exposed pipes should be insulated; flooring and other surfaces should be non-slippery. The toilet and shower should be wheelchair-accessible and have ample room for two caregivers to assist the patient. The emergency call cord should be within easy reach of a seated or standing patient or one who has fallen. The bathroom should be well ventilated and acoustically insulated, with nighttime lighting and a door that can be opened from the outside.

o   An attractive inpatient lounge offers a change of scene and can encourage patients to get out of bed as part of the recovery process. It should be centrally located and designed to accommodate a variety of activities, with subspaces that can be defined by room dividers or moveable furnishings. A glass panel in or beside the door should allow patients to see inside the lounge before entering. There should also be a dedicated inpatient lounge for teenagers, with age-appropriate features such as a graffiti wall.

o   Family and visitors often spend long hours in a healthcare facility, providing important assistance and emotional support to patients. They need comfortable spaces and practical amenities to help them through such stressful situations. In the patient room they require at least one comfortable chair; a table for writing, eating meals, and using digital devices; and secure storage space for coats and personal belongings. Overnight accommodations, such as a cot or sofa bed, should be available in a private inpatient room. A family lounge, which may also be adaptable for overnight stays, offers a needed change of scene. It should be furnished with comfortable chairs, tables, areas for eating, beverage facilities, and perhaps a kitchenette. A children's area and a TV area should be provided. Both should be physically or at least acoustically separated from quieter portions of the space. Visitors need places to use and charge digital devices. Restrooms and family showers should be nearby. Laundry facilities are desirable, particularly on extended-stay patient floors.

○ The design of an ICU should act together with medical technology, healthcare staff, and hospital policies to create a humane setting for patients and families in this particularly stressful environment. Important provisions for patient privacy include solid partitions and glass doors to separate patients from one another, arrangements to shield patients from public view, acoustical privacy for confidential conversations, and a space for staff to confer, away from but close by, the patient area.

○ Sensory overload and challenges of maintaining family support can be addressed by providing ample space and comfortable bedside chairs for family and visitors, minimizing contact with machinery, providing a clear view to the outside, including sky and ground, providing space for get-well cards and personal possessions, and avoiding visual elements that can be confusing, such as abstract art and patterned curtains. Every effort should be made to keep noise levels as low as possible. Temperature and lighting should be adjustable.

○ Each ICU area should have its own comfortable, amply-sized waiting area that provides both group spaces and private areas, including sleeping accommodations. Each ICU should have a private consultation or grieving room. Patient families should have opportunities to participate in patient care.

DISCUSSION QUESTIONS

1. What considerations and criteria determine the optimal size and layout of an inpatient room? What are some ways of analyzing room size?

2. What design features support visual privacy for patients?

3. What criteria should be considered in providing patients with a view to the outside?

4. What design features should be included on controls for the bed, nurse-call button, light, and television?

5. What are some design requirements for patient chairs?

6. What design elements enhance safety and accessibility in the patient bathroom?

7. Why are inpatient lounges desirable, and what design elements make them effective?

8. What design features are important in accommodating families and visitors on inpatient units?

9. What is "intensive care unit syndrome"? What design features can help mitigate it?

10. What design features can enhance patient privacy in the ICU?

11. What design features support the role of family and visitors in the ICU?

Design Review Questions

Acute Care Inpatient Rooms

Size and Layout

☐ Will full-scale mock-ups be developed to systematically evaluate proposed designs of acute care and ICU patient rooms?

☐ When deciding among room layouts for inboard, outboard, or nested bathrooms, and headwall or footwall placement, will the needs of patients and staff be considered for each unit? (Pati et al., 2009)

☐ Will acuity-adaptable patient room design, related space, and organizational needs be considered?

☐ Will decision-makers consider the pros and cons of placing the doorway in line with the foot of the bed versus placing it in line with the head of the bed?

☐ Will there be ample circulation space so medical emergency teams and equipment can easily reach patients?

☐ Will rooms be sized and arranged to maximize patient mobility, rehabilitation, weight-bearing exercise, and ambulation potential? (Facility Guidelines Institute, 2014)

☐ Will an easily accessible handwashing sink be provided at the entrance of each patient room? (Cahnman, 2010; Facility Guidelines Institute, 2014)

☐ Will ample space be provided for the bed, wardrobe, bedside stand, overbed table, and patient chair?

☐ Will patient rooms contain zones for staff, patient, and family?

☐ Will ample space be provided around the bed so visitors can place their chairs on either side?

☐ Will a well-lit, clear path be provided between the patient bed and the bathroom? (McCullough, 2010)

☐ Will decision-makers consider providing a ceiling-mounted lift system between bed and bathroom?

☐ Will ample, unobstructed circulation space be provided for wheelchairs, rolling IV poles, and walkers?

☐ Will space and accommodations be provided for a visitor to spend the night?

Number of Occupants

☐ Will both private and semi-private rooms be available?

☐ Will multiple-bed suites be available for patients hospitalized for extended periods of time?

Control Over Social Contact

Visual Privacy

☐ If a door-side window is provided, will patients be able to control its covering?

☐ For ground-level rooms with views to a courtyard or other exterior space, will tinted exterior windows or private porch areas outside patient rooms preserve patient privacy and prevent views into patient rooms? (Sherman et al., 2005)

☐ In a side-by-side bed scheme, will design decision-makers consider the lack of window view for the bed closer to the hallway and the lack of clear territory for visitors? (Reizenstein and Grant, 1981 [unpub. No. 1])

☐ In a toe-to-toe bed scheme, will design decision-makers consider the negative effects of having patients face each other? (Reizenstein and Grant, 1981 [unpub. No. 1])

☐ Will decision-makers consider providing motorized cubicle curtains with remote controls in areas other than ICUs where patients are most likely to be non-ambulatory and hospitalized for extended periods of time?

☐ Will measures be taken to protect the patient's medical information, including positioning medical charts and digital devices in nurses' stations or on charting carts so passersby cannot view them? (Dubbs, 2003)

☐ Will digital devices use screensavers or programs that time-out quickly?

Acoustical Privacy

☐ Will decision-makers consider providing walls between patients, rather than curtains, in order to promote acoustical privacy? (Barlas et al., 2001; Malcolm, 2005; Olsen and Sabin, 2003)

☐ In situations when staff need visual access to patients, will sound barriers rather than walls be considered in order to provide acoustical privacy? (Mazer, 2005)

☐ Will sound-attenuating materials be used in patient room walls? (Leibrock, 1990)

☐ Will fire-retardant, easily washable wall fabrics be considered in order to muffle sounds and protect walls from wheelchair abrasion? (Hiatt, 1991; Leibrock, 1990)

☐ Will a private room or setting be available where patients, visitors, and staff can hold confidential conversations? (Dubbs, 2003; Malcolm, 2005)

Design That Cares: Planning Health Facilities for Patients and Visitors, third edition, by Janet R. Carpman and Myron A. Grant. ©2016 by Jossey-Bass.

☐ Will only quiet functions be located near patient rooms?

☐ Will nurse and physician work areas be acoustically contained on patient floors?

Color

☐ Will colors be chosen based on the intended use of the space? (Tofle et al., 2004)

☐ Will geographic locations, user characteristics (such as age and culture), lighting sources, and size and shape of the room be considered in choosing colors? (Tofle et al., 2004)

☐ Will the personal preferences of design decision-makers be avoided when selecting colors? (Beach et al., 1988; Tofle et al., 2004; Young, 2007)

Lighting

☐ Will general room lighting be adjustable by multiple switching and/or rheostats? (Beck and Meyer, 1982; Fong, 2003; Fong and Nichelson, 2006; Hayward, 1974)

☐ Will the reflective properties of wall coverings, floors, and furnishings be considered in order to reduce glare? (Brainard, 1995; Fong and Nichelson, 2006)

☐ Will windows have blinds, shades, or drapes to reduce brightness or glare? (Fong, 2003; Fong and Nichelson, 2006)

☐ Will lighting controls be placed within easy reach of both staff and patients? (Fong and Nichelson, 2006)

☐ Will a reading light be available above or close to the patient's bed? (Beck and Meyer, 1982; Fong, 2003; Fong and Nichelson, 2006; Lam, 1977; Rosenfeld, 1971)

☐ Will light fixtures allow patients to adjust the light upward and downward? (Fong, 2003; Fong and Nichelson, 2006; Lam, 1977; Rosenfeld, 1971)

☐ Will nighttime lighting be provided to illuminate the path between the bed and the bathroom?

☐ Will lighting be avoided that casts shadows or lends an unnatural tone to the patient's skin? (Fong, 2003)

☐ Will a single lamp color be chosen for patient areas in order to maintain diagnostic consistency when staff assess skin color? (Fong, 2003; Fong and Nichelson, 2006)

☐ Will examination and general room lighting have color characteristics as close as possible to natural daylight? (Beck and Meyer, 1982)

☐ Will a lamp color with a Color Rendering Index in the mid-80,000s and color temperature between 3,000 and 3,500 degrees Kelvin be chosen in order to provide neutral lighting that brings out the true colors of objects? (Fong and Nichelson, 2006)

☐ Will daylight and indirect artificial lighting be integrated into patient rooms? (Fong, 2003; Fong and Nichelson, 2006)

☐ Will indirect lighting, such as lights with dimmers, recessed downlights, or wallwashers, be provided in patient rooms? (Boyce, 1981; Fong and Nichelson, 2006; Rosenfeld, 1971)

☐ Will a mix of fluorescent and incandescent lighting be considered? (Boyce, 1981)

Inpatient Room Furnishings
Patient Beds and Chairs

☐ Will controls for the bed, nurse-call button, light, and television be easy to understand and operate by patients who are lying flat or sitting upright? (Carpman and Grant, 1984 [unpub. No. 25]; Soloman and Gaudette, 1984)

☐ Will controls be lighted for nighttime use? (Carpman and Grant, 1984 [unpub. No. 25]; Soloman and Gaudette, 1984)

☐ Will controls be operable with either hand? (Carpman and Grant, 1984 [unpub. No. 25]; Soloman and Gaudette, 1984)

☐ Will pressure-sensitive control buttons be available for patients who have difficulty with hand manipulation? (Carpman and Grant, 1984 [unpub. No. 25]; Soloman and Gaudette, 1984)

☐ Will standing assists, such as bedrails, be provided? (Carpman and Grant, 1984 [unpub. No. 25]; Facility Guidelines Institute, 2014; Soloman and Gaudette, 1984)

☐ Will the telephone be easy to reach and manipulate with either hand? (Carpman and Grant, 1984 [unpub. No. 25]; Soloman and Gaudette, 1984)

☐ Will patient chairs be comfortable for extended periods? (Carpman and Grant, 1984 [unpub. No. 25]; Soloman and Gaudette, 1984)

☐ Will patient chairs provide back and lumbar support? (Carpman and Grant, 1984 [unpub. No. 25]; Soloman and Gaudette, 1984)

☐ Will patient chairs be easy to get into and out of? (Carpman and Grant, 1984 [unpub. No. 25]; Soloman and Gaudette, 1984)

☐ Will patient chairs have sturdy and comfortable arms? (Carpman and Grant, 1984 [unpub. No. 25]; Soloman and Gaudette, 1984)

☐ Will patient chairs be easy to move? (Carpman and Grant, 1984 [unpub. No. 25]; Soloman and Gaudette, 1984)

☐ Will patients be able to elevate their feet while sitting in the chair? (Carpman and Grant, 1984 [unpub. No. 25]; Lowry, 1989; Soloman and Gaudette, 1984)

☐ Will trip hazards, such as separate footstools or ottomans, be avoided? (Carpman and Grant, 1984 [unpub. No. 25]; Facility Guidelines Institute, 2014; Soloman and Gaudette, 1984)

☐ Will chair coverings be easy to clean and comfortable to sit on? (Baier, 1989; Carpman and Grant, 1984 [unpub. No. 25]; Reizenstein, Vaitkus, and Grant, 1982; Soloman and Gaudette, 1984)

☐ Will patient chairs be adjustable in order to accommodate patients who vary in size, weight, and physical condition? (Carpman and Grant, 1984 [unpub. No. 25]; Soloman and Gaudette, 1984)

☐ Will chairs have legs that do not extend laterally or forward beyond the chair seat? (Carpman and Grant, 1984 [unpub. No. 25]; Facility Guidelines Institute, 2014; Soloman and Gaudette, 1984)

☐ To facilitate ease of sitting and rising, will chairs have armrests extending to the front edge of the chair and open space below the front for placement of the patient's feet? (Carpman and Grant, 1984 [unpub. No. 25])

☐ Will chairs be available that can accommodate obese patients? (Carpman and Grant, 1984 [unpub. No. 25]; Soloman and Gaudette, 1984)

Storage for Belongings: Overbed Tables

☐ Will the overbed table be stable and easy to operate by people with limited dexterity? Will it be easily adjustable to various heights?

☐ Will staff be trained to show patients and visitors how to use overbed tables?

☐ Will storage space be provided inside the overbed table, with easy access from both sides?

☐ Will the overbed table contain an adjustable mirror that can be used from either side?

☐ Will the drawer and mirror be located inside the overbed table, easy to manipulate by people with limited dexterity?

☐ Will the overbed table be usable as a writing surface when the patient is sitting in a chair? (Carpman and Grant, 1984 [unpub. No. 25]; Soloman and Gaudette, 1984)

Design That Cares: Planning Health Facilities for Patients and Visitors, third edition, by Janet R. Carpman and Myron A. Grant. ©2016 by Jossey-Bass.

Storage for Belongings: Bedside Stands

☐ Will bedside stands provide easy access by bedridden patients to the top surface and drawers?

☐ Will the drawers of the bedside stand be easy to open by patients with limited dexterity? (Carpman and Grant, 1984 [unpub. No. 25]; King et al., 1982; Soloman and Gaudette, 1984)

Storage for Belongings: Wardrobes

☐ Will wardrobes have sufficient capacity to store winter outerwear, shoes or boots, some clothing, underwear, a suitcase, and other small possessions?

☐ Will a lockable drawer be provided within the wardrobe?

☐ Will the wardrobe be easily opened and closed by people with limited dexterity?

☐ Will the clothes rod be accessible by wheelchair users?

☐ Will the wardrobe be located so it will not impede circulation or other patient room functions?

☐ Will the wardrobe contain hooks for bathrobes and other clothing? (Reizenstein and Grant, 1982)

Storage for Belongings: Other

☐ Will a tackboard be provided so patients can display cards and mementos? (Reizenstein et al., 1982)

☐ Will a shelf be provided for displaying flowers and other personal items? (Reizenstein et al., 1982)

☐ Will the flower shelf be wide enough and have sufficient vertical clearance to accommodate large flower arrangements? (Reizenstein et al., 1982)

☐ Will the flower shelf be positioned so it will not be bumped?

☐ Will the flower shelf be free of sharp corners? (Reizenstein et al., 1982)

☐ Will hooks be available for visitors' coats behind the door or in some other location that will not obstruct views or circulation? (Reizenstein et al., 1982)

Televisions

☐ Will television services be available that include on-demand, patient-education programs and interactive features?

☐ Will individual televisions be provided in semi-private rooms?

☐ Will personal audio devices be provided, such as pillow speakers or earphones?

Clocks

☐ Will a clock be placed in each patient room? Will it be visible from the bed, yet not directly in the patient's line of sight?

☐ If analog clocks are used, will they have clear numbers, as well as hour, minute, and second hands legible from the bed?

☐ Will patient clocks reflect the dominant culture, by using either 12-hour or 24-hour systems?

Artwork

☐ Will an art cart program be available so patients can choose the artwork in their rooms? (Carpman and Grant, 1984 [unpub. No. 32]; Nanda et al., 2007; Nanda et al., 2008)

☐ Will locations for hanging artwork be selected so patients can see artwork from their beds? (Carpman and Grant, 1984 [unpub. No. 32]; Nanda, 2006)

☐ Will artwork be available with nature-related subjects and settings? (Carpman and Grant, 1984 [unpub. No. 32]; Miller and Goldman, 1984; Nanda, 2006; Nanda et al., 2008)

☐ Will representational art be available? (Carpman and Grant, 1984 [unpub. No. 32]; Miller and Goldman, 1984; Nanda et al., 2008)

☐ Will photographs or reproductions be available? (Carpman and Grant, 1984 [unpub. No. 32])

☐ Will texturally complex images be available? (Carpman and Grant, 1984 [unpub. No. 32])

☐ Will mobiles be available? (Carpman and Grant, 1984 [unpub. No. 32])

☐ Will the following types of artwork be avoided: urban scenes, portraits, muted or dark colors, posters with words? (Carpman and Grant, 1984 [unpub. No. 32])

☐ When selecting artwork, will decision-makers consider differences between designers' and patients' preferences? (Nanda et al., 2008)

☐ Will virtual skylights or virtual windows depicting nature settings be considered for windowless rooms? (Corcoran, 2007)

An Outside View

☐ Will patient room windows be as large as possible?

☐ Will window sills be ~20–30 inches (~50.8–76.2 centimeters) high to allow outside views by patients in beds and wheelchairs? (Cooper Marcus and Barnes, 1999)

☐ Will windows be positioned so bedridden patients can see both sky and ground? (Cooper Marcus and Barnes, 1999; Verderber and Reuman, 1987)

☐ Will angling the bed be considered, so patients can easily see out of the window? (Zeit, 2013)

☐ Will the potential be minimized for views from the outside into ground-floor patient rooms? (Cooper Marcus and Barnes, 1999)

☐ Will tinted windows and private porch areas outside ground-floor patient rooms be considered in order to preserve privacy? (Sherman et al., 2005)

☐ Will there be views to street-level activities? (Verderber and Reuman, 1987)

☐ Will there be unobstructed visual access to the window? (Verderber and Reuman, 1987)

☐ Will window coverings be easily manipulated by patients and visitors? Can patients control window coverings from the bed? (Cullinan and Wolf, 2010)

☐ Will window coverings allow the room to be completely darkened at night? (Patient Rooms, 2014)

☐ Will windows avoid undue heat gain?

Reducing Noise on Acute Care Units

☐ Will efforts be made to reduce noise in the acute care unit, including insulating rooms, installing hydraulic door closers and rubber pads on door frames, lowering the volume of phones and medical equipment, and using padded charts and chart racks? (Cmiel et al., 2004; Grumet, 1993; Mazer, 2005)

☐ Will sound-absorbing materials be used in patient rooms? (Hiatt, 1991; Leibrock, 1990)

☐ Will patient rooms be located near quiet, rather than noisy, work areas?

☐ Will staff work areas on patient floors be acoustically contained?

Using Music Therapeutically

☐ Before music is offered to patients, will the patient's history and medical condition be assessed to determine potential adverse effects of music? (Brown and Theorell, 2005)

☐ Will music be considered as a supplementary pain management method and as a way to reduce anxiety in patients recovering from surgery?

☐ Will patients be offered guided imagery, with or without music, and other relaxation techniques?

☐ Will patients be able to choose from a variety of music selections?

☐ Will cultural preferences be considered in the type of music offered?

☐ Will the known effects of different types of music be considered?

☐ Will music known to increase anxiety not be offered to patients?

☐ Will staff ensure that music is not too loud or played for too long? (Cardozo, 2004; Cooke et al., 2005; Henry, 1995)

☐ Will individual music-listening devices with headphones be available (as opposed to using piped-in music)?

☐ Will accommodations be made to provide access to music for people with hearing limitations?

Inpatient Bathrooms

☐ Will easy access be provided from the bathroom threshold to the sink, toilet, and shower for patients using walkers, wheelchairs, or IV poles? (Heulat, 1991)

☐ Will ample space be available for staff to assist patients?

☐ Will the bathroom door swing allow sufficient clearance?

☐ Will the bathroom door be openable from the outside?

☐ Will nighttime lighting be provided?

☐ Will the bathroom be well ventilated, with a mechanical ventilation system that meets code or provides approximately ten air changes per hour? (Facility Guidelines Institute, 2014)

☐ Will the bathroom be acoustically insulated to help ensure privacy?

Sink Area

☐ To accommodate both ambulatory patients and those using wheelchairs, will the sink be at least 34½ inches (~87.6 centimeters) and no more than 36½ inches (~92.7 centimeters) high? Will it meet all applicable codes? (Kira, 1977)

☐ Will sink undersides be smooth and free from obstructions? (Kira, 1977)

☐ Will exposed pipes be insulated in order to prevent burns and other injuries? (Kira, 1977)

☐ Will the sink be large enough to accommodate a small basin?

☐ Can water-control levers or knobs be reached and operated by patients with little strength or grasping ability?

☐ Will water-control levers or knobs be labeled clearly?

☐ Will the mirror be selected and positioned (or adjusted) so it can be seen by tall or ambulatory patients as well as by wheelchair users, short, or seated patients?

☐ Will electrical outlets for hair dryers and shavers be located in close, yet safe, proximity to the sink and mirror? (Bergstrom et al., 1985)

☐ Will electrical outlets be positioned so they can be reached by wheelchair users or seated patients?

☐ Will storage shelves be large enough to hold patients' toiletries? (Reizenstein et al., 1982)

☐ Will storage shelves be free from sharp corners? (Reizenstein et al., 1982)

☐ Will shelves be positioned so they can be easily reached by wheelchair users? (King et al., 1982)

☐ Will towel racks be strong enough to support a patient's weight?

☐ Will towel racks be large enough to hold a washcloth and face towel for each patient?

Shower Area

☐ Will nonslip flooring be installed? (Bergstrom et al., 1985; Kira, 1977)

☐ Will a portable or foldable seat be provided? (King et al., 1982; Kira, 1977)

☐ Will the shower seat be comfortable and non-slippery?

☐ Will space in the shower area be provided for two caregivers to assist a patient?

☐ Will the shower area be designed so a patient can transfer between a wheelchair and a shower seat?

☐ Will grab bars provide support as patients rise from a shower seat, transfer from a wheelchair, or stand?

☐ Will shower controls and the shower head be operable by patients with little strength or grasping ability?

☐ Will shower controls be easy to read and understand by patients standing a few feet away?

☐ Will patients be able to reach shower controls and the nozzle from both seated and standing positions? (Kira, 1977)

☐ Will a handheld shower head be provided? (King et al., 1982; Kira, 1977)

☐ Will an emergency call cord be within easy reach of a seated or standing patient or one who has fallen? Will a soap dish and a space for shampoo be within easy reach of a seated or standing patient? (Bergstrom et al., 1985)

☐ Will hooks for clothing and towels be available in close proximity to the shower, but outside the spray area? (Bergstrom et al., 1985; King, et al., 1982)

Toilet Area

☐ Will ample space be provided in front of and directly alongside the toilet for two caregivers to assist a patient transferring from a wheelchair? (Bergstrom et al., 1985; Kira, 1977)

☐ Will the toilet area be designed so a patient can sit on the toilet and use the sink? (Bergstrom et al., 1985; Hickler, 1969)

☐ Will grab bars be provided as supports for patients sitting and rising? (Bergstrom et al., 1985)

☐ Will toilets be high enough to facilitate easy wheelchair transfer and comfortable use by older patients?

☐ Will the toilet paper dispenser be within easy reach of a patient seated on the toilet? (Bergstrom et al., 1985; King et al., 1982)

☐ Will the toilet flushing lever be positioned within easy reach of a patient seated on the toilet? (King et al., 1982; Kira, 1977)

☐ Will the toilet flushing lever be operable by patients with little strength or grasping ability? (King et al., 1982; Kira, 1977)

☐ Will patients be able to reach an emergency call cord from the toilet? (Bergstrom et al., 1985)

☐ Will there be a storage area easily reached from the toilet? (Bergstrom et al., 1985; Kira, 1977)

Inpatient Lounges

☐ Will inpatient lounges be centrally located? (Chaudhury et al., 2005; Joseph, 2006b; Spear, 1997)

☐ Will inpatient lounges be designed to accommodate all the activities that will occur there? (Chaudhury et al., 2005; Spear, 1997)

Design That Cares: Planning Health Facilities for Patients and Visitors, third edition, by Janet R. Carpman and Myron A. Grant. ©2016 by Jossey-Bass.

☐ Will subspaces be easily formed using furnishings or dividers? (Chaudhury et al., 2005; Janssen et al., 2000)

☐ Will glass panels be provided in doors or walls to allow patients to see inside lounges before entering? (Pease, 2002)

☐ Will a dedicated inpatient lounge be provided for teenagers? (St. Louis Children's Hospital, 2014)

Accommodating Visitors

☐ Will at least one comfortable, moveable chair be provided for visitors, positioned within easy conversational distance of the bedridden patient?

☐ Will secure storage space be provided for visitors' coats and personal belongings?

Providing for Mealtimes

☐ Will visitors have a comfortable place to sit and eat in the patient room? (Reizenstein and Grant, 1981 [unpub. No. 2])

Providing a Place to Spend the Night

☐ Will a cot or pull-out sofa bed be available for visitors who wish to spend the night? (Arneill and Frasca-Beaulieu, 2003)

☐ Will a family shower and changing room be available in the facility? (Facility Guidelines Institute, 2014)

Family Lounges

☐ Will family lounges be located near patient units?

☐ Will family lounges include areas for eating and food preparation?

☐ Will family lounges provide Wi-Fi and electrical outlets for charging digital devices?

☐ Will restrooms be located nearby?

☐ Will the TV area be separated from quieter portions of the space?

☐ Will visitor laundry facilities be available on extended-stay patient floors?

☐ Will child-friendly areas be available; separate from quieter areas of the lounge but visually connected with it?

Intensive Care Units

Providing Control Over Social Contact

☐ Will sliding-glass doors (for visual monitoring) and solid partitions or walls be considered in order to separate patients from one another and provide acoustical privacy? (Barlas et al., 2001; Hickler, 1969; Malcolm, 2005; Olsen and Sabin, 2003)

☐ Will patients be shielded from public view, as desired? (Clipson and Wehrer, 1973)

☐ Will acoustical privacy be provided for patients so they can have confidential conversations? (Barlas et al., 2001; Clipson and Wehrer, 1973; Dubbs, 2003; Malcolm, 2005)

☐ To ensure confidentiality and decrease anxiety, will space be availabe for staff to confer away from, but close by, the patient area? (Clipson and Wehrer, 1973)

☐ Will acoustical and visual privacy be provided for patients using the bedpan or commode? Will this equipment be stored out of sight? (Clipson and Wehrer, 1973)

☐ Will digital screens and medical records in nurses' stations and on charting carts be positioned so passersby cannot view them? (Dubbs, 2003)

Addressing Sensory Overload and Challenges of Maintaining Family Support

☐ Will ample space and comfortable bedside chairs be provided for families and visitors? (Clipson and Wehrer, 1973; Relman, 2014)

☐ Will there be ways for patients and staff to keep each other within view? (Clipson and Wehrer, 1973; Sturdavant, 1960)

☐ When a patient is well enough to receive and make calls, will a telephone be available within easy reach of the bed? (Clipson and Wehrer, 1973)

☐ Will a large clock and a calendar be in clear view, but not directly in front of each patient? (Kornfeld, 1972; Task Force on Guidelines, 1988)

☐ Will each patient have a clear view to the outside and will this view include sky and ground? (Clipson and Wehrer, 1973; Hickler, 1969; Keep, 1977; Keep et al., 1980; Popkin, 1980)

☐ Will patient contact with machinery be minimized? (Clipson and Wehrer, 1973; Duffy and Florell, 1990; Zubatkin, 1980)

☐ Will patients be able to display personal possessions or cards by their bedsides? (Clipson and Wehrer, 1973)

Design That Cares: Planning Health Facilities for Patients and Visitors, third edition, by Janet R. Carpman and Myron A. Grant. ©2016 by Jossey-Bass.

☐ Will paintings or other artwork be available?

☐ Will design elements that can be confusing, such as abstract art or patterned curtains, be avoided? (Williams, 1991)

Reducing Noise in ICUs

☐ Will staff be periodically reminded to reduce ambient noise, particularly at night?

☐ Will noise attenuation be considered in the design of the ICU (for example, locating nurses' stations and reception areas away from patient rooms, creating fully enclosed patient rooms, and so on)? (Joseph and Ulrich, 2007; Kam et al., 1994; Petterson, 2000)

☐ Will sound-absorbing ceiling tiles be installed? (Berg, 2001; Joseph and Ulrich, 2007)

☐ Will hallways, nurses' stations, and patient rooms be insulated? (Kam et al., 1994)

☐ Will there be a dedicated service corridor? (Wang et al., 2013)

☐ Will acoustical standards be established and followed when decision-makers select new medical equipment? (Mazer, 2006)

☐ Will the volume of telephones and medical equipment alerts be set to the lowest level consistent with good care? (Cmiel et al., 2004; Hilton, 1985; Task Force on Guidelines, 1988)

☐ Will cell phones or wireless communication devices, rather than potentially noisy pagers, be carried by staff? (Joseph and Ulrich, 2007)

☐ Will there be padding at the bottom of patient chart holders, medical carts, and receptacles of pneumatic tubing systems? (Cmiel et al., 2004)

☐ Will maintenance activities (for example, floor cleaning) be scheduled to minimize sleep disturbances? (Snyder-Halpern, 1985; Whitfield, 1975)

Music in ICUs

☐ If patients wish to listen to music, will there be a variety of music choices and individual listening devices available?

Patient Comfort in ICUs

☐ Will windows be provided in ICU patient rooms? Will patients have exposure to sunlight or other sources of bright light?

☐ Will window shades, dimmers, and other controls be available so patients can adjust lighting? (Clipson and Wehrer, 1973; Fong, 2003; Fong and Nichelson, 2006)

☐   Will windows and light fixtures be free of glare? (Clipson and Wehrer, 1973; Fong and Nichelson, 2006)

☐   Will lighting at the nurses' station be designed so it does not disturb resting patients? (Clipson and Wehrer, 1973)

☐   Will nighttime lighting be positioned so staff can monitor sleeping patients without disturbing them? (Clipson and Wehrer, 1973)

☐   Will ICU room temperatures be adjustable in order to accommodate patients' needs and preferences? (Clipson and Wehrer, 1973)

☐   Will a relative humidity level of 50 percent be maintained in patient areas? (Hickler, 1969)

☐   Will a comfortable chair be located near the patient bed? (Clipson and Wehrer, 1973)

Addressing ICU Visitors' Needs

☐   Will each ICU area have its own visitor waiting area?

☐   Will the ICU waiting area be comfortable and large enough to accommodate visitors and families?

☐   Will the ICU waiting area offer group spaces and private areas?

☐   Will couches or fold-out beds be available?

☐   Will visitors in the waiting area have access to information about their patient?

☐   Will family members be able to participate in ICU patient care?

☐   Will each ICU area have its own private consultation or grieving room?

Design That Cares: Planning Health Facilities for Patients and Visitors, third edition, by Janet R. Carpman and Myron A. Grant. ©2016 by Jossey-Bass.

References

Alexander, M. E. No windows. *Lancet* 1(7802):549, March 10, 1973.

Arneill, B., and Frasca-Beaulieu, K. Healing environments: Architecture and design conducive to health. In S. Frampton, L. Gilpin, and P. Charmel, editors. *Putting Patients First: Designing and Practicing Patient-Centered Care*, 163–90. San Francisco: Jossey-Bass, 2003.

Baier, S. Patient perspective. In Proceedings from the First Annual National Symposium on Health Care Interior Design. *Journal of Health Care Design* 1:13–17, 1989.

Bakalar, N. Sleeping through noise, but still feeling its effects. *New York Times*, March 4, 2008, p. D6.

Balling, J. D., and Falk, J. H. Development of visual preference for natural environments. *Environment and Behavior* 14(1):5–28, 1982.

Balogh, D., Kittinger, E., Benzer, A., and Hackl, J. M. Noise in the ICU. *Intensive Care Medicine* 19(6):343–46, 1993.

Barker, M. People-oriented design. *Hospital Forum* 35:36, July–August 1985.

Barlas, D., Sama, A. E., Ward, M. F., and Lesser, M. L. Comparison of the auditory and visual privacy of emergency department treatment areas with curtains versus those with solid walls. *Annals of Emergency Medicine* 38(2):135–39, August 2001.

Barnason, S., Zimmerman, L., and Nieveen, J. The effects of music interventions on anxiety in the patient after coronary artery bypass grafting. *Heart and Lung* 24(2):124–32, March–April 1995.

Baron, J. H., and Greene, L. Art in hospitals. *British Medial Journal* 289(22):1731–37, December 1984.

Battisto, D., and Allison, D. A patient room prototype: Bridging design and research. *Practicing Architecture / Knowledge Communities*. 2014. www.aia.org/practicing/groups/kc/AIAS076322.

Beach, L. R., Wise, B., and Wise, J.A. The human factors of color in environmental design [microform]: A critical review. Moffett Field, CA: National Aeronautics and Space Administration, Ames Research Center, 1988.

Beauchemin, K. M., and Hays, P. Dying in the dark: Sunshine, gender and outcomes in myocardial infarction. *Journal of the Royal Society of Medicine* 91(7):352–54, July 1998.

_____. Sunny hospital rooms expedite recovery from severe and refractory depressions. *Journal of Affective Disorders* 40(1–2):9–51, September 9, 1996.

Beck, W., and Meyer, R. *The Health Care Environment: The User's Viewpoint.* Boca Raton, FL: CRC Press, 1982.

Beckman, R. Getting up and getting out: Progressive patient care. *Progressive Architecture* 55(11):64–68, November 1974.

Ben-Abraham, R., Keller, N., Szold, O., Vardi, A., Weinberg, M., Barzilay, Z., et al. Do isolation rooms reduce the rate of nosocomial infections in the pediatric intensive care unit? *Journal of Critical Care* 17(3):176–80, September 2002.

Benedetti, F. Morning sunlight reduces length of hospitalization in bipolar depression. *Journal of Affective Disorders* 62(3):221–23, February 2001.

Benya, J. R. Lighting for healing. In Proceedings from the First Annual National Symposium on Health Care Interior Design. *Journal of Health Care Design* 1:55–58, 1989.

Berg, S. Impact of reduced reverberation time on sound-induced arousals during sleep. *Sleep* 24(3):289–92, 2001.

Bergstrom, E., Cooper, D., and Simonsson, J. Bathrooms, for the disabled. *Nursing Mirror* 160(25):21–24, June 1985.

Bernardo, J. R. What color reveals: A therapist's point of view. *Color Research and Application* 8(1):5–11, 1983.

Birren, F. Human response to color and light. *Hospitals* 53(14):93–96, July 16, 1979.

Blumberg, R., and Devlin, A. S. Design issues in hospitals: The adolescent client. *Environment and Behavior* 38(3):293–317, May 2006.

Bobrow, M. L., and Thomas, J. Achieving quality in hospital design. *Hospital Forum* 19(4):4–6, September 1976.

Boyce, P. R. *Human Factors in Lighting.* New York: Macmillan, 1981.

Brainard, G. The future is now: Implications of the effect of light on hormones, brain, and behavior. *Journal of Healthcare Design* 7:49–56, 1995.

Brown, S., and Theorell, T. The social uses of background music for personal enhancement. In S. Brown and U. Volgsten, editors. *Music and Manipulation: On the Social Uses and Social Control of Music,* 126–60. New York: Berghahn Books, 2005.

Bunker-Hellmich, L. Interiors: Patient focus. *Health Facilities Management.* March 1, 2010. www .hfmmagazine.com/display/HFM-news-article.dhtml?dcrPath=/templatedata/HF_Common /NewsArticle/data/HFM/Magazine/2010/Mar/1003HFM_FEA_Interiors.

Cahnman, S. F. Key considerations in patient room design: 2010 update. *Healthcare Design.* July 31, 2010. www.healthcaredesignmagazine.com/article/key-considerations-patient-room-design-2010-update.

Cardozo, M. Harmonic sounds: Complementary medicine for the critically ill. *Journal of Nursing* 13(22):1321–24, 2004.

Carpman, J. R., and Grant, M. A. Hospital patient room furnishings mock-ups. Unpublished research report No. 25. Patient and Visitor Participation Project, Office of Hospital Planning, Research and Development, University of Michigan, Ann Arbor, 1984.

_____. Inpatient preferences for hospital room artwork. Unpublished research report No. 32, Patient and Visitor Participation Project, Office of the Replacement Hospital Program, University of Michigan, Ann Arbor, 1984.

_____. TVs in hospitals: Behavior and preferences. Unpublished research report No. 11, Patient and Visitor Participation Project, Office of Hospital Planning, Research and Development, University of Michigan, Ann Arbor, 1984.

Cepeda, M. S., Carr, D. B., Lau, J., and Alvarez, H. Music for pain relief. *Cochrane Database of Systematic Reviews* 4, 2006.

Chan, M. F., Wong, O. C., Chan, H. L., Fong, M. C., Lai, S. Y., Lo, C. W., et al. Effects of music on patients undergoing a C-clamp procedure after percutaneous coronary interventions. *Journal of Advanced Nursing* 53(6), 669–79, March 2006.

Chaney, P. S. Décor reflects environmental psychology. *Hospitals* 47(11):61–66, June 1, 1973.

Changing the Concept of Families as Visitors. Institute for Patient- and Family-Centered Care. 2014. www.ipfcc.org/advance/topics/family-presence.html.

Chapman, J. S. The relation between auditory stimulation of short gestation infants and their gross motor limb activity. Unpublished PhD diss. New York University, New York City, 1975. [Available from ProQuest, 789 E. Eisenhower Parkway, Ann Arbor, MI 48108.]

Chaudhury, H., Mahmood, A., and Valente, M. Advantages and disadvantages of single- versus multiple-occupancy rooms in acute care environments. A review and analysis of the literature. *Environment and Behavior* 37(6):760–86, November 2005.

Chlan, L. L. Music therapy as a nursing intervention for patients supported by mechanical ventilation. *AACN Advanced Critical Care* 11(1):128–38, 2000.

Clipson, C. W., and Wehrer, J. I. *Planning for Cardiac Care: A Guide to the Planning and Design of Cardiac Care Facilities.* Ann Arbor, MI: Health Administration Press, 1973.

Cmiel, C. A., Karr, D. M., Gasser, D. M., Oliphant, L. M., and Neveau, A. J. Noise control: A nursing team's approach to sleep promotion: Respecting the silence creates a healthier environment for your patients. *American Journal of Nursing* 104(2):40–48, February 2004.

Collins, B. L. *Windows and People: A Literature Survey.* Washington, DC: US Government Printing Office, 1975.

Cooke, M., Chaboyer, W., and Hiratos, M. A. Music and its effect on anxiety in short waiting periods: A critical appraisal. *Journal of Clinical Nursing* 14(2):145–55, February 2005.

Cooper Marcus, C., and Barnes, M. *Healing Gardens: Therapeutic Benefits and Design Recommendations.* New York: Wiley, 1999.

Corcoran, S. The art of nature and the nature of art. *Healthcare Design* 7(8):78–79, October 2007.

Craig, R., Cioni, D., and Morrison, C. Families of your surgical patients. *Journal of Post Anesthesia Nursing* 1(3):170–74, August 1986.

Cullinan, K., and Wolf, M. The patient room: What is the ideal solution? *Design Dilemma DEA 4350.* November 8, 2010. http://iwsp.human.cornell.edu/file_uploads/iwsp_4530_2010_dilemma_wolf -callinan.pdf.

D'Alessio, A. Marshall Erdman's art program: Art as medicine. *Group Practice Journal,* 72–80, September–October 1986.

Detsky, M. E., and Etchells, E. Single-patient rooms for safe patient-centered hospitals. *Journal of the American Medical Association* 300(8):954–56, 2008.

Dubbs, D. Privacy please! *Health Facilities Management* 16(8):20–24, August 2003.

Duffy, T. M., and Florell, J. M. Intensive care units. In Proceedings from the Second Symposium on Health Care Interior Design. *Journal of Health Care Design* 2:167–79, 1990.

Dyer, I. D. Meeting the needs of visitors: A practical approach. *Intensive Care Nursing* 7:135–47, 1991.

Edge, K. J. Wall color of patient's room: Effects on recovery. Unpublished master's thesis. University of Florida, 2003.

Edwards, K. The environment inside the hospital. *Practitioner* 222(1332):746–51, June 1979.

Evans, D. The effectiveness of music as an intervention for hospital patients: A systematic review. *Journal of Advanced Nursing* 37(1):8–18, January 2002.

Facility Guidelines Institute. *Guidelines for Design and Construction of Hospitals and Outpatient Facilities.* Dallas, TX: American Institute of Architects/Facility Guidelines Institute, 2014.

Ferenc, J. A new vision of care. *Health Facilities Management.* February 3, 2014. www.hfmmagazine .com/display/HFM-news-article.dhtml?dcrPath=/templatedata/HF_Common/NewsArticle/data /HFM/Magazine/2014/Feb/0214HFM_FEA_Interview.

Flaherty, J. What would the ideal hospital look like in 2020? *Wired.* July 19, 2013. www.wired.com /2013/07/hospital-of-the-future/.

Fong, D. B. Illuminating thoughts: Devising lighting strategies for clinical spaces. *Health Facilities Management*, July 2003, 24–29.

Fong, D. B., and Nichelson, K. Evidence-based lighting design. *Healthcare Design*, September 2006, 6(5), 50–53.

Fontaine, D. K., Briggs L. P., and Pope-Smith, B. Designing humanistic critical care environments. *Critical Care Nursing Quarterly* 24:21–34, 2001.

Freedman, N. S., Gazendam, J., Levan, L., Pack, A. I., and Schwab, R. J. Abnormal sleep/wake cycles and the effect of environmental noise on sleep disruption in the intensive care unit. *American Journal of Respiratory Critical Care Medicine* 163(2):451–57, February 2001.

Freedman, N. S., Kotzer, N., and Schwab, R. J. Patient perception of sleep quality and etiology of sleep disruption in the intensive care unit. *American Journal of Respiratory Critical Care Medicine* 159(4):1155–62, April 1999.

Frellick, M. Innovators design hospital room of the future. *Medscape Medical News*. March 3, 2014. www.medscape.com/viewarticle/821339.

Gabor, J. Y., Cooper, A. B., Crombach, S. A., Lee, B., Kadikar, N., Bettger, H. E., et al. Contribution of the intensive care unit environment to sleep disruption in mechanically ventilated patients and health subjects. *American Journal of Respiratory and Critical Care Medicine* 167:708–15, 2003.

Gallant, D., and Lanning, K. Streamlining patient care processes through flexible room and equipment design. *Critical Care Nursing Quarterly* 24(3):59–76, November 2001.

Gowan, N. I. The perceptual world of the intensive care unit: An overview of some environmental considerations in the helping relationship. *Heart and Lung* 8(2):340–44, March–April 1979.

Grumet, G. W. Pandemonium in the modern hospital. *New England Journal of Medicine* 1993, 328(6), 433–37, February 11.

Guidelines/Practice Parameters Committee of the American College of Critical Care Medicine, Society of Critical Care Medicine. Guidelines for intensive care unit design. *Critical Care Medicine* 23:582–88, 1995.

Halpin, L. S., Spier, A. M., CapoBianco, P., and Barnett, S. D. Guided imagery in cardiac surgery. *Outcomes Management* 6(3):132–37, July-September 2002.

Hamilton, D. N. Patient lounge study. Unpublished research report No. 1, Saskatoon Hospital Evaluation Project, University of Saskatchewan, Canada, 1983.

Hansell, H. The behavioral effects of noise on man: The patient with "intensive care unit psychosis." *Heart and Lung* 13(1):59–65, January 1984.

Hardy, J. No hidden patient: Facility design for safety. *Patient Safety and Quality Healthcare*. September–October 2006. psqh.com/sepoct06/facility-design.html.

Haslam, P. Noise in hospitals: Its effect on the patient. *Nursing Clinics of North America* 5(4):715–24, December 1970.

Hayward, C., and members of the AIA Committee on Architecture for Health, Programming Subcommittee. *A Generic Process for Projecting Health Care Space Needs.* Washington, DC: AIA Committee, October 1985.

Hayward, D. G. Psychological factors in the use of light and lighting in buildings. In J. Lang, C. Burnette, W. Moleski, and D. Vachen, editors. *Designing for Human Behavior: Architecture and the Behavioral Sciences*, 120–29. Stroudsburg, PA: Dowden, Hutchinson and Ross, 1974.

Heerwagen, J. The psychological aspects of windows and window design. Symposium on Windows, Windowlessness and Simulated View. Richard Wener, convener. EDRA21, 269–80. Brooklyn: Polytechnic Institute of New York, 1990.

Henry, L. L. Music therapy: A nursing intervention for the control of pain and anxiety in the ICU: A review of the research literature. *Dimensions of Critical Care Nursing* 14(6):295–304, November–December 1995.

Heulat, J. Current trends in cancer center design. In Proceedings from the Third Symposium on Health Care Interior Design. *Journal of Health Care Design* 3:9–16, 1991.

Hewitt, J. Psycho-affective disorder in intensive care units: A review. *Journal of Clinical Care Nursing* 11(5):575–84, September 2002.

Hiatt, L. H. Breakthroughs in long term care design. In Proceedings from the Third Symposium on Health Care Interior Design. *Journal of Health Care Design* 3:205–15, 1991.

Hickler, F. D. Symposium on design and function of the operating room suite and special areas. *Journal of Anesthesiology* 31(2):103–6, August 1969.

Hilton, B. A. Noise in acute patient care areas. *Research in Nursing and Health* 8:283–91, 1985.

Hoover, M. I. Intensive care for relatives. *Hospitals* 53(14):219–22, July 16, 1979.

Horwitz-Bennett, B. Patient bathroom designs balance style and safety. *Healthcare Design.* June 25, 2014. www.healthcaredesignmagazine.com/article/patient-bathroom-designs-balance-style-and-safety.

Hospital room of the future. *Wall Street Journal*, November 17, 1013. http://online.wsj.com/news/articles/SB10001424052702303442004579119922380316310.

Howell, S., Epp, G., Reizenstein, J., and Albright, C. *Shared Spaces in Housing for the Elderly.* Cambridge: Massachusetts Institute of Technology, Department of Architecture, 1976.

Hurst, T. W. Is noise important in hospital? *International Journal of Nursing Studies* 3:125–35, 1966.

It's the right thing to do: The campaign to modernize inpatient rooms. Riverview Medical Center. Sebastian Cook Valley Health. 2014. http://sebasticookvalleyhealth.org/assets/0/284/312/988/994/bf154c5a-cd2f-40c8–995a-cb50fb768708.pdf.

Janssen, P. A., Klein, M. C., Harris, S. J., Soolsma, J., and Seymour, L. C. Single room maternity care and client satisfaction. *Birth* 27(4):235–43, December 2000.

Jenna, J. Toward the patient-driven hospital. *Healthcare Forum* 22–59, July–August 1986.

Jolley, S. Single rooms and patient choice. *Nursing Standard* 20(9):41–48, November 9, 2005.

Joseph, A. The impact of light on outcomes in healthcare settings. Center for Health Design, Issue Paper No. 2:1–12, August 2006a.

_____. The role of the physical and social environment in promoting health, safety, and effectiveness in the healthcare workspace. Center for Health Design, Issue Paper No. 3:1–17, November 2006b.

Joseph, A., and Ulrich, R. Sound control for improved outcomes in healthcare settings. Center for Health Design, Issue Paper No. 4, January 2007.

Kam, P.C.A., Dam, A. C., and Thompson, J. F. Noise pollution in the anaesthetic and intensive care environment. *Anaesthesia* 49(11):982–86, November 1994.

Kaplan, R., and Kaplan, S. *The experience of nature: A psychological perspective.* Cambridge: Cambridge University Press, 1989 (Republished by Ann Arbor, MI: Ulrich's, 1995).

Keep, P. J. Stimulus deprivation in windowless rooms. *Anesthesia* 32(7):598–602, July–August 1977.

Keep, P. J., James, J., and Inman, M. Windows in the intensive therapy unit. *Anesthesia* 35(3):257–62, March 1980.

Kemper, K. J., and Danhauer, S. C. Music as therapy. *Southern Medical Journal* 98(3), 282–288, March 2005.

Kenny, C., and Canter, D. Findings from the development of USEP. Report, Department of Psychology, University of Surrey, Guildford, Surrey, September 1978.

King, J., Marans, R. A., and Solomon, L. A. Pre-construction evaluation: A report on the full scale mock-up and evaluation of hospital rooms. Ann Arbor: Architectural Research Laboratory, University of Michigan, 1982.

Kira, A. *The Bathroom.* New York: Bantam Books, 1977.

Kornfeld, D. S. The hospital environment: Its impact on the patient. *Advances in Psychosomatic Medicine* 8:252–70, 1972.

Kshettry, V., Carole, L. F., Henly, S. J., Sendelbach, S., and Kummer, B. Complementary alternative medical therapies for heart surgery patients: Feasibility, safety, and impact. *Annals of Thoracic Surgery*, 2006, 81(1), 201–5.

Kwan, M. A. Acuity-adaptable nursing care: Exploring its place in designing the future patient room. *Health Environments Research and Design Journal.* October 31, 2011. www.herdjournal.com/article/acuity-adaptable-nursing-care-exploring-its-place-designing-future-patient-room.

Lam, W.M.C. *Perception and Lighting as Formgivers for Architecture.* New York: McGraw-Hill, 1977.

Laufman, H., ed. *Hospital Special-Care Facilities: Planning for User Needs.* New York: Academic Press, 1981.

Leibrock, C. A. Design prescriptions for the disabled. In Proceedings from the Second Symposium on Health Care Interior Design. *Journal of Health Care Design* 2:153–58, 1990.

Leske, J. S. Needs of relatives of critically ill patients: A follow-up. *Heart and Lung* 15(2):189–93, March 1986.

Locsin, R. G. The effect of music on the pain of selected post-operative patients. *Journal of Advanced Nursing* 6:19–25, 1981.

Lowry, M. Are you sitting comfortably? Good seating requirements in a patient care setting. *Professional Nurse* 162–64, December 1989.

Malcolm, H. A. Does privacy matter? Former patients discuss their perceptions of privacy in shared hospital rooms. *International Journal for Healthcare Professionals* 12(2):156–66, March 2005.

Malin, S. New rural surgery center is designed to support inpatient and outpatient care. *Healthcare Building Ideas.* March 1, 2011. www.hcalthcaredesignmagazine.com/building-ideas/new-rural-surgery-center-designed-support-inpatient-and-outpatient-care.

Malkin, J. Designing a better environment. In S. O. Marberry, editor. *Improving Healthcare with Better Building Design*, 109–24. Chicago: Health Administration Press, 2006.

Marberry, S., and Zagon, L. *The Power of Color: Creating Healthy Interior Spaces.* New York: Wiley, 1995.

Martin, C. Interior design for hospitals: Preferences of patients and staff for color in the patient room environment. PhD diss. Oklahoma State University, Stillwater, OK, 1992. [Available from ProQuest, 789 E. Eisenhower Parkway, Ann Arbor, MI 48108.]

Maze, C. Inboard, outboard, or nested? A look inside the great toilet room debate. *Healthcare Design.* March 1, 2009. www.healthcaredesignmagazine.com/article/inboard-outboard-or-nested?page=4.

Mazer, S. E. Increase patient safety by creating a quieter hospital environment. *Biomedical Instrumentation and Technology* 40(2):145–46, March-April 2006.

Mazer, S. E. Speech privacy: Beyond architectural solutions. Paper presented at Noise Conference, Minneapolis, MN, October 17–19, 2005.

McCraty R., Barrios-Choplin B., Atkinson M., and Tomasino D. The effects of different types of music on mood, tension, and mental clarity. *Alternative Therapies in Health and Medicine* 4(1):75–84, January 1998.

McCullough, C. S. Evidence-based design. In *Evidence-Based Design for Healthcare Facilities*, 1–18. Indianapolis: Sigma Theta Tau International, 2010.

McLaughlin, A., McLaughlin, B., Elliot, J., and Campalani, G. Noise levels in a cardiac surgical intensive care unit: A preliminary study conducted in secret. *Intensive Care and Critical Care Nursing* 12:226–30, 1996.

Medina, A. Q. A visual assessment of children's and environmental educators' urban residential preference patters. Unpublished PhD diss. University of Michigan, Ann Arbor, 1983.

Meyer, T. J., Eveloff, S. E., Bauer, M. S., Schwartz, W. A., Hill, N. S., and Millman, R. P. Adverse environmental conditions in the respiratory and medical ICU settings. *Chest* 105(4):1211–16, April 1994.

Miller, D. B., and Goldman, L. Selecting paintings for the nursing home. *Nursing Homes* 12–16, January–February 1984.

Miller, N. O., Friedman, S. B., and Coupey, S. M. Adolescent preferences for rooming during hospitalization. *Journal of Adolescent Health* 23(2):89–93, August 1998.

Minato, S. Color in industrial design. F. W. Billmeyet and G. Wyszecki, editors. AIC Color Proceedings of the Third Congress of the International Colour Association. Bristol: Adam Hilger 1977, 199–207.

Minckley, B. B. A study of noise and its relationship to patient discomfort in the recovery room. *Nursing Research* 17(3):247–50, May–June 1968.

Molter, N. C. Needs of relatives of critically ill patients: A descriptive study. *Heart and Lung* 8(2):332–39, March–April 1979.

Moore, J. D. Jr. Designed to heal: Architecture of Swedish clinic is about more than medicine. *Modern Healthcare* 30(47):32–34, Novmber 2000.

Morgan, V. R., Mathison, J. R., Rice, J. C., and Clemmer, D. I. Hospital falls: A persistent problem. *American Journal of Public Health* 75(7):775–77, July 1985.

Murtha, D. M. Environmental requirements for a community room on a patient care unit: Recommendations. Unpublished report, Nurse Utilization Project. Milwaukee, WI: St. Mary's Hospital, 1970.

Nanda, U. Evidence base on healing art. *American Art Resources,* unpublished research report, 2006, 1–5.

Nanda, U., Eisen, S., and Baladandayuthapani, V. Patients' art preferences different than design students'. *Environment and Behavior* 40(2):269–301, 2008.

Nanda, U., Hathorn, K., and Neumann, R. The art-cart program at St. Luke's Episcopal Hospital, Houston. *Healthcare Design*, 10–12, September 2007.

Nilsson, U., Rawal, N., Enqvist, B., and Unosson, M. Analgesia following music and therapeutic suggestions in the PACU in ambulatory surgery: A randomized controlled trial. *ACTA Anaesthesiologica Scandinavica* 47:278–83, 2003.

Noble, A., and Dixon, R. Ward evaluation: St. Thomas Hospital. Unpublished report, Medical Architecture Research Unit, Polytechnic of North London, December 1977.

Noise and Hearing Loss. *NIH Consensus Statement* 8(1):1–24, January 22–24, 1990.

Novaes, M.A.F.P., Aronovich, A., Ferraz, M. B., and Knobel, E. Stressors in ICU: Patients' evaluation. *Intensive Care Medicine* 23, 1282–85, 1997.

Olsen, J. C., and Sabin, B. R. Emergency Department patient perceptions of privacy and confidentiality. *Journal of Emergency Medicine* 25(3), 329–33, October 2003.

Olsen, R. V. The effect of the hospital environment: Patient reactions to traditional versus progressive care settings. *Journal of Architectural Planning Research* 1:121–136, 1984.

Olsen, R. V., Pershing, A., and Winkel, G. A patient and staff evaluation of the Scanmural lounges. Unpublished research report, Environmental Design Program, Bellevue Hospital Center and Environmental Psychology Program, City University of New York, 1984.

Owens, L. D. The effects of music on the weight loss, crying, and physical movement of newborns. *Journal of Music Therapy* 16:83–90, 1979.

Parthasarathy, S., and Tobin, M. J. Sleep in the intensive care unit. *Intensive Care Medicine* 30(2):197–206, February 2004.

Pati, D., Harvey, T. E. Jr., Reyers, E., Evans, J., Waggener, L., Serrano, M., Saucier, R., and Nagle, T. A multidimensional framework for assessing patient room configurations. *Health Environments and Research Journal.* February 1, 2009. www.herdjournal.com/article /multidimensional-framework-assessing-patient-room-configurations.

Patient Rooms. *The new hospital.* Rush University Medical Center. 2014. http://transforming.rush.edu /NewHospital/Pages/Patient-Rooms.aspx.

Patient room design: The same-handed, mirror-image debate. Research Summary, 2011. http://www .hermanmiller.com/MarketFacingTech/hmc/research/research_summaries/assets/wp_Same_vs _Mirror.pdf

Pease, N.J.F. Do patients and their relatives prefer single cubicles or shared wards? *Palliative Medicine* 16(5):445–46, September 2002.

Petterson, M. Reduced noise levels in ICU promote rest and healing. *Critical Care Nurse* 20(5):104, October 2000.

Popkin, S. Form must follow function. *Michigan Hospitals* 16(9):9–11, September 1980.

Prototype hospital room provides privacy and amenities. *Contract,* 92–93, February 1985.

Public Health, Madison and Dane County. Potential health effects of noise exposure. June 7, 2013. www .epa.gov/history/topics/noise/01.html.

Rabin, M. Medical-facility colors reduce patient stress. *Contract* 23(2):78–83, February 1981.

Redding, J. S., Hargest, T. S., and Minsky, S. H. How noisy is intensive care? *Critical Care Medicine* 5(6):275–76, November–December 1976.

Reid, E. Factors affecting how patients sleep in the hospital environment. *British Journal of Nursing,* 2001, 10(14), 912–15.

Reiling, J., Hughes, R. G., and Murphy, M. R. The impact of facility design on patient safety. *Patient Safety and Quality: An Evidence-Based Handbook for Nurses,* chap. 28. 2008. www.ncbi.nlm.nih.gov/books /NBK2633/.

Reizenstein, J. E., and Grant, M. A. Color, cubicle curtains, handrails. Unpublished research report No. 23. Patient and Visitor Participation Project, Office of Hospital Planning, Research and Development, University of Michigan, Ann Arbor, 1981.

_____. From hospital research to hospital design. Patient and Visitor Participation Project, Office of Hospital Planning, Research and Development, University of Michigan, Ann Arbor, 1982.

_____. Patient activities and schematic design preferences. Unpublished research report No. 2, Patient and Visitor Participation Project, Office of Hospital Planning, Research and Development, University of Michigan, Ann Arbor, 1981.

_____. Schematic design of the inpatient room. Unpublished research report No. 1. Patient and Visitor Participation Project, Office of Hospital Planning, Research and Development, University of Michigan, Ann Arbor, 1981.

_____. Spontaneous design suggestions by patients and visitors. Unpublished research report No. 6. Patient and Visitor Participation Project, Office of Hospital Planning, Research and Development, University of Michigan, Ann Arbor, 1981.

Reizenstein, J. E., Vaitkus, M. A., and Grant, M. A. Patient belongings. Unpublished research report No. 9. Patient and Visitor Participation Project, Office of Hospital Planning, Research and Development, University of Michigan, Ann Arbor, 1982.

_____. Visitor activities and schematic design preferences. Unpublished research report No. 4. Patient and Visitor Participation Project, Office of Hospital Planning, Research and Development, University of Michigan, Ann Arbor, 1981.

Relman, A. On breaking one's neck. *New York Review of Books.* February 6, 2014. www.nybooks.com /articles/archives/2014/feb/06/on-breaking-ones-neck/?pagination=false&src=longreads.

Renzi, C., Peticca, L., and Pescatori, M. The use of relaxation techniques in the perioperative management of proctological patients: Preliminary results. *International Journal of Colorectal Disease* 15(5–6):313–16, November 2000.

Robert Wood Johnson University Hospital. *Patient Guide: About Your Stay.* August 21, 2008. www .rwjuh.edu/patient_guide/guide_about_your_stay.html.

Rosenfeld, N. Indirect lighting improves outlook for everyone. *Modern Hospital* 117(2):78–80, August 1971.

Scalise, D. Shhh, quiet please! *Hospitals and Health Networks* 78(5):16–17, May 2004.

Scalise, D., Thrall, T. H., Haugh, R., and Runy, L. A. The patient room. *Hospitals and Health Networks* 78(5):34–38, 40, 49–51, May 2004.

Shepley, M., Gerbi, R., Watson, A., Imgrund, S., and Sagha-Zadeh, R. The impact of daylight and windows on ICU patients and staff. *Health Environments Research & Design Journal.* March 2012. www .herdjournal.com/article/impact-daylight-and-views-icu-patients-and-staff.

Sherman, S. A., Varni, J. W., Ulrich, R. S., and Malcarne, V. L. Post-occupancy evaluation of healing gardens in a pediatric cancer center. *Landscape and Urban Planning* 73(2–3):167–83, 2005.

Shertzer, K. E., and Keck, J. F. Music and the PACU environment. *Journal of PeriAnesthesia Nursing* 16(2):90–102, April 2001.

Simpson, T. The family as a source of support for the critically ill adult. *AACN Clinical Issues in Critical Care Nursing* 2(2):229–35, May 1991.

Snyder-Halpern, R. The effect of critical care unit noise on patient sleep cycles. *Critical Care Quarterly* 7(4):41–51, March 1985.

Solomon, L. A., and Gaudette, R. Adult general hospital bed and furniture evaluation. Unpublished report, Office of Hospital Planning, Research and Development, University of Michigan, Ann Arbor, 1984.

Spear, M. Current issues: Designing the universal patient care room. *Journal of Healthcare Design* 9:81–83, 1997.

Spork, C. Patients' wishes regarding sickrooms. *Nursing Times* 86(20):53, May 16, 1990.

St. Louis Children's Hospital. *Child Life Teen Lounge.* 2014. www.stlouischildrens.org/our-services.

Stanchina, M. L., Abu-Hijleh, M., Chaudhry, B. K., Carlisle, C. C., and Millman, R. P. The influence of white noise on sleep in subjects exposed to ICU noise. *Sleep Medicine* 6(5):423–28, September 2005.

Standley, J. Music research in medical/dental treatment: Meta-analysis and clinical applications. *Journal of Music Therapy* 23(2):56–122, Summer 1986.

Storlie, F. J. Does urban noise represent a hazard to health? PhD diss. Portland State University, Portland, OR, 1976.

Stouffer, J. Same-handed rooms. *Healthcare Design.* December 1, 2010. www.healthcaredesignmagazine.com/article/same-handed-rooms.

Sturdavant, M. Intensive nursing service in circular and rectangular units compared. *Hospitals* 34(14):46–48, 71–78, July 16, 1960.

Task Force on Guidelines of the Society of Critical Care Medicine. Recommendations for critical care unit design. *Critical Care Medicine* 16(8):796–806, 1988.

Taylor, E. M. 2009 Survey of design research in healthcare settings: The use and impact of evidence-based design. The Center for Health Design, 2009. www.healthdesign.org/chd/research/2009-survey-design-research-healthcare-settings-use-and-impact-evidence-based-design.

Tofle, R. R., Schwarz, B., Yoon, S.-Y., and Max-Royale, A. *Color in Healthcare Environments: A Critical Review of the Research Literature.* Coalition of Health Environments Research (CHER), 2004.

Topf, M. Noise pollution in the hospital [letter]. *New England Journal of Medicine* 309(1):53–54, July 7, 1983.

Topf, M., and Davis, J. E. Critical care unit noise and rapid eye movement (REM) sleep. *Heart and Lung* 22(3):52–58, May–June 1993.

Topf, M., and Thompson, S. Interactive relationships between hospital patients: Noise-induced stress and other stress with sleep. *Heart and Lung* 30(4):237–43, July–August 2001.

Topf, M., Bookman, M., and Arand, D. Effects of critical care unit noise on the subjective quality of sleep. *Journal of Advanced Nursing* 24(3): 545–51, September 1996.

Torrice, A. F. Color for healing. In Proceedings from the First Annual National Symposium on Health Care Interior Design. *Journal of Health Care Design* 1:35–43, 1989.

Tusek, D. L., Church, J. M., Strong, S. A., Grass, J. A., and Fazio, V. W. Guided imagery: A significant advance in the care of patients undergoing elective colorectal surgery. Paper presented at the meeting of the American Society of Colon and Rectal Surgeons, Seattle, WA, June 9–14, 1996.

US Environmental Protection Agency. Information on levels of environmental noise requisite to protect public health and welfare with an adequate margin of safety. No. 550/9–74–004. Washington, DC: US Government Printing Office, 1974.

Ulrich, R. S. Effects of interior design on wellness: Theory and recent scientific research. In Proceedings from the Third Symposium on Health Care Interior Design. *Journal of Health Care Design* 3:97–109, 1991.

_____. View through a window may influence recovery from surgery. *Science* 224(4647):420–21, April 27, 1984.

Ulrich, R. S., and Gilpin L. Healing arts: Nutrition for the soul. In S. Frampton, L. Gilpin, and P. Charmel, editors. *Putting Patients First: Designing and Practicing Patient-Centered Care*, 117–46. San Francisco: Wiley, 2003.

Ulrich, R., Quan, X., Zimring, C., Joseph, A., and Choudhary, R. The role of the physical environment in the hospital of the twenty-first century: A once-in-a-lifetime opportunity. Report to the Center for Health Design, September 2004.

Ulrich, R. S., Zimring, C., Quan, X., and Joseph, A. The environment's impact on stress. In S. O. Marberry, editor. *Improving Healthcare with Better Building Design*, 37–62. Chicago: Health Administration Press, 2006.

Van Enk, R. Modern hospital design for infection control. *Healthcare Design*, 10–14, September 2006.

Verderber, S. Dimensions of person–window transactions in the hospital environment. *Environment and Behavior* 18(4):450–66, July 1986.

Verderber, S., and Reuman, D. Windows, views and health status in hospital therapeutic environments. *Journal of Architectural and Planning Research* 4(2):120–33, 1987.

Vogelsang, J. Effect of visitors on patient behavior in the postanesthesia period. *Dimensions in Critical Care Nursing* 7(2):91–100, March–April 1988.

Walch, J. M., Rabin, B. S., Day, R., Williams, J. N., Choi, K., and Kang, J. D. The effect of sunlight on postoperative analgesic medication use: A prospective study of patients undergoing spinal surgery. *Psychosomatic Medicine* 67:156–63, 2005.

Wallace, J., Robins, J., Alvord, L. S., and Walker, J. M. The effect of earplugs on sleep measures during exposure to simulated intensive care unit noise. *American Journal of Critical Care* 8(4):210–19, July 1999.

Wang, Z., Downs, B., Farell, A., Cook, K., Hourihan, P., and McCreery, S. Role of a service corridor in ICU noise control, staff stress, and staff satisfaction: Environmental research of an academic medical center. *Health Environments Research and Design Journal* 6(3):80–84, Spring 2013. www.ncbi.nlm.nih.gov/pubmed/23817908.

Whitfield, S. Noise on the ward at night. *Nursing Times* 71:408–12, March 13, 1975.

Williams, M. Design for therapeutic outcome. Paper presented at the Fourth Symposium on Healthcare Design, Boston, November 14–17, 1991.

Williams, M. A. Physical environment of the intensive care unit and elderly patients. *Critical Care Nursing Quarterly* 12(1):52–60, 1989.

Williams, M., and Murphy, J. Noise in critical care units: A quality assurance approach. *Journal of Nursing Care Quality* 6(1):53–59, 1991.

Wilson, L. M. Intensive care delirium: The effect of outside deprivation in a windowless unit. *Archives of Internal Medicine* 130:225–26, August 1972.

Winter M., Paskin S., and Baker T. Music reduces stress and anxiety of patient in the surgical holding area. *Journal of Post Anesthesia Nursing*, 9, 340–43, 1994.

Wong, H., Lopez-Nahas, V., and Molassiotis, A. Effects of music therapy on anxiety in ventilator-dependent patients. *Heart and Lung* 30(5): 376–87, September-October 2001.

Wunsch, H., Gershengorn, H., Mayer, S. A., and Claassen, J. The effect of window rooms on critically ill patients with subarachnoid hemorrhage admitted to intensive care. *Critical Care* 15:R81, 2011.

Young, J. M. A summary of color in healthcare environments: A critical review of the research literature. *Healthcare Design* 7(7):22–23, September 2007.

Yung, P., Chui-Kam, S., French, P., and Chan, T. A controlled trial of music and pre-operative anxiety in Chinese men undergoing transurethral resection of the prostate. *Journal of Advanced Nursing* 39(4):352–59, August 2002.

Zagon, L. Design technology: Selecting appropriate colors for healthcare. *Journal of Healthcare Design* V:135–41, 1993.

Zeit, K. D. Patient-centered design: Next steps. *Healthcare Design*. January 14, 2013. www.healthcare -designmagazine.com/blogs/kristin-zeit/patient-centered-design-next-steps.

Zimring, C., Ulrich, R., Joseph A., and Quan X. The environment's impact on safety. In S. O. Marberry, editor. *Improving Healthcare with Better Building Design,* 63–79. Chicago: Health Administration Press, 2006.

Zubatkin, A. D. Psychological impact of medical equipment on patients. *Journal of Clinical Engineering* 5(3):250–55, July–September 1980.

CHAPTER 8

ACCESS TO NATURE

Patients, visitors, and staff at healthcare facilities use out-door areas for a variety of reasons. Some need solitude. Some need a place to hold a private conversation, talk on the phone, or work on a digital device. Others need a com-fortable place to have lunch with companions. Outdoor areas might also be used for larger functions, such as staff meetings, special events, performances, and community gatherings (Cooper Marcus and Barnes, 1999).

Several studies reveal the significant value people place on outdoor spaces at hospitals, whether or not they actually spend time in them (Olsen, n.d.; Whitehouse et al., 2001). People like to know outdoor spaces are available in case they want to visit them. Others enjoy the view of these spaces from inside. One study found that respon-dents felt more relaxed just walking by the hospital's park. For these "visual users," the park served as a focal point, a pleasant place for one's mind to wander. The research-ers concluded that the park benefited a much larger group than just those who entered it (Olsen, n.d.). Similarly, benefits have been documented for views to nature from inside a hospital. (See the section on "Bringing the Out-doors In.")

In a post-occupancy evaluation of a garden at a hospi-tal in Southern California, 90 percent of the respondents, including those who had never used it, said that gardens are important elements of hospitals (Whitehouse et al., 2001). Although this particular garden was found to be underutilized, particularly in the morning and late after-noon, the researchers explained that the value of outdoor spaces may not be accurately represented by their physical utilization. (Discussed in Research Box 8.2.)

LEARNING OBJECTIVES
- Become familiar with the ways in which nature can contribute to healing.
- Know some of the ways nature can be incorporated into the design and planning of a healthcare facility.
- Identify characteristics of outdoor areas for healthcare facilities preferred by patients and visitors.

Kimberley B. Phalen, PhD, contributed to this chapter.

Patients, visitors, and staff likely to use outdoor courtyards or parks are diverse in age and ability. Although it might seem surprising, even inpatients may be users of an outdoor space. In one study, 91 percent of the inpatients sampled at a tertiary-care hospital said they would like to use an outdoor space (Reizenstein and Grant, 1981 [unpub. No. 2]). Because more than two-thirds of these patients reported walking to at least one place—at distances from ~25 feet (~7.6 meters) to well over ~1,000 feet (~304.8 meters) from their rooms—patients' use of an outdoor space seems possible. The fact that many patients are eager for a change of scenery makes it likely that they would go outdoors, given no medical restrictions, good weather, and an outdoor space that accommodates their needs.

An outdoor space that serves a wide range of inpatients, outpatients, and visitors has particular design requirements not necessarily met by a typical urban courtyard. In addition, outdoor areas that will be used as play spaces for children—both sick and well—need to follow certain guidelines (Alcock, 1978; Henneberry and Robertson, 1983; Cooper Marcus and Sachs, 2013; Moore, Cohen, and McGinty, 1979; Moore et al., 1979; Olds and Daniel, 1987; Sherman et al., 2005; Whitehouse et al., 2001). This broad spectrum of would-be users requires thoughtful, responsive design.

The Importance of Nature in Healthcare Facilities

For most of us, nature holds deep meaning; it is a place of refuge, peace, and tranquility and a symbol of life and growth (Alexander, Ishikawa, and Silverstein, 1977; Wohlwill, 1983). It is not surprising, then, that people gain a great deal of pleasure from contact with nature. We surround ourselves with plants, we hang photographs and paintings of natural scenes, we travel to mountains and seashores as a way of "getting away from it all." Nature has long been considered an integral part of a healing process.

However, the benefits reaped from natural scenes go beyond simple pleasure. Many research studies have shown that spending time in nature, or even simply viewing photographs of nature, has positive health effects (Frumkin, 2001; Gerlach-Spriggs, Kaufman, and Warner, 1998; Irvine and Warber, 2002; Sternberg, 2010; Ulrich, 1979, 1981). Nature has been associated with reduced anxiety, increased relaxation, and improvements in the ability to think clearly (Berman, Jonides, and Kaplan, 2008; Canin, 1991; Cimprich, 1993; Hartag, Mang, and Evans, 1991; R. Kaplan, 2001; Taylor, Kuo, and Sullivan, 2001; Tennessen and Cimprich, 1995; Ulrich, 1979, 1981; Wells, 2000). These studies suggest that the availability of nature, in views from windows and use of accessible outdoor spaces, can be restorative for people experiencing stress and mental fatigue.

Stress and mental fatigue are not the same thing. Stress is a physiological and psychological reaction to a harmful or threatening situation (S. Kaplan, 1995). Mental fatigue is the result of overworking the part of the brain needed to concentrate. For example, staff members are more likely to suffer from mental fatigue, rather than stress, as a result of a hard day's work in a job that is, for the most part, predictable, manageable, and within their competence level. Patients and family members experience stress because of uncertainty and threatening health concerns, often in addition to mental fatigue. Access to nature can be used as a strategy to help address both of these problems.

Research findings support the importance of nature. Evidence of the pleasure associated with nature emerges from a number of empirical studies in which participants consistently preferred photographs of natural views dominated by vegetation or water over urban scenes (R. Kaplan, 1983; Reizenstein and Grant, 1981 [unpub. No. 2]; Ulrich, 1983).

Several researchers have conducted post-occupancy evaluations of outdoor spaces to assess the fit among the design, intended use, and actual use (Cooper Marcus and Barnes, 1995, 1999; Olsen, n.d.; Sherman et al., 2005; Whitehouse et al., 2001). (See Research Box 8.2 later in the chapter.) A landmark study was conducted in the late 1990s that evaluated outdoor spaces in more than 70 hospitals in order to inform design recommendations for hospital outdoor spaces (Cooper Marcus and Barnes, 1999). This study provides a collection of examples and photographs of healthcare gardens in the United States, Canada, and England.

The majority of studies on the physiological and emotional effects of nature compare the extremes: pristine wilderness or parklike settings versus urban settings devoid of nature elements (Ulrich, 1979, 1981; Ulrich et al., 1991). Additional research is needed to evaluate the physiological and emotional effects of natural features within urban, suburban, and rural settings.

Facilitating Recovery from Stress

According to some researchers, when a stressed individual views an attractive natural scene, that scene will be considered soothing because it "elicits feelings of pleasantness, holds interest, and blocks or reduces stressful thoughts" (Ulrich, 1983). The stress response, an individual's response to a threatening or harmful situation, involves both psychological changes (for example, fear, anger, and sadness) and physiological changes (for example, increases in sweating, pulse rate, muscle tension, and blood pressure). Researchers have found that exposure to nature is associated with faster and more complete stress recovery and more positive emotional states than exposure to urban settings with little or no vegetation (Ulrich, 1979, 1981; Ulrich et al., 1991).

Facilitating Recovery from Mental Fatigue

There is some evidence that the benefits of exposure to nature extend beyond reducing stress to resting the part of the brain used to focus or concentrate (S. Kaplan, 1995). Patients and family members are often inundated with new information about disease, injuries, conditions, and related treatment options. They face difficult decisions that require balancing risks and implications, planning ahead, and making difficult life changes, all of which require the ability to concentrate (Cimprich, 1993). The emotional intensity and mental effort associated with these situations can be draining. Even after patients come to terms with a diagnosis, they may have trouble adhering to treatment regimens and appointment schedules, remembering to take medications, and being productive at their jobs.

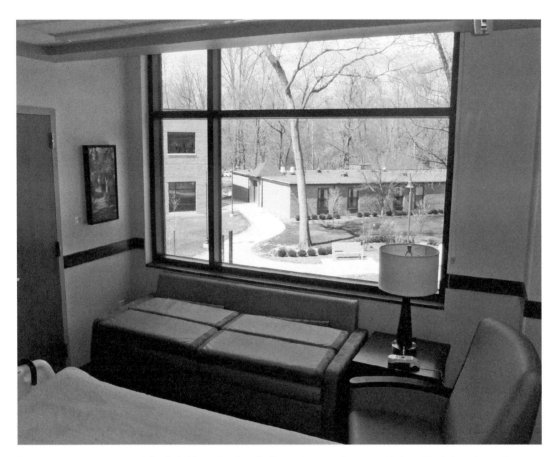

Everyone in a patient room, especially a bedridden patient, benefits from seeing an outdoor area with views of both sky and ground.
Photo credit: Courtesy of St. Joseph Mercy Chelsea

It is important for patients to have frequent opportunities to rest their minds. This is critical for maintaining mental clarity, coping with conditions, treating injuries, and managing a disease. Family members caring for patients also are in need of mental rest. Numerous studies show that spending time in nature is one way to attain this needed mental rest (Berman et al., 2008; Canin, 1991; Cimprich, 1993; Hartag et al., 1991; R. Kaplan, 2001; Taylor et al., 2001; Tennessen and Cimprich, 1995; Wells, 2000). (See Research Box 8.1.) People find that elements of nature, such as swaying leaves, floating clouds, and flowing water, attract and compel attention. Because this fascination is automatic, it allows rest in the part of the mind used to concentrate on tasks (S. Kaplan, 1995; R. Kaplan and Kaplan, 1995). Studies on attention-deficit disorders and cognitive functioning in children provide additional support for the positive effects of nature on attention (Taylor et al., 2001; Wells, 2000).

RESEARCH BOX 8.1 IMPROVING CONCENTRATION IN CANCER PATIENTS THROUGH NATURE ACTIVITIES

Research indicates that attention problems are common in patients with cancer. Distractibility, loss of concentration, and fatigue have been observed during and after cancer treatments. Patients may also have trouble remembering self-care instructions following discharge. With a view to developing nursing interventions to help patients improve their abilities to pay attention, a researcher evaluated the effectiveness of participation in relaxing activities during the early phase of cancer treatment (Cimprich, 1993).

Thirty-two women undergoing treatment for stage I or II breast cancer were randomly assigned to one of two groups. A control group received standard self-care instructions following discharge. An activity group received self-care instructions plus an individually designed plan for regular participation in activities that could help improve their abilities to focus and concentrate. Members of the activity group chose activities they thought would be relaxing, interesting, enjoyable, and physically easy to do, such as making arts and crafts objects, reading interesting books or stories, and viewing or spending time in nature by bird watching, tending to flowers or plants, walking, or sitting in a park, garden, or backyard. Quiet activities involving nature were chosen most often. Participants performed the activity for 20–30 minutes at least three times a week for the length of the study (90 days post-surgery).

The activity group showed greater improvements than the control group in attention tests administered between 3 and 90 days after surgery. Researchers measured attention using multiple standardized tests and collected patients' self-ratings of their attention. Participants in the activity group reported consistent improvement in their abilities to function on tasks requiring attention, such as planning, deciding, and concentrating on details.

Although this preliminary study is limited in its generalizability, due in part to a small sample size, the findings support the notion that quiet activities in nature can be effective in improving people's abilities to focus and concentrate. The study did not examine the specific effects of nature activities versus other relaxing activities. It is possible that any effort that enhances patients' participation in self-care programs could lead to similar improvements.

Improving the Productivity and Satisfaction of Caregivers

The issue of mental fatigue applies to caregivers as well as patients. Staff can feel mentally worn out as a result of their everyday job demands. Many of their tasks, including monitoring patient care, thinking on their feet, maintaining vigilance, and resisting distractions, require significant concentration.

Research indicates that spending time in nature benefits caregivers. In a study of 200 AIDS caregivers, one researcher found that caregivers who frequently participated in leisure activities involving active movement in nature (for example, walking, biking, boating, hiking, and the like) reported a better ability to perform tasks requiring concentration than did caregivers who frequently spent their leisure time watching TV (Canin, 1991). Other activities associated with similar benefits were reading, listening to music, visiting quietly with friends and family, attending cultural activities (movies, plays, and museums, and the like), community volunteering, and attending religious services. Other fatigued caregivers reported frequent involvement in shopping for pleasure and watching or playing sports.

In a study of outdoor spaces in hospitals, many staff respondents noted feeling "more productive" after spending time in nature (Cooper Marcus and Barnes, 1999). Even mini-exposures to nature, such as walking through or viewing nature, may help users feel more focused and satisfied (R. Kaplan, 2001).

Findings suggest that outdoor spaces in hospitals may even help with staff recruitment and retention (Cooper Marcus and Barnes, 1995; Cooper Marcus and Sachs, 2013; Sherman et al., 2005; Ulrich et al., 2006; Whitehouse et al., 2001). In a study of four San Francisco–area hospitals, staff members were the most frequent users of outdoor spaces, compared with patients or visitors (Cooper Marcus, 2002; Cooper Marcus and Barnes, 1995). One surgeon noted that the existence of a garden at the hospital was a large factor in the decision to accept a position there (Cooper Marcus, 2002). These findings suggest that outdoor spaces can play an important role in addressing the well-documented problems of high staff turnover, shortage of nurses, and low job satisfaction in the healthcare industry (Ulrich et al., 2006).

One study described a hospital policy that prohibited staff members from using the horticulture therapy gardens during their breaks (Heath, 2004). Although the reasoning behind this policy is not fully understood, evidence of the positive effects of nature on concentration and mental clarity presents a strong argument against implementing such a policy. Potential privacy concerns can be addressed by designing gardens with distinct "rooms" benefiting patients and visitors as well as staff (Cooper Marcus and Sachs, 2013). Moreover, the particular restorative benefits of outdoor spaces for staff suggest that, whenever possible, at least one outdoor space should be provided that is accessible only to staff (Cooper Marcus and Sachs, 2013). In these areas, which should be located near lunchrooms and other places where breaks are taken, staff are briefly freed from the necessity of interacting with patients or visitors and can meet with each other, talk on the phone, and relax. Although most health facility nature settings are considered beneficial for patients and visitors, they also hold great promise for improving staff productivity and well-being.

Encouraging Physical Activity

Outdoor spaces can encourage physical activity by providing attractive places for walking or other forms of exercise. In fact, two literature reviews examining the relationship between environmental attributes and walking found that aesthetically pleasing environments, such as settings with attractive natural features, were positively associated with walking (Humpel, Owen, and Leslie, 2002; Owen et al., 2004).

Given the health problems associated with the rise in obesity and widespread lack of physical activity in the United States, fitness centers and exercise programs associated with healthcare facilities are becoming more popular. With an increased awareness of the role of fitness in maintaining health, health-facility decision-makers are realizing that they too can be part of the solution by designing spaces that support physical activity, providing classes, and encouraging participation in fitness programs.

Creating a Positive Image

An attractive outdoor space has important symbolic value. The design of outdoor spaces in and around healthcare facilities can create a positive image, showing both users and the community that the healthcare organization is sensitive to user experience and that it understands that comfort and beauty, as well as technical competence, are part of the healing process. In fact, studies have revealed that the existence of designed outdoor spaces affected people's perceptions of a hospital's quality of care (Olsen, n.d.; Whitehouse et al., 2001). For example, the establishment of an outdoor space at a New York hospital was seen as evidence that the hospital cared about staff, patients, and visitors (Olsen, n.d.). (See also Research Box 8.2.) These findings have important marketing implications. Creating outdoor spaces and including them in marketing materials and campaigns may attract patients and foster good feelings about the healthcare facility.

Valuing Access to Nature in Healthcare Facilities

A growing number of hospital decision-makers recognize the value of access to nature in providing needed relief and respite for patients, family members, visitors, and staff. As a result, they have commissioned outdoor spaces that provide soothing and inviting opportunities to "get away," at least psychologically, from pressures inside the facility. These spaces also offer places for exercise, physical rehabilitation, social support, and privacy (Cooper Marcus and Barnes, 1999; Cooper Marcus and Sachs, 2013; Sherman et al., 2005; Stigsdotter and Grahn, 2003).

Outdoor spaces at healthcare facilities come in many forms, including courtyards, rooftop gardens, and "vest-pocket" parks. Many facilities refer to these spaces as "gardens," a term used widely to refer to almost any type of outdoor space designed for use and consisting of some nature elements. Another common term used in practice and in the literature is "healing garden." The term arose from a trend toward viewing health more holistically, to include the body, mind, and spirit. "Healing gardens" are typically designed with the whole person in mind. They are intended to improve overall well-being, reduce stress, and provide relief from physical symptoms (Cooper Marcus and Barnes, 1999; Cooper Marcus and Sachs, 2013). (See Research Box 8.2.)

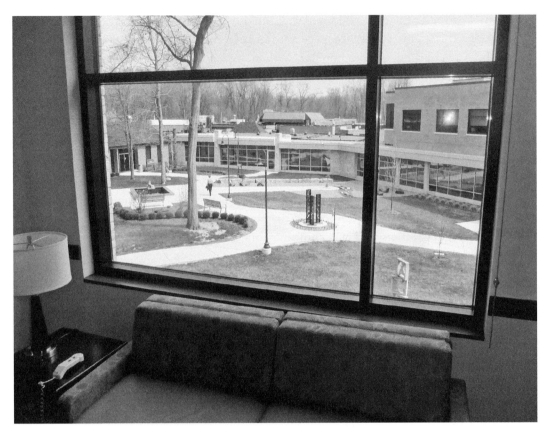

Views from a patient room to a courtyard can provide patients with positive distraction and preview a destination they may wish to explore.
Photo credit: Courtesy of St. Joseph Mercy Chelsea

RESEARCH BOX 8.2 EVALUATING A HOSPITAL GARDEN

An outdoor garden for patients, staff, and visitors was created at a children's hospital in southern California as part of an effort to create a caring environment. The garden was geared toward children and included a sculpture of a dinosaur, a seahorse-shaped fountain, a windmill, fish murals, colorful tiles and walls, and spaces scaled for children. Palms and deciduous trees created areas of shade and shadow. Planter walls, large rocks, and colorful benches with wheels (resembling flower carts) provided seating. Overall, there was a greater proportion of hardscape elements than natural elements (Whitehouse et al., 2001).

Researchers conducted a post-occupancy evaluation to determine whether the garden accomplished what the designers intended, including reducing stress, restoring energy, and increasing consumer satisfaction. Researchers observed the patterns of use and types of users in the garden. They administered surveys and interviews with adult users and non-users to gain insight into their knowledge of the garden's existence, perceptions of the garden, preferred features, and the impact of the garden on mood and satisfaction. Children at the hospital were also interviewed. The sample included patients, families, and staff from a variety of departments.

Over a two-week period, more than 200 people were observed visiting the garden. Families represented the largest percentage of users. They typically talked while their children played. Other adults sat quietly or walked around. Staff used the garden for lunch breaks, talking with one another, or spending quiet time alone. Nearly half of all visitors spent less than five minutes in the garden.

The researchers found that respondents perceived the garden to be a relaxing place. Ninety percent of adult users reported a positive change in mood after visiting the garden. Consistent with other studies, respondents noted an increase in customer satisfaction and, for some respondents, a perceived increase in quality of care (Olsen, n.d.). In their view, the choice to have a garden indicated that hospital decision-makers valued the well-being of patients.

Although 90 percent of respondents indicated the importance of providing outdoor spaces in hospitals, the outdoor space was not used as much as researchers had expected. In fact, 48 percent of family members and 80 percent of the children did not know the garden existed. Additionally, there was uncertainty about the purpose of the garden and its intended users. The researchers recommended informing staff about how to incorporate the garden into patient care and providing informational brochures, posters, and maps to encourage its use. Subsequently, plentiful signage in both English and Spanish was added inside the hospital (Cooper Marcus and Sachs, 2013).

Respondents recommended changes to the garden itself. For those who used the garden, 50 percent requested more trees, vegetation, and greenery. Others wanted more private spaces screened by vegetation. Children requested more interactive activities such as gardening, watering plants, picking flowers, and making things, such as signs to identify plants, needs that were later addressed by the construction of a more conventional playground area on the roof of a new building (Cooper Marcus and Sachs, 2013). Wheelchair access and facilities to accommodate IV poles and other medical devices were needed for patients requiring more intensive levels of care. The bumpy transition between the concrete approach and the garden path bothered some patients.

Numerous outdoor functions can be accommodated when a healthcare facility has ample space and conditions. If a single, large, optimally located space is not available, it may be advantageous to provide several smaller spaces that relate well to the building areas they are near. For instance, exterior space near the cafeteria could accommodate staff and visitors having lunch outside during warm weather. An outdoor area near a major public space like the

Main Lobby might be suitable for a children's play area and for a parklike area where visitors could walk or sit. If patients and visitors can receive text messages or use pagers, outdoor areas near waiting areas could be used by people waiting for appointments or news about loved ones (Cooper Marcus and Sachs, 2013). Large, centrally located spaces could accommodate special events such as ceremonies, performances, and meetings. Quiet, protected, easily accessible areas near inpatient units could provide opportunities for bedridden and ambulatory patients to get outside or simply to view nature.

Providing outdoor spaces at a healthcare facility is not the only way to offer access to nature. In some cases, hospitals may be located near local parks, gardens, or trails. Healthcare staff can help patients, visitors, and workers take advantage of nearby nature settings by providing maps and directions to these places. Shuttle bus services or stops on existing shuttle routes also could increase access to nearby nature opportunities.

Designing Outdoor Spaces for Healthcare Facilities

Although people enjoy contact with nature and welcome outdoor spaces associated with healthcare facilities, not all outdoor spaces are similar. Each site has its own particular attributes and limitations. The design of a parklike space that works well in one area may not be appropriate for a different site. In addition, user needs and preferences may differ from one area to another. Consequently, we suggest a participatory approach to outdoor space design. (See Research Box 8.3.) Paying heed to the preferences of future users allows design decision-makers to develop a plan that balances user preferences with site demands and other constraints. (See chapter 11.)

RESEARCH BOX 8.3 ENABLING USERS TO PARTICIPATE IN THE DESIGN OF AN OUTDOOR COURTYARD

Each outdoor site comes with a slightly different set of parameters, such as size, climate, and adjacent spaces. Outdoor space design also needs to reflect the characteristics and preferences of its eventual users.

As part of a multi-year research effort at the University of Michigan Medical Center, one study focused on design elements of an outdoor courtyard (Reizenstein and Grant, 1981 [unpub. No. 10]). Two hundred randomly sampled patients and visitors were interviewed about their preferences for different planting densities, seating arrangements, and other issues.

As part of the interview process, patients and visitors indicated their preferences for photographs showing various outdoor spaces. Photographs used in this study were taken of a specially constructed architectural model that could be rearranged to show different design alternatives for the proposed courtyard. Participants rated 27 photos, indicating how much they thought they would like to go to the place shown in the photograph.

The responses showed that patients and visitors preferred:

- Dense rather than sparse tree plantings
- An opportunity to choose from among several different seating options
- Seating areas designed to let people sit directly or diagonally across from each other while talking, rather than on benches arranged in a straight line
- Private seating areas surrounded by both shrubs and trees, rather than by little or no vegetation
- Benches with both armrests and backs

The findings of the study allowed researchers to make a number of design recommendations based directly on the preferences of respondents who were similar to eventual users.

Planning and Designing Outdoor Areas during New Construction

The design of healthcare facility outdoor spaces should occur concurrently with site planning and building design. Landscape architects should be on board at this time, so they can determine the location, orientation, function, and potential uses of outdoor spaces. They also can assess soil conditions and microclimates to inform the choice and placement of plants and other garden features (Cooper Marcus and Barnes, 1999).

Consider the following guidelines when planning and designing outdoor spaces for new construction:

- Consider a garden at the beginning of site planning and building design (Cooper Marcus and Barnes, 1999).

- Involve a landscape architect trained in the design of therapeutic gardens (Cooper Marcus and Barnes, 1999; Cooper Marcus and Sachs, 2013).

- Seek input from potential users of the space.

- When determining building placement, take advantage of views and access to existing green space (Cooper Marcus and Barnes, 1999).

- Design the building(s) so the main garden is readily visible and accessible from the main public spaces of the building, such as the Main Lobby (Cooper Marcus and Sachs, 2013).

- Locate gardens away from food exhaust vents so as to minimize cooking odors (Cooper Marcus and Sachs, 2013).

- Design the main garden to receive an optimal amount of sunlight (Cooper Marcus and Sachs, 2013).

- Provide surface grading that is as level as possible (Cooper Marcus and Barnes, 1999).

- Create courtyards at least ~30 feet (~9.1 meters) wide if there are windows, to prevent a "fishbowl" effect for people in the courtyard and to provide privacy to the people inside adjacent buildings. A distance of ~30 feet (~9.1 meters) between buildings helps ensure that people at one window cannot see into a window across the courtyard (Cooper Marcus and Barnes, 1999).

- In spaces enclosed by buildings, design the relationship between the width of the open space and the height of the adjacent buildings at a ratio between 1:3 and 1:2, to create a human scale and to allow sunlight to enter (Cooper Marcus and Sachs, 2013).

- In spaces enclosed by buildings, select and locate trees within the space to create a canopy that brings the space down to human scale (Cooper Marcus and Barnes, 1999).

Creating a Preferred Nature Setting

Just as most people hold strong preferences for natural settings over urban scenes, some natural areas are preferred over others. Researchers have described characteristics of places that are highly preferred: understandable and harmoniously composed, with a degree of complexity and a sense of enclosure. People are more likely to enter settings that look easy to navigate and offer opportunities for exploration. For example, gently winding paths with partially obstructed views offer direction and promote curiosity about what is to come (S. Kaplan and Kaplan, 1978, 1983; R. Kaplan, Kaplan, and Ryan, 1998).

People seek scenes that are inviting and offer enough complexity to attract them and maintain their interest (S. Kaplan and Kaplan, 1978, 1983; R. Kaplan et al., 1998). For instance, a densely planted area that appears orderly and consists of an assortment of plants provides greater visual interest than a sparsely planted one. The densely planted area offers more to look at and a greater variety of textures. Similarly, an area of lawn where people are sitting or walking is more visually interesting than an area planted with ground cover that prevents people from using it (Paine, 1984).

An outdoor space not only needs to be complex, it must also maintain a sense of order and coherence for it to be preferred by users (S. Kaplan and Kaplan, 1978, 1983; R. Kaplan et al., 1998; Nassauer, 1995). Creating boundaries between plant masses and mowing edges of tall grasses, for example, can contribute to a sense of structure and signify that the space is cared for (R. Kaplan et al., 1998; Nassauer, 1995). Orderliness is especially important when native landscaping is used in places where people are more accustomed to manicured landscaping (Nassauer, 1995). People tend to like spaces that are understandable, where there is no question of how one element relates to another. They tend not to enjoy elements in the landscape that "float" or seem disconnected and alone, like single trees in planters (Grant, 1979).

People also have strong preferences about what they like to look at (R. Kaplan, 1983). Though attitudes toward landscapes are to some extent culturally conditioned and thus cannot be universally generalized, one study found that healthcare facility courtyard scenes with a greater number of trees were consistently rated higher than those with fewer trees. The ratings increased in a linear fashion as the number of trees increased. Trees were seen as a source of visual interest as well as a source of beauty, shade, and color. Conversely, the absence of plantings was characterized as "bare" and "boring" by some respondents (Reizenstein and Grant, 1981 [unpub. No. 10]).

Water features are known to be highly preferred landscape elements (R. Kaplan and Kaplan, 1995). Moving water can provide soothing sights and sounds, although care must be taken that the sounds remain comforting and natural (Cooper Marcus and Sachs, 2013; Tetlow, 1989). Water features should also be designed to be attractive in all seasons and conditions, including when dry (Cooper Marcus and Sachs, 2013).

Many people enjoy a sense of enclosure when they are outdoors (S. Kaplan and Kaplan, 1978, 1983). A seating area surrounded by trees, adjacent to an open circulation or activity area, provides a sense of enclosure. It lets users look through trees to a visible open space, allowing them to people-watch. Although the mere presence of vegetation is likely to be appreciated, it is also important for trees and other planting materials to be arranged in a way that gives users a sense of enclosure.

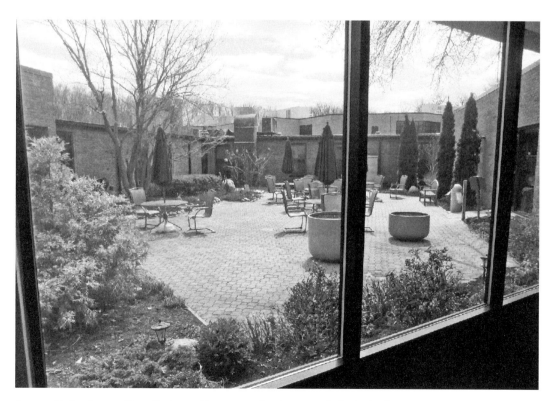

A memorable view from a public corridor to an outdoor space can function as a wayfinding landmark.
Photo credit: Courtesy of St. Joseph Mercy Chelsea

Several studies have identified the importance of private spaces surrounded by vegetation (Cooper Marcus and Barnes, 1999; Paine, 1984; Reizenstein and Grant, 1981 [unpub. No. 10]; Sherman et al., 2005; Whitehouse et al., 2001). In one study, patients and visitors were asked to choose among private seating areas surrounded by shrubs, trees, or both shrubs and trees. They preferred the greatest amount of vegetation possible (Reizenstein and Grant, 1981 [unpub. No. 10]). The option showing "shrubs and trees" was most preferred, "trees only" was a close second choice, and "shrubs only" was the third choice. This preference for enclosure was also affirmed in a study of seating behavior in hospital courtyards, where one of the most popular areas to sit—particularly with couples looking for privacy—was screened by a planter (Paine, 1984). (See also Research Box 8.2.)

Consider these guidelines for designing health facility outdoor spaces that patients, visitors, and staff will find inviting, pleasant, and interesting:

- Provide clearly marked paths, signs, and landmarks for easy wayfinding (Cooper Marcus and Barnes, 1999; R. Kaplan et al., 1998).

- Provide long-distance and partially obstructed views to encourage exploration and curiosity (Cooper Marcus and Barnes, 1999; R. Kaplan et al., 1998).

- Design gardens with a ratio of approximately 30 percent hardscape (steps, walls, paving, and so on) to 70 percent vegetation (Cooper Marcus and Barnes, 1999).

- Choose trees and shrubs that provide different colors and fragrances throughout the year (Cooper Marcus and Barnes, 1999).

- Provide distinct boundaries between areas (R. Kaplan et al., 1998).

- Provide as many trees as possible (Reizenstein and Grant, 1981 [unpub. No. 10]).

- Select some plants with moving foliage (Cooper Marcus and Barnes, 1995, 1999; R. Kaplan and Kaplan, 1995).

- Consider including a water feature, such as a fountain, pond, waterfall, or stream (Cooper Marcus and Barnes, 1999).

- Consider offering interactive design features and activities such as watering and weeding plants, planting flowers, and making crafts.

- Choose plants and garden features that attract butterflies, birds, chipmunks, and squirrels and promote animal-watching (Cooper Marcus and Barnes, 1999).

- Provide a range of seating arrangements and locations, from public to private (Reizenstein and Grant, 1981 [unpub. No. 10]).

- Arrange some seating and planting areas so that users' views to and from the seating are through the trees and shrubs, in order to provide a sense of enclosure and privacy.

- Design comfortable seating areas as settings for conversation and people-watching (Reizenstein and Grant, 1981 [unpub. No. 10]).

- Provide some open lawn for active use (Cooper Marcus and Barnes, 1999; Paine, 1984).

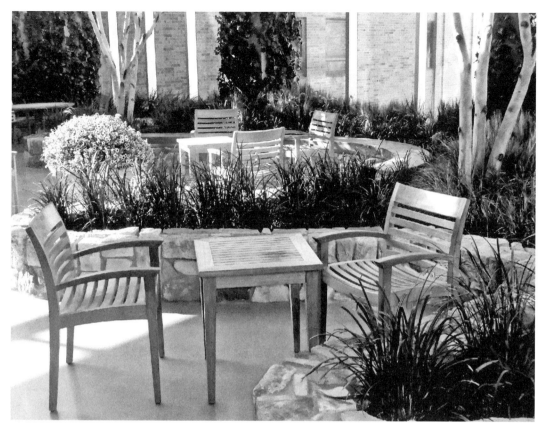

This courtyard provides a variety of seating options, from public to private. Seats that face inward, like this, create a cozy setting for conversation.

Photo credit: Courtesy of St. Joseph Mercy Ann Arbor

Location and Access

Patients, visitors, and staff can use outdoor spaces only when they know these spaces exist and how to access them. Some health-facility gardens are not used to their full potential. In fact, several post-occupancy evaluations found that many staff, family members, and patients did not know the gardens were there (Cooper Marcus and Barnes, 1995, 1999; Heath, 2004; Whitehouse et al., 2001). In one study, researchers found that only 3 of 70 hospitals provided directional signs with messages guiding people to outdoor areas (Cooper Marcus, 2002).

One study comparing the uses of different hospital courtyards found that the most fre-quently used courtyard was visible from a main circulation area (Paine, 1984). Courtyards that could be seen and entered only from a particular unit were not as widely used. Moreover, pro-viding seating near windows has been found not only to facilitate visual access to nature, but also to encourage the active use of outdoor spaces (Rodiek and Fried, 2004). Thus, the location of the outdoor space and its adjacency to other spaces or buildings affects how readily patients and visitors use it.

Consider these guidelines:

- Provide visual access to outdoor spaces from main public spaces and circulation areas (Cooper Marcus and Barnes, 1999; Paine, 1984).

- Provide direct access to outdoor spaces from public areas, including dining areas (Cooper Marcus and Barnes, 1999; Paine, 1984).

- Provide seating and a canopy, roof, or other shelter at the entrance to the main garden (Cooper Marcus and Sachs, 2013).

- Promote outdoor spaces by showing them on maps, providing related messages on directional signs, and including them on facility tours (Cooper Marcus and Barnes, 1999).

- Provide indoor seating near windows with nature views (Rodiek and Fried, 2004).

- Light outdoor spaces to enhance their nighttime safety and aesthetics (Cooper Marcus and Barnes, 1999; Paine, 1984; Souhrada, 1989).

- Offer patients and visitors pagers or text messaging in waiting areas so that they can use adjacent gardens while they wait (Cooper Marcus and Sachs, 2013).

Some users of a healthcare facility's outdoor spaces may have difficulty walking or have limited upper-body strength. Some may use wheelchairs, walkers, or crutches. Some may have limited vision or hearing. Some may be carrying babies or pushing strollers. Patients and visitors may need reassurance and a feeling of security before they venture outside. Consider these design features:

- Avoid specifying heavy doors that take considerable strength to open or that have a raised threshold (Paine, 1984).

- Use automatic doors at entrances to outdoor spaces in order to ensure easy access for everyone (Cooper Marcus and Barnes, 1999; Paine, 1984).

- Avoid using self-locking doors (Paine, 1984).

- Provide visual access to the outdoor space, so patients and visitors can decide whether or not they want to use it (Cooper Marcus and Barnes, 1999; Paine, 1984).

- Provide staff with the ability to monitor the outdoor space from indoors (Cooper Marcus and Barnes, 1999).

Walkways

The look and condition of walkways should encourage use of a health facility's outdoor spaces. It is easy to imagine a pleasant outdoor space with winding brick or stone pathways; however, uneven or bumpy surfaces, or even moderate grades would subject many patients and visitors to unnecessary discomfort. In order to accommodate all users, circulation surfaces should allow wheeled equipment to proceed smoothly. There should also be some physical support, such as handrails, to make it easier for frail patients to enjoy the outdoors. In addition, there should be places where non-ambulatory patients can inconspicuously situate themselves near friends seated on benches.

These design features can facilitate use of outdoor walkways:

• Provide walkway surfaces that can be easily and smoothly negotiated by stretchers, gurneys, wheelchairs, walkers, strollers, and other wheeled equipment. Avoid brick and other uneven surfaces. Make control joints as flat as possible (Cooper Marcus and Barnes, 1999; Cooper Marcus and Sachs, 2013; Paine, 1984; Whitehouse et al., 2001).

• Provide curbs along main pathways to make it easier for people using wheeled equipment (Cooper Marcus and Sachs, 2013).

• Avoid ramps at doorways that inhibit movement of patients and visitors using wheeled equipment (Cooper Marcus and Barnes, 1999; Paine, 1984).

• Provide continuous handrails on both sides of walkways on sloped and flat areas.

• When metal handrails are used, coat them with a material that prevents them from becoming cold, hot, or slippery (Koncelik, 1976).

• Make walkways wide enough for two gurneys to pass and for three or four people to walk side by side (Cooper Marcus and Barnes, 1999).

• Keep walkways clear of leaves, ice, and snow.

• In regions where winter weather is severe, consider installing melting devices below the surface of walkways in order to prevent ice and snow buildup (Cooper Marcus and Barnes, 1999).

• Consider smooth, permeable surfaces to decrease water runoff and improve groundwater recharge.

Outdoor Seating

Given a wide variety of potential activities, users of outdoor spaces will appreciate having seating options. Seating layout and design influence the degree of available privacy and ease of conversing. For example, when having a conversation, people usually prefer to sit directly or diagonally across from each other. With a single straight bench, people have to turn their bodies or heads in order to talk. Conversation is easier when two or three short benches or chairs face one another at a comfortable distance.

Seating orientation may also affect comfort. Seats should be oriented to allow users to take advantage of or to shield themselves from the sun. Some patients may be particularly bothered by wind and cooler temperatures and need sheltered seating located in maximum sunlight (Paine, 1984). Some medical conditions, treatments, and medications increase sun sensitivity, leading some patients to seek shaded areas (Cooper Marcus and Barnes, 1999).

Consider the following guidelines for the design of outdoor seating arrangements:

• Provide a variety of seating types ranging from chairs to benches.

• Provide some seating that allows for groups of five or six and some seating for one or two.

- Provide seating that users can arrange in groups or move to a more comfortable location.

- Provide seating that enables people to see and talk with each other.

- Provide some seating that is usually in sunlight and some that is usually in shade. In addition, provide some seating that is sheltered from the wind (Cooper Marcus and Barnes, 1999; Paine, 1984).

- Provide some seating along major circulation paths to encourage people-watching.

- Provide some seating that gives users a feeling of enclosure and separation from the mainstream.

- Place the majority of seating against a comforting backing such as a wall or plantings (Cooper Marcus and Sachs, 2013).

- Provide some seating around tables (Paine, 1984).

- Provide places for patients on stretchers or in wheelchairs to situate themselves among seating for ambulatory people. Make these areas accessible from a major walkway.

Bench size and design are also important considerations. How seating is designed (for example, how high it is and whether it has armrests or a back) affects comfort and use. Some ambulatory patients, especially older people, have trouble getting up from low seats. Benches with backs give needed support, and armrests help patients and visitors lower themselves comfortably and rise more easily and safely.

Seating capacity should be considered when outdoor furniture is selected. For instance, one study of responses to photos of various outdoor seating options found that respondents considered a small bench holding one to three people "too small" (Reizenstein and Grant, 1981 [unpub. No. 10]). Some respondents said that this bench might force them to sit uncomfortably close to someone else. They considered the large benches holding six to seven people "too large." Respondents felt comfortable only with the medium-sized bench holding three to five people. (This study did not examine preferences for sitting in individual chairs.)

Bench materials also make a difference. A bench that looks comfortable is more likely to be used than one that looks hard, hot in the summer, or cold in the winter. In one study, in which patients and visitors were shown drawings of bench designs using various materials (wood, concrete, and wire mesh), with various types of back support and with or without armrests, their perceptions of comfort became clear. The two most-preferred styles were made of wood and had backrests, whereas the concrete bench without arms or a backrest was one of the least-preferred options (Reizenstein and Grant, 1981 [unpub. No. 10]).

Consider the following guidelines when selecting seating for outdoor areas (see also Research Box 8.3):

- Provide seating with backs and armrests.

- Provide some seating with higher-than-usual seat heights in order to assist people, including some older patients and visitors, who have difficulty sitting and rising.

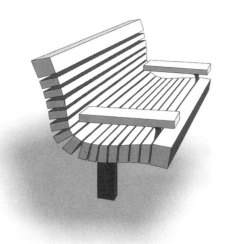

Wooden benches with backs were preferred in a study of outdoor seating.

- Provide seating users will consider comfortable for an hour or more at a time.
- Consider seating materials other than concrete.
- Provide seating that is considered attractive by most patients and visitors.

RESEARCH BOX 8.3   EVALUATING OUTDOOR SEATING OPTIONS

Several seating types were considered for a courtyard being designed for the University of Michigan Medical Center. In order to make an informed decision, planners sought information from potential users about comfort and aesthetics (Reizenstein and Grant, 1983 [unpub. No. 22]). Four seats were considered: two wire mesh outdoor chairs and two wooden outdoor chairs. Seat A was portable and was made of white metal mesh. Seat B had a curved wooden back and seat, with metal arms. Seat C consisted of heavy, dark-green wire mesh. Seat D, like seat B, had a curved wooden back and seat, but had wooden arms.

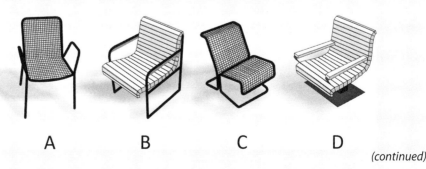

A   B   C   D

(continued)

RESEARCH BOX 3.5. (*Continued*)

The four seats were placed in the hospital cafeteria, where patients, visitors, and staff were asked to sit in them and fill out a short questionnaire. The questionnaire asked the 320 participants to indicate their preferences for the various seats on the basis of comfort and aesthetics. Seat D (curved wood with wooden arms) was the overwhelming favorite. It ranked consistently high on the various comfort and aesthetic criteria as well as on overall evaluation. The researchers recommended that only this seat be selected for the courtyard.

Outdoor Amenities

A number of design features are necessary in order to accommodate diverse uses of outdoor spaces. Mundane, yet important everyday functions include getting a drink of water, properly disposing of trash, and charging a digital device. Consider these guidelines:

- Provide drinking fountains that can be used by children and wheelchair users, as well as by ambulatory adults of all heights.
- Provide trash receptacles that are attractive and yet obvious about their function.
- Install covered electrical outlets near tables and benches.
- Install hose bibs closest to those plantings that require hand watering or that are most used for horticultural therapy (Cooper Marcus and Sachs, 2013).

If outdoor spaces will be used for gatherings, meetings, performances, ceremonies, or community events, consider the following design elements:

- Include a stage or other open area that will accommodate performances and gatherings.
- Install covered electrical outlets near stage areas.
- Provide lighting in stage or presentation areas.
- Provide moveable furnishings (for example, seating, tables, umbrellas) to accommodate different types of large gatherings.
- Provide storage for moveable furnishings.

Additional Considerations

When designing outdoor spaces for healthcare facilities, decision-makers need to consider issues relating to medical emergencies, security, maintenance, and conflicting uses.

Medical emergencies can occur anywhere and may be more likely in and around healthcare facilities. Thus, outdoor spaces need to be equipped with emergency phones or other well-marked and easily used communication systems. Decision-makers may want to consider

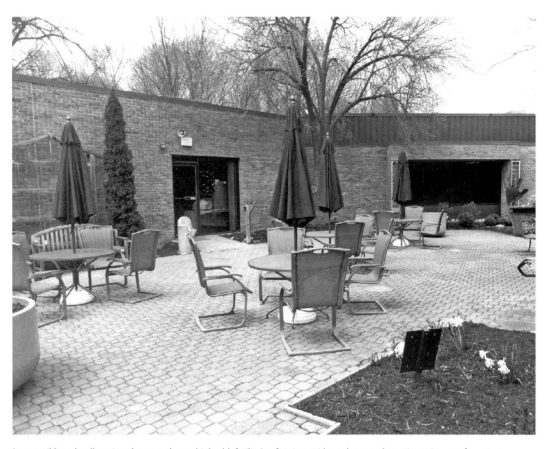

An accessible and well-equipped courtyard near this health facility's cafeteria provides a pleasant, alternative eating area for patients, visitors, and staff. It could also function as a gathering space or small performance venue.

Photo credit: Courtesy of St. Joseph Mercy Chelsea

providing some form of supervision for patients who are outside, because many patients who would benefit from visiting an outdoor area may not be able to leave their unit without assistance (Cooper Marcus and Barnes, 1999; Paine, 1984).

It is important to consider safety when selecting garden elements such as railings. Obviously, poisonous plants should be avoided. Water features present a number of challenges, and the landscape architect should be in early contact with the infection control officer and the facility manager, in order to mitigate potential problems. Issues include easy routine maintenance, the avoidance of spray, which can carry airborne bacteria, and a water feature's interactive potential, which can be either desirable or problematic (Cooper Marcus and Sachs, 2013).

Although a healthcare facility's outdoor space is likely to be more heavily used during the day, it may also be used at night when there may be greater risk of assaults. By following some simple principles, however, planners can design outdoor spaces that discourage crime (Newman,

1975). Lighting should be carefully designed so that there are no unlit areas providing potential hiding places. The location and shape of plantings are critical for security, as well.

Maintenance plays a critical role in preventing hazardous conditions. Winter weather may discourage active use of outdoor spaces at facilities located in cold and snowy climates, but there are always people who use outdoor spaces in all kinds of weather, if only in transit. Icy patches can be treacherous and should be prevented by regular snow removal. In addition, wet leaves can cause slippery surfaces. Walkways need to be kept clear in all seasons.

Regular maintenance is important for keeping outdoor areas looking attractive, encouraging their use, and preserving a positive image. Lawns need to be mowed, plants pruned and watered, and walkways cleared on a regular basis. The selection of plant materials, the design of landscape architectural details, and the provision of a watering system require careful consideration of maintenance ease (Cooper Marcus and Barnes, 1999).

Conflicting user needs are a potential problem in any space. One area of possible conflict in outdoor spaces is between those who want to be social and those who want to be quiet. For instance, large gatherings in the outdoor space could be distracting or disturbing to people using the space for reflection or private conversations. Fountains are one type of design feature that may provide acoustical privacy and buffer noise between areas with potentially conflicting uses.

Smoking has been identified as a source of conflict among users of outdoor spaces at hospitals (Cooper Marcus and Barnes, 1999). Although most campuses are now smoke-free, some places still allow smoking, particularly facilities such as veterans' hospitals, where going for a smoke may be a valuable motivator for patient exercise and socializing (Cooper Marcus and Sachs, 2013). When smoking is banned inside, however, smokers must find outdoor spaces where they can smoke. And as in one study of a patio garden at an AIDS facility, non-smokers tend to avoid such areas due to the concentration of smokers at the entrance and in the seating area (Shepley and Wilson, 1999). It is essential to provide separate outdoor areas for smokers and non-smokers. Smoking-related policies in both indoor and outdoor spaces need to be clearly communicated.

Environmentally Friendly Landscape Design

Given the rising cost of energy and shortages of water in some regions, healthcare-facility designers need to consider environmental impacts when designing outdoor spaces. The US Environmental Protection Agency provides valuable resources on environmentally beneficial landscaping practices (US Environmental Protection Agency, 2008a, 2008b).

The following design practices can reduce costs and minimize the demand on natural resources:

- Consider environmental impacts in the selection of plants and materials (US Environmental Protection Agency, 2008a, 2008b).

- Select plants native to the region to match soil and climate conditions, thereby minimizing water consumption, maintenance, fertilizer, and pesticide use (Phalen, 2008).

- Select low-maintenance or slow-growing plants (Phalen, 2008).

- Group plants according to water and soil needs (Phalen, 2008).

- Plant trees strategically so as to provide shade and a wind barrier, possibly reducing heating and cooling costs in nearby buildings (Phalen, 2008).

- Purchase benches, deck materials, and signs made of environmentally safe materials (Phalen, 2008).

- Purchase recycled gardening equipment such as plastic hoses, garden borders, and planters (Phalen, 2008).

- Recycle materials and packaging when possible (Phalen, 2008).

Another way to be environmentally responsible is to design healthcare facilities with rooftop vegetation (a "green" roof). Green roofs can provide pleasant views from higher floors in adjacent buildings that otherwise might not have access to nature. Green roofs can also provide building insulation, thereby reducing noise as well as heating and cooling costs. They have been shown to last twice as long as traditional roofs, saving maintenance and replacement costs. Green roofs can diminish the "urban heat island" effect of increased city temperatures resulting from heat reflecting off pavements and rooftops. Green roofs also reduce storm-water runoff, which can improve the quality of nearby water bodies (US Environmental Protection Agency, 2015).

Bringing the Outdoors In

Atriums, greenhouses, planters, and window boxes bring nature indoors, providing psychological benefits similar to those gained from access to nature outdoors (Tetlow, 1989). Plants are soothing and restful; they symbolize life, growth, and hope, and they can provide interest and diversion (Hughes and Bryden, 1983; McDuffie, 1984; Wasserman, 1974). The number of people who bring plants or flowers to sick friends or relatives indicates nature's powerful symbolic value (Reizenstein, Vaitkus, and Grant, 1982 [unpub. No. 9]). Plants have been used as a therapeutic tool for psychiatric, pediatric, geriatric, and rehabilitation patients. Some hospitals have incorporated horticulture therapy in their treatment programs (Allison, 1998; Irvine and Warber, 2002; Sempik, Aldridge, and Becker, 2005). Horticulture therapy provides the opportunity for physical activity and social interaction. One study found patient improvements in motor skills, mood, and self-confidence following horticulture therapy sessions (Sempik et al., 2005). For people with vision disabilities, including seniors, it provides an absorbing activity that does not cause eyestrain (Flourney, 1975; Relf, 1978; Spelfogel and Modrzakowski, 1980; Sullivan, 1979).

Design considerations for horticulture therapy gardens include:

- Leave space in the garden or provide planters for residents to do their own gardening (Heath, 2004).

- Accommodate patients with functional limitations by providing ground-level beds, raised beds, handrails, freestanding plant containers, and shelves for the collection of plants in pots (Allison, 1998).

Plants do have their limitations. They are not appropriate in every space and they require maintenance. Because they catch dust and provide a moist growing environment, plants should not be placed in sterile environments such as surgical suites and recovery rooms (Schultz, 1979). It is also possible that funds allocated for the maintenance of indoor plantings may be cut if the administration is not firmly committed to a landscaped interior.

Indoor water features, such as fountains, pools, aquariums, and flowing water, can help create an attractive setting with soothing sights and sounds and can also serve as useful way-finding landmarks. Specialized design is necessary, however, because the Facility Guidelines Institute no longer permits unsealed (open) water features inside a hospital or a licensed outpatient health care occupancy area (Facility Guidelines Institute, 2014).

Views to the Outdoors

Views of outdoor spaces are important, especially if patients are unable to go outside. Attractive views can provide relief, pleasure, and mental rest for both patients and visitors. For long-term and critically ill inpatients, outdoor views provide important "reality cues," reminding them of the season, time of day, and weather. When visual access is provided to an outdoor space, a greater number of users can benefit from it (Cooper Marcus and Barnes, 1999; Paine, 1984).

The content of the outdoor view matters, according to studies conducted in a number of settings, including hospitals, homes, prisons, and workplaces (R. Kaplan, 1993, 2001; Moore, 1981; Tennessen and Cimprich, 1995; Ulrich, 1984; Verderber, 1986). One study, comparing nature views with views of buildings, provided evidence that nature views can increase a patient's sense of well-being and decrease recovery time and the need for pain relief medication. (See Research Box 8.4.) In another study, students in dorm rooms with a nature view performed better on attention measures than students with a view of buildings (Tennessen and Cimprich, 1995).

RESEARCH BOX 8.4 EFFECTS OF OUTSIDE VIEWS ON RECOVERY

Outside views in healthcare facilities offer patients a variety of benefits, from increased orientation to decreased stress. It is also important to consider how windows in patient rooms affect patient outcomes.

One researcher studied the records of patients in a 200-bed suburban hospital in Pennsylvania, where, after standard gall bladder surgery, patients were assigned to rooms with a large window facing either a small stand of trees or a plain brown brick wall (Ulrich, 1984). The study examined whether patients in the two types of rooms differed on several post-surgical outcomes: length of stay, doses and strength of analgesics and anti-anxiety medication (including tranquilizers and barbiturates), post-surgical minor complications (such as headache and nausea), and nurses' notes about the patient's condition and course of recovery.

Researchers examined records of 46 surgical patients who met the selection criteria and could be matched by age, gender, smoking, weight, previous hospitalization, year of surgery, floor level, and room color. Surgical methods during the period were sufficiently similar to allow valid matching.

Seven of the 23 pairs were also matched for physician, and among the rest, patients' physicians and room assignments (made as available) were well mixed. There were 15 female pairs and 8 male pairs, ages 20–69, all without serious complications from the surgery or histories of pathology.

The analysis of patient records turned up significant differences between the pairs on three of the five measures. Patients having a view of trees stayed in the hospital after surgery less time on the average than those with a view of the brick wall (7.96 versus 8.70 days per patient).

Most important, between the second and fifth days following surgery, the tree-view patients received fewer than half the number of strong and moderate doses of analgesics and more than twice as many doses of weak medications (for example, aspirin and acetaminophen) than did wall-view patients.

Nurses' notes, written during the first seven days following surgery, were classified as negative or positive (poor or good conditions, respectively) by a nurse who was "blind" to the patients' room assignments. Again, patients with the landscape view had many fewer negative comments in their records than did the wall-view patients (1.13 versus 3.96 per patient). Tree-view patients also had more positive comments, but the difference was not statistically significant.

On the two other measures, tree-view patients fared better than wall-view patients, but the differences were not significant. They took on average fewer anti-anxiety drugs than the wall-view patients and had fewer post-surgical complications. However, an interaction effect apparently existed between the two types of medication, such that the narcotic analgesics taken by the wall-view patients probably lessened the need for anti-anxiety drugs and diminished the likelihood of minor complications.

In summary, patients with a tree view needed less medication and recovered more quickly than those whose views were of a brick wall. The researcher does not speak to the possibility that nurses may tend to give better quality of care to patients in rooms with tree views than they do to those in rooms with brick-wall views or that nurses may tend to perceive patients in rooms with tree views to be in better condition than patients in rooms with brick-wall views.

Studies comparing responses to videos of nature settings versus videos of urban scenes show similar results to the study in Research Box 8.4 (Ulrich et al., 1991; Ulrich, Simons, and Miles, 2003). For example, in one study, researchers found stress recovery was faster and more complete for subjects viewing nature videos than for those viewing urban videos. Nature viewers had lower anger, less fear, and higher positive emotions than did urban viewers (Ulrich et al., 1991).

Consider the following guidelines when planning nature views:

- Provide windows in patient rooms and staff offices to maximize associated benefits.

- Consider providing floor-to-ceiling windows with nature views in high-traffic corridors (Cooper Marcus and Barnes, 1999).

Summary

○ Nature confers not only pleasure but also positive health effects. It has been associated with reduced anxiety, increased relaxation, improvements in the ability to think clearly, and generally, with facilitating recovery from stress and mental fatigue. These benefits are experienced by patients, staff, and other caregivers and can contribute to staff productivity, well-being, and retention. Outdoor spaces can encourage physical activity and support the role of physical fitness in maintaining health. Additionally, attractive outdoor spaces send a message that the facility cares about its customers and can, in turn, affect perceptions of quality care. These outdoor spaces can help attract patients and foster good feelings about a healthcare facility.

○ Outdoor spaces at healthcare facilities come in many forms, from large, centrally located spaces to courtyards, rooftop gardens, vest-pocket parks, and the like. Nearby nature settings such as parks, gardens, and trails can also be considered as resources, especially when patients, visitors, and staff are made aware of them. The many uses of outdoor spaces include exercise, solitude, quiet conversation, work, checking and sending digital messages, children's play, eating, and attending events and performances, as well as "visual uses" such as providing views or a focal points for contemplation. Users include the full range of patients, visitors, and staff.

○ The design of outdoor spaces should begin at the start of the site-planning and building design process, with landscape architects providing expertise about location, orientation, soil, microclimates, water features, plant materials, outdoor furniture, and maintenance, as well as providing budget estimates. Input should be sought from facility managers and potential users of the spaces. Buildings should be designed to take advantage of views and access to outdoor areas.

○ Research into user preferences for outdoor spaces in healthcare facilities confirms the desirability of trees, water features, and plantings, with both long-distance and partially obstructed views, as well as clear signs and landmarks for easy wayfinding. Visual access should be provided from main public spaces and circulation areas. Direct access from public areas, particularly eating areas, is desirable. Accessibility requirements must be met regarding use by people with functional limitations. Seating should be comfortable but also varied, offering choices of location and arrangement. Amenities such as trash receptacles and drinking fountains should be provided. Safety must be a high priority for all users, and especially children and people with functional limitations, and designers should consider environmental impacts and strive for environmentally friendly design. Nature can also be brought indoors by means of therapy gardens, plants, and by providing visual access to outdoor views.

DISCUSSION QUESTIONS

1. What are some physical and psychological benefits derived from including nature in the design of healthcare facilities?

2. What are some options for including nature in healthcare-facility design?

3. What is the meaning of the term "healing garden"? Why has it come into common use?

4. What are important design process considerations regarding healthcare-facility outdoor spaces?

5. How can outdoor areas be designed to be accessible to people with functional limitations? What safety measures should be considered?

6. What design issues should be considered in the creation of seating options and walkway construction?

7. What factors are important in achieving environmentally friendly design of outdoor spaces?

8. What are some options for "bringing the outdoors in"?

Design Review Questions
The Importance of Nature in Healthcare Facilities

☐ Will access to nature be provided to all who can benefit, including patients, family members, visitors, and staff?

Facilitating Recovery from Mental Fatigue
Encouraging Physical Activity

☐ Will decision-makers consider ways in which the design of outdoor spaces can support physical activity?

Creating a Positive Image

☐ Will the facility's marketing materials highlight the availability of outdoor spaces?

Valuing Access to Nature in Healthcare Facilities

☐ Will the health facility offer accessible outdoor spaces?

☐ Will nearby parks, gardens, and trails be identified? Will decision-makers provide maps, directions, and a shuttle service to nearby outdoor activity sites?

☐ Will the needs of all users of the outdoor space be considered, including active, passive, and visual users?

☐ Will the needs of people of all ages and abilities be considered?

☐ Will there be an effort to include at least one outdoor space available only to staff?

☐ Will the purposes for and benefits of outdoor spaces be clearly communicated to staff, patients, and visitors? (Whitehouse et al., 2001)

☐ Will staff be encouraged to integrate the use of outdoor spaces in patient care? (Whitehouse et al., 2001)

Designing Outdoor Spaces for Healthcare Facilities

☐ Will a participatory approach be used in designing outdoor spaces?

Planning and Designing Outdoor Areas during New Construction

☐ In new construction, will the design of outdoor areas be incorporated into the early phases of site planning and design? (Cooper Marcus and Barnes, 1999)

☐ Will a landscape architect be selected who is trained in the design of therapeutic gardens? (Cooper Marcus and Barnes, 1999; Cooper Marcus and Sachs, 2013)

☐ Will views and access to nature be considered during the planning and design process, especially with regard to building locations? (Cooper Marcus and Barnes, 1999)

☐ Will the main garden (outdoor space) be visible and accessible from major circulation paths and other interior public spaces? (Cooper Marcus and Sachs, 2013)

☐ Will gardens be located away from food exhaust vents? (Cooper Marcus and Sachs, 2013)

☐ Will the main garden be designed so it receives an optimal amount of sunlight? (Cooper Marcus and Sachs, 2013)

☐ Will paths and sidewalks be as level as possible? (Cooper Marcus and Barnes, 1999)

☐ Will courtyards be at least ~30 feet (~9.1 meters) wide, if they are located between walls with windows? (Cooper Marcus and Barnes, 1999)

☐ In spaces enclosed by buildings, will the relationship between the width of the open space and the height of the adjacent buildings be at a ratio between 1:3 and 1:2? (Cooper Marcus and Sachs, 2013)

☐ In areas enclosed by buildings, will trees be selected and located to create a space at "human scale"? (Cooper Marcus and Barnes, 1999)

Creating a Preferred Nature Setting

☐ Will clearly marked walkways and landmarks be provided? (Cooper Marcus and Barnes, 1999; R. Kaplan et al., 1998)

☐ Will long-distance and partially obstructed views be provided? (Cooper Marcus and Barnes, 1999; R. Kaplan et al., 1998)

☐ Will there be a ratio of approximately 30 percent hardscape (steps, walls, paving, and so on) to 70 percent vegetation? (Cooper Marcus and Barnes, 1999)

☐ Will trees, shrubs, and flowers be chosen to provide outdoor spaces with different colors and fragrances throughout the year? (Cooper Marcus and Barnes, 1999)

☐ Will the space be organized with distinct boundaries between areas? (R. Kaplan et al., 1998)

Design That Cares: Planning Health Facilities for Patients and Visitors, third edition, by Janet R. Carpman and Myron A. Grant. ©2016 by Jossey-Bass.

☐ Will outdoor spaces be designed to have as many trees and shrubs as possible? (Reizenstein and Grant, 1981 [unpub. No. 10])

☐ Will soothing design features be considered such as water features and plants whose foliage moves easily? (Cooper Marcus and Barnes, 1995, 1999; R. Kaplan and Kaplan, 1995)

☐ Will interactive design features and activities be considered, such as allowing users to water and weed plants, plant flowers, and make crafts?

☐ Will plants and garden features be selected to attract butterflies, birds, chipmunks, and squirrels and promote animal-watching by indoor viewers and outdoor users? (Cooper Marcus and Barnes, 1999)

☐ Will a range of seating arrangements and locations be provided, from public to private? (Reizenstein and Grant, 1981 [unpub. No. 10])

☐ Will some seating and planting areas be designed to provide a sense of enclosure and privacy, with views to and from the seating through trees and shrubs?

☐ Will plantings and bench arrangements be designed to provide comfortable settings for conversation and people-watching? (Reizenstein and Grant, 1981 [unpub. No. 10])

☐ Where appropriate, will some open lawn be available for active use? (Cooper Marcus and Barnes, 1999; Paine, 1984)

Location and Access

☐ Will visual access to outdoor spaces be provided from main public circulation spaces and patient rooms? (Cooper Marcus and Barnes, 1999; Paine, 1984)

☐ Will indoor seating be available near windows with nature views? (Rodiek and Fried, 2004)

☐ Will direct access be available to outdoor spaces from public areas and dining areas? (Cooper Marcus and Barnes, 1999; Paine, 1984)

☐ Will seating and a canopy, roof, or other shelter be available at the entrance to the main garden? (Cooper Marcus and Sachs, 2013)

☐ Will outdoor spaces be labeled on maps? (Cooper Marcus and Barnes, 1999; Paine, 1984)

☐ Will the location of outdoor spaces be included in directional sign messages? (Cooper Marcus and Barnes, 1999)

☐ Will outdoor spaces be included in facility tours? (Cooper Marcus and Barnes, 1999; Paine, 1984)

☐ Will exterior lighting enhance safety and security and be aesthetically pleasing? (Cooper Marcus and Barnes, 1999; Paine, 1984; Souhrada, 1989)

☐ In waiting areas, will pagers or text messaging be offered so patients and visitors can use adjacent gardens while waiting? (Cooper Marcus and Sachs, 2013)

☐ Will heavy or self-locking doors be avoided at entrances to outdoor spaces? (Paine, 1984)

☐ Will automatic doors be provided at the entrances to outdoor spaces to ensure easy access for all users? (Cooper Marcus and Barnes, 1999; Paine, 1984)

☐ Will there be visual access to outdoor spaces, so patients and visitors can decide if they want to use them? (Cooper Marcus and Barnes, 1999; Paine, 1984)

☐ Will staff be able to monitor outdoor spaces from indoors? (Cooper Marcus and Barnes, 1999)

Walkways

☐ Will sidewalk surfaces facilitate smooth rides for people using stretchers, gurneys, wheelchairs, strollers, and other wheeled equipment? Will control joints be as flat as possible? (Cooper Marcus and Barnes, 1999; Cooper Marcus and Sachs, 2013; Paine, 1984; Whitehouse et al., 2001)

☐ Will curbs be provided along main pathways, for ease of users with wheeled equipment? (Cooper Marcus and Sachs, 2013)

☐ Will ramps be avoided at doorways, so as not to impede the movement of patients and visitors using wheeled equipment? (Cooper Marcus and Barnes, 1999; Paine, 1984)

☐ Will continuous handrails be provided along both sides of walkways in both sloped and flat areas?

☐ If metal handrails are used, will they be coated with a material that prevents them from becoming hot, cold, or slippery? (Koncelik, 1976)

☐ Will walkways be wide enough for two gurneys to pass or for three or four people to walk side-by-side? (Cooper Marcus and Barnes, 1999)

☐ Will walkways be kept clear of leaves, ice, and snow?

☐ In regions where winter weather is severe, will melting devices in the concrete be provided to prevent ice and snow on walkways? (Cooper Marcus and Barnes, 1999)

☐ Will permeable surfaces be used in order to decrease water runoff and improve groundwater recharge?

Outdoor Seating

☐ Will a variety of seating types be provided, including benches and chairs? (Reizenstein and Grant, 1981 [unpub. No. 10])

☐ Will seating arrangements accommodate groups of different sizes and allow for conversation? (Reizenstein and Grant, 1981 [unpub. No. 10])

☐ Will some moveable seating be available?

☐ Will seating be oriented to allow users choices about facing or facing away from the wind and sun? (Cooper Marcus and Barnes, 1999; Paine, 1984)

☐ Will the majority of the seating be placed against a comforting backing, such as a wall or plantings? (Cooper Marcus and Sachs, 2013)

☐ Will some seats be placed along major circulation paths so users can people-watch?

☐ Will some seats be placed so users feel a sense of enclosure and privacy?

☐ Will some seating be available around tables? (Paine, 1984)

☐ Will some seating areas allow for patients on gurneys, on stretchers, or in wheelchairs?

☐ Will seating have backs and armrests?

☐ Will some seating be provided with higher-than-usual seat heights in order to assist people who have difficulty sitting and rising?

☐ Will seating be comfortable for a long period?

☐ Will concrete seating be avoided?

☐ Will seating be considered attractive by most patients and visitors?

Outdoor Amenities

☐ Will drinking fountains be usable by all patients and visitors?

☐ Will attractive, identifiable trash receptacles be available?

☐ Will the outdoor space accommodate large public gatherings, performances, and presentations?

☐ Will covered electrical outlets be available near tables, benches, and stage areas?

☐ Will lighting be available in stage or presentation areas?

☐ Will hose bibs be installed closest to plantings that require hand watering or that are used for horticulture therapy? (Cooper Marcus and Sachs, 2013)

☐ Will moveable furnishings (for example, seating, tables, umbrellas) be available to accommodate different types of gatherings?

☐ Will storage be available for moveable furnishings?

Additional Considerations

☐ Will an emergency communication system be provided?

☐ Will safety be considered when decision-makers choose garden elements, such as railings, water features, and non-poisonous plants? (Heath, 2004)

☐ Will lighting be provided to facilitate wayfinding and discourage crime?

☐ Will trees and shrubs be selected and arranged for safety? (Newman, 1975)

☐ Will outdoor spaces be maintained, including mowing lawns, pruning and watering plants, and clearing walkways of snow, ice, and debris?

☐ Will plants, watering systems, and other design elements be selected to facilitate ease of maintenance?

☐ Will a fountain or other water feature be provided between areas with potentially conflicting uses to buffer noise and provide acoustical privacy?

☐ Will the smoking policy be clearly indicated in both outdoor and indoor areas?

Environmentally Friendly Landscape Design

☐ Will environmental impacts be considered in the selection of plants and materials? (US Environmental Protection Agency, 2008a, 2008b)

☐ Will local plants and trees native to the region be selected to match soil and climate conditions? (Phalen, 2008)

☐ Will low-maintenance or slow-growing plants be selected? (Phalen, 2008)

☐ Will plants be grouped according to soil and water needs? (Phalen, 2008)

☐ Will trees be placed strategically with regard to shade on buildings, in order to reduce heating and cooling costs? (Phalen, 2008)

☐ Will benches, deck materials, and signs be made of environmentally safe materials? (Phalen, 2008)

☐ Will recycled gardening equipment (such as hoses, garden borders, planters) be used? (Phalen, 2008)

☐ Will materials and packaging be recycled when possible? (Phalen, 2008)

☐ Will a green roof or rooftop garden be considered? (US Environmental Protection Agency, 2015)

Bringing the Outdoors In

☐ Will plants be considered as a therapeutic tool for patients? (Allison, 1998; Flourney, 1975; Irvine and Warber, 2002; Relf, 1978; Sempik et al., 2005; Spelfogel and Modrzakowski, 1980; Sullivan, 1979)

☐ Will space be provided for patients to do their own gardening? (Heath, 2004)

☐ Will ground-level beds, raised beds, handrails, free-standing plant containers, and shelves for collection of plants in pots be provided to accommodate patients with a variety of abilities? (Allison, 1998)

☐ Will sealed indoor water features be considered? (Facility Guidelines Institute, 2014)

Views to the Outdoors

☐ Will windows in patient rooms, staff offices, lounges, waiting areas, lobbies, food-services areas, and corridors maximize exterior views?

☐ Will floor-to-ceiling windows with nature views be considered in high-traffic corridors? (Cooper Marcus and Barnes, 1999)

References

Alcock, D. Developing an outdoor playground. *Dimensions in Health Service* 55:32–37, 1978.

Alexander, C., Ishikawa, S., and Silverstein, M. *A Pattern Language.* New York: Oxford University Press, 1977.

Allison, P. C., et al., The anatomy of a healing garden. *Journal of Healthcare Design* 10:101–12, 1998.

Berman, M., Jonides, J., and Kaplan, S. The cognitive benefits of interacting with nature. *Psychological Science 19*(12):1207–12, 2008.

Canin, L. H. Psychological restoration among AIDS caregivers: Maintaining self-care. Unpublished PhD diss., University of Michigan, Ann Arbor, 1991. [Available from ProQuest, 789 E. Eisenhower Parkway, Ann Arbor, MI 48108.]

Cimprich, B. Development of an intervention to restore attention in cancer patients. *Cancer Nursing* 16(2):83–92, 1993.

Cooper Marcus, C. Great greenery: Some basic advice on creating a healing garden. *Health Facilities Management* 15(5); 20–23, May 2002.

Cooper Marcus, C., and Barnes, M. Gardens in healthcare facilities: Uses, therapeutic benefits, and design recommendations. Center for Health Design, 1995.

_____. *Healing Gardens: Therapeutic Benefits and Design Recommendations.* New York; Wiley, 1999.

Cooper Marcus, C., and Sachs, N. A. *Therapeutic Landscapes: An Evidence-Based Approach to Designing Healing Gardens and Restorative Outdoor Spaces.* Hoboken, NJ: Wiley, 2013.

Facility Guidelines Institute. Major additions and revisions. *2014 FGI Guidelines for Hospitals and Outpatient Facilities.* www.fgiguidelines.org/guidelines2014_HOP.php.

Flourney, R. L. Gardening as therapy: Treatment activities for psychiatric patients. *Hospital and Community Psychiatry* 26(2):75–76, February 1975.

Frumkin, H. Beyond toxicity: Human health and the natural environment. *American Journal of Preventive Medicine* 20(3):234–40, 2001.

Gerlach-Spriggs, N., Kaufman, R. E., and Warner, S. B. *Restorative Gardens: The Healing Landscape.* New Haven, CT: Yale University Press, 1998.

Grant, M. A. Structured participatory input. Master's thesis, University of Michigan, Ann Arbor, 1979.

Hartag, T., Mang, M., and Evans, G. W. Restorative effects of natural environment experiences. *Environment and Behavior* 23(1):3–26, 1991.

Heath, Y. Evaluating the effect of therapeutic gardens. *American Journal for Alzheimer's Disease and Other Dementias* 19(4):239–42, July–August 2004.

Henneberry, I., and Robertson, P. Free in the sun: An outdoor program in a health care setting. *Children's Health Care* 12(1):37–40, Summer 1983.

Hughes, E. F., and Bryden, M. C. The development of an occupational therapy program in a solarium area. *Canadian Journal of Occupational Therapy* 50(1):15–19, February 1983.

Humpel, N., Owen, N., and Leslie, E. Environmental factors associated with adults' participation in physical activity: A review. *American Journal of Preventive Medicine* 22(3), 188–199, 2002.

Irvine, K. N., and Warber, S. L. Greening healthcare: Practicing as if the natural environment really mattered. *Alternative Therapies in Health and Medicine* 8(5):76, 2002.

Kaplan, R. The nature of the view from home: Psychological benefits. *Environment and Behavior* 33(4): 507–42, 2001.

———. The role of nature in the context of the workplace. *Landscape and Urban Planning* 26(1–4): 193–201, 1993.

———. The role of nature in the urban context. In I. Altman and J. F. Wohlwill, editors. *Human Behavior and Environment: Advances in Theory and Research.* Vol. 6. New York: Plenum, 1983.

Kaplan, R., and Kaplan, S. *The Experience of Nature: A Psychological Perspective.* Cambridge: Cambridge University Press, 1989. (Republished by Ulrich's Bookstore located in Ann Arbor, Michigan, 1995)

Kaplan, R., Kaplan, S., and Ryan, R. L. *With People in Mind: Design and Management of Everyday Nature.* Washington, DC: Island Press, 1998.

Kaplan, S. The restorative benefits of nature: Toward an integrative framework. *Journal of Environmental Psychology* 15(3):169–82, 1995.

Kaplan, S., and Kaplan, R. *Cognition and Environment: Functioning in an Uncertain World.* New York: Praeger, 1983.

———, editors. *Humanscape: Environments for People.* Belmont, CA: Duxbury, 1978.

Koncelik, I. A. *Designing the Open Nursing Home.* Stroudsburg, PA: Dowden, Hutchinson and Ross, 1976.

McDuffie, R. F. The greening of interiors. *Interior Landscape Industry* 1(6):29–31, June 1984.

Moore, E. O. A prison environment's effect on health care service demands. *Journal of Environmental Systems, 1981–1982* (11):17–34, 1981.

Moore, G., Cohen, U., and McGinty, T. *Planning and Design Guidelines: Child Care Centers and Outdoor Play Environments.* 7 vols. Milwaukee: Center for Architecture and Urban Planning Research, University of Wisconsin, Milwaukee, 1979.

Moore, G., Cohen, U., et al., *Designing Environments for Handicapped Children.* New York: Educational Facilities Laboratory, 1979.

Nassauer, J. I. Messy ecosystems, orderly frames. *Landscape Journal* 14(2):161–70, 1995.

Newman, O. *Design Guidelines for Creating Defensible Space.* Washington, DC: US Government Printing Office, 1975.

Olds, A., and Daniel, P. *Child Health Care Facilities: Design Guidelines and Literature Review.* Washington, DC: Association for the Care of Children's Health, 1987.

Olsen, R. V. A user evaluation of a hospital park. Unpublished report. Environmental Design Program, Bellevue Hospital Center, New York, n.d.

Owen, N., Humpel, N., Leslie, E., Bauman, A., and Sallis, J. F. Understanding environmental influences on walking: Review and research agenda. *American Journal of Preventive Medicine* 27(1), 67–76, 2004.

Paine, R. Design guidelines for hospital open space: Case studies of three hospitals. Master's thesis, University of California, Berkeley, 1984.

Phalen, K. B. Personal communication, December 12, 2008.

Reizenstein, J. E., and Grant, M. A. Outdoor seating evaluation. Unpublished research report No. 22. Patient and Visitor Participation Project, Office of Hospital Planning, Research and Development, University of Michigan, Ann Arbor, 1983.

_____. Patient activities and schematic design preferences. Unpublished research report No. 2. Patient and Visitor Participation Project, Office of Hospital Planning, Research and Development, University of Michigan, Ann Arbor, 1981.

_____. Patient and visitor preferences for outdoor courtyard design. Unpublished research report No. 10. Patient and Visitor Participation Project, Office of Hospital Planning, Research and Development, University of Michigan, Ann Arbor, 1981.

Reizenstein, J. E., Vaitkus, M. A., and Grant, M. A. Patient belongings. Unpublished research report No. 9. Patient and Visitor Participation Project, Office of Hospital Planning, Research and Development, University of Michigan, Ann Arbor, 1982.

Relf, P. D. Horticulture as a recreational activity. *Journal of American Health Care Association* 4(5): 68–71, September 1978.

Rodiek, S. D., and Fried, J. T. Access to the outdoors: Using photographic comparison to assess preferences of assisted living residents. *Landscape and Urban Planning*, 2004. DOI:10.1016/j .landurbplan.2004.11.006.

Schultz, I. K. Plants in OR harbor potential contaminants. *Association of Operating Room Nurses Journal* 29(5):898–99, April 1979.

Sempik, J., Aldridge, J., and Becker, S. *Health, Well-Being, and Social Inclusion: Therapeutic Horticulture in the UK.* Bristol: Policy Press, University of Bristol, 2005.

Shepley, M. M., and Wilson, P. Designing for persons with AIDS: A post-occupancy study at the Bailey-Boushay House. *Journal of Architectural and Planning Research* 16(1):17–32, Spring 1999.

Sherman, S. A., Varni, J. W., Ulrich, R. S., and Malcarne, V. L. Post-occupancy evaluation of healing gardens in a pediatric cancer center. *Landscape and Urban Planning, 73*(2–3):167–83, 2005.

Souhrada, L. Lighting decisions affect image, morale, efficiency. *Health Facilities Management* 2(5): 19–27, May 1989.

Spelfogel, B., and Modrzakowski, M. Curative factors in horticultural therapy in a hospital setting. *Hospital and Community Psychiatry* 31(8):572–73, August 1980.

Sternberg, E. M. *Healing Spaces: The Science of Place and Well-Being.* Cambridge, MA: Belknap Press, 2010.

Stigsdotter, U., and Grahn, P. Experiencing a garden: A healing garden for people suffering from burnout diseases. *Journal of Therapeutic Horticulture* XIV:38–49, 2003.

Sullivan, M. E. Horticultural therapy: The role gardening plays in healing. *Journal of the American Health Care Association* 5(3):3–8, May 1979.

Taylor, A. F., Kuo, F. E., and Sullivan, W. C. (2001). Coping with ADD: The surprising connection to green play settings. *Environment and Behavior* 33(1):54–77, 2001.

Tennessen, C. M., and Cimprich, B. Views to nature: Effects on attention. *Journal of Environmental Psychology* 15(1):77–85, 1995.

Tetlow, K. Healing abroad. *Interiors,* 90–93, December 1989.

US Environmental Protection Agency. GreenScapes. 2008a. www.epa.gov/greenscapes/.

US Environmental Protection Agency. U.S. EPA's 2008 Report on the Environment (Final Report). U.S. Environmental Protection Agency, Washington, DC: EPA/600/R-07/045F (NTIS PB2008–112484), 2008b.

US Environmental Protection Agency. Using Green Roofs to Reduce Heat Islands. 2015. https://www
.epa.gov/heat-islands/using-green-roofs-reduce-heat-islands.

Ulrich, R. S. Aesthetic and affective response to natural environment. In I. Altman and J. F. Wohlwill,
editors. *Human Behavior and Environment: Advances in Theory and Research*. Vol. 6. New York:
Plenum, 1983.

_____. Natural versus urban scenes: Some psychological effects. *Environment and Behavior* 13(5):
523–56, September 1981.

_____. View through a window may influence recovery from surgery. *Science* 224(4647):420–21, April 27,
1984.

_____. Visual landscapes and psychological well-being. *Landscape Research* 4(1):17–23, Spring 1979.

Ulrich, R. S., Simons, R. F., Losito, B. D., Fiorito, E., Miles, M. A., and Zelson, M. Stress recovery during
exposure to natural and urban environments. *Journal of Environmental Psychology* 11(3):201–30,
1991.

Ulrich, R. S., Simons, R. F., and Miles, M. A. Effects of environmental simulations and television on blood
donor stress. *Journal of Architectural and Planning Research* 20(1): 38–47, 2003.

Ulrich, R. S., Zimring, C., Quan, X., and Joseph, A. The environment's impact on stress. In S. O. Marbury,
editor. *Improving Healthcare with Better Building Design*, 47–59. Chicago: Health Administration
Press, 2006.

Verderber, S. Dimensions of person–window transactions in the hospital environment. *Environment
and Behavior* 18(4):450–66, July 1986.

Wasserman, B. Greening the corner where you are. *Dental Management* 14(12):65–71, December 1974.

Wells, N. M. At home with nature: Effects of "greenness" on children's cognitive functioning. *Environment and Behavior* 32(6):775–95, 2000.

Whitehouse, S., Varni, J. W., Seid, M., Cooper Marcus, C., Ensberg, M. J., Jacobs, J. R., et al. Evaluating
a children's hospital garden environment: Utilization and consumer satisfaction. *Journal of Environmental Psychology* 21(3):301–14, 2001.

Wohlwill, J. F. The concept of nature: A psychologist's view. In I. Altman and J. F. Wohlwill, editors. *Human
Behavior and Environment: Advances in Theory and Research*. Vol. 6. New York: Plenum, 1983.

CHAPTER 9

USERS WITH DISABILITIES

Every patient and visitor is unique and has particular needs and preferences with regard to the physical environment and related features of healthcare facilities. Moreover, changes in ability occur naturally throughout a person's lifetime. As the World Health Organization (WHO) emphasizes, this is not something that happens to only a minority: whether for the short term or the long term, experiencing a decrement in health and a resulting disability (or multiple disabilities) is a universal human experience (WHO, 2002). In addition, the incidence of neurological, emotional, cognitive, and developmental conditions has risen significantly. Therefore, when considering the various needs and preferences of patients and visitors, it is essential to factor in the people for whom physical, mental, and sensory conditions play an even more important role than usual in how they experience health facilities. (We will use the terms *disabilities* and *limitations* synonymously in this chapter.)

Statistics tell the story: in 2012, there were more than 37 million people in the United States with hearing disabilities, almost 21 million with vision disabilities, and more than 35 million with a physical functioning difficulty (CDC/National Center for Health Statistics, 2015). Add to these the large numbers of people who are *temporarily* disabled at any given time because of injury, illness, post-operative recovery, pregnancy, or other reasons, and it is clear that there is tremendous need for supportive design in healthcare and other types of facilities.

LEARNING OBJECTIVES
- Become familiar with the concept of disability, the principles of Universal Design, and US federal legislation on disability rights.
- Understand the design features necessary to ensure equal access to and participation in healthcare services by people with mobility limitations, people who are blind or have low vision, and people who are deaf or hard of hearing.
- Become familiar with the physiological, social, emotional, and psychological changes associated with aging and the design-related needs of older patients and visitors.
- Learn about design requirements related to obese patients and visitors.

The authors thank Valerie Fletcher, Christopher Hart, and Ruth Super of the Institute for Human Centered Design for significant contributions to this chapter.

The Principles of Universal Design were conceived and developed by The Center for Universal Design at The North Carolina State University. Use or application of the Principles in any form by an individual or organization is separate and distinct from the Principles and does not constitute or imply acceptance or endorsement by The Center for Universal Design for the use or application.

In this chapter, we take a look at the design-related needs of people with disabilities related to mobility, hearing, and vision; older people; and obese people.

Statistics Regarding Users with Disabilities

Issues related to accessibility for people with mobility disabilities are likely to affect a large number of healthcare consumers. Consider these figures from the US Census Bureau's 2010 national breakdown of the non-institutionalized population ages 15 and older (Brault, 2012):

– 30.6 million (12.6%) had limitations associated with ambulatory activities of the lower body.
– 23.9 million (9.9%) had difficulty walking a quarter of a mile.
– 22.3 million (9.2%) had difficulty climbing a flight of stairs.
– 11.6 million (4.8%) used a cane, crutches, or walker to assist with mobility.
– 3.6 million (1.5%) used a wheelchair.
– 8.1 million (3.3%) had difficulty seeing words, including 2 million who were blind or unable to see.
– 7.6 million (3.1%) experienced a hearing difficulty, including 1.1 million who had severe difficulty hearing.
– 15.2 million (6.3%) experienced difficulty with some kind of cognitive, mental, or emotional functioning. About 10.6 million (4.4%) had a condition that limited mental or cognitive functioning, such as a learning disability or Alzheimer's disease, senility, or dementia. (Brault, 2012, pp. 8–9)

If these statistics aren't sobering enough, of the 51.5 million adults with a disability in at least one disability category (also called "domains"—communicative, mental, or physical), 30.3 million had a disability in one category, 15.8 million had disabilities in two categories, 4.0 million had disabilities in all three categories, and ~1.3 million adults had a disability for which a category wasn't identified (Brault, 2012).

Thus, it is important for healthcare-facility planners and designers to be concerned with issues of accessibility and usability for people with disabilities, whether visible or hidden, temporary or permanent. As a US Department of Justice publication emphasizes:

Accessibility of doctors' offices, clinics, and other health care providers is essential in providing medical care to people with disabilities. Due to barriers, individuals with disabilities are less likely to get routine preventative medical care than people without disabilities. Accessibility is not only legally required, it is important medically so that minor problems can be detected and treated before turning into major and possibly life-threatening problems. (US Department of Justice, 2010 [Access to Medical], p. 1)

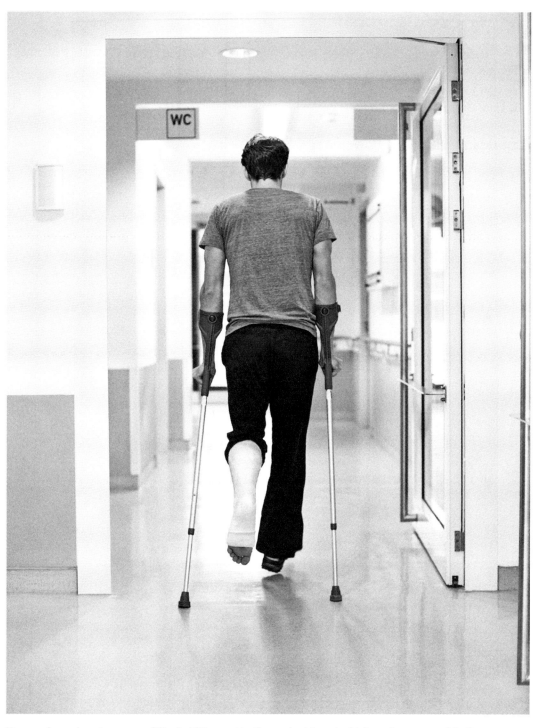

Many people experience temporary mobility disabilities, requiring the use of crutches, wheelchairs, walkers, canes, and the like.

Federal Legislation on Disability Rights

American healthcare providers and health-facility design decision-makers need to be familiar with federal legislation that addresses the rights and requirements of people with disabilities. Pertinent legislation includes the Americans with Disabilities Act (ADA), the Patient Affordable Care Act, and the Section 504 of the Rehabilitation Act of 1973.

Americans with Disabilities Act

The Americans with Disabilities Act of 1990 (ADA):

> prohibits discrimination and ensures equal opportunity for persons with disabilities in employment, State and local government services, public accommodations, commercial facilities, and transportation. It also mandates the establishment of TDD/telephone relay services. The current text of the ADA includes changes made by the ADA Amendments Act of 2008 (P.L. 110–325), which became effective on January 1, 2009. The ADA was originally enacted in public law format and later rearranged and published in the United States Code.
>
> On Friday, July 23, 2010, Attorney General Eric Holder signed final regulations revising the Department's ADA regulations, including its ADA Standards for Accessible Design. The official text was published in the Federal Register on September 15, 2010 (corrections to this text were published in the Federal Register on March 11, 2011).
>
> The revised regulations amend the Department's 1991 title II regulation (State and local governments), 28 CFR Part 35, and the 1991 title III regulation (public accommodations), 28 CFR Part 36. Appendix A to each regulation includes a section-by-section analysis of the rule and responses to public comments on the proposed rule.
>
> These final rules went into effect on March 15, 2011, and were published in the 2011 edition of the Code of Federal Regulations (CFR). (Information and Technical Assistance on the Americans with Disabilities Act, n.d.)

(See Box 9.1.)

BOX 9.1. CONTENTS OF THE US DEPARTMENT OF JUSTICE 2010 ADA STANDARDS FOR ACCESSIBLE DESIGN

Chapter 1. Application and Administration

Chapter 2. Scoping Requirements

Chapter 3. Building Blocks

Chapter 4. Accessible Routes

Chapter 5. General Site and Building Elements

Chapter 6. Plumbing Elements and Facilities

Chapter 7. Communication Elements and Features

Source: US Access Board, 2012 [2010 ADA Standards].

The ADA Standards for Accessible Design provide health facility planners and designers with detailed, cross-referenced information. Some key requirements include:

– Multi-story buildings containing medical offices must have at least one accessible route or elevator serving each floor (US Access Board [Scoping §206.2.3]).

– Ten percent of patient and visitor parking spaces provided to serve hospital outpatient facilities must be accessible and comply with Section 502 parking requirements (US Access Board [Scoping §208.2.1]).

– Twenty percent of patient and visitor parking spaces provided to serve rehabilitation facilities specializing in treating conditions that affect mobility and outpatient physical therapy facilities must be accessible and comply with Section 502 parking requirements (US Access Board [Scoping §208.2.2]).

– Accessible passenger loading zones must be provided at medical care and long-term-care facilities (US Access Board [Scoping §209.3]).

– Every effort must be made to disperse accessible patient bedrooms by medical specialty (US Board [Scoping §§223–223.2.1], Advisory §223.1.1).

– For facilities specializing in treating conditions affecting mobility, all patient sleeping rooms must provide mobility features complying with Section 805 (US Access Board [Scoping §§223–223.2.1], [Scoping §§805–805.4]).

– For facilities not specializing in treating conditions affecting mobility, at least 10 percent, but no fewer than one inpatient room(s) and resident sleeping room(s) must provide turning space, clear floor space on each side of the bed, and where provided, no fewer than one accessible toilet, lavatory, and tub/shower (US Access Board [Scoping §223.2.1], [Scoping §§805–805.4]).

Patient Protection and the Affordable Care Act

People with disabilities have had long-standing concerns over the accessibility of medical equipment, including transfer heights, leg rests and armrests, padding, seat width, and the like. To fill this critical gap in the ADA accessibility standards, the Medical Diagnostic Equipment (MDE) Accessibility Standards Advisory Committee of the United States Access Board issued a report in December 2014 on accessibility standards for medical diagnostic equipment under the "Patient Protection and Affordable Care Act." Once finalized by the Access Board, the standards will be up for adoption by the enforcing authorities, including the US Department of Health and Human Services and the US Department of Justice:

> The proposed standards contain minimum technical criteria to ensure that medical diagnostic equipment, including examination tables, examination chairs, weight scales, mammography equipment, and other imaging equipment used by health care providers for diagnostic purposes, are accessible to and usable by individuals with disabilities. The standards will allow independent entry to, use of, and exit from the equipment by individuals with disabilities to the maximum extent possible. The standards do not impose any mandatory requirements on health care providers or medical device manufacturers. However, other agencies, referred to as an enforcing authority in the standards, may issue regulations or adopt policies that require health care providers subject to their jurisdiction to acquire accessible medical diagnostic equipment that conforms to the standards. (US Access Board 2012 [Proposed Accessibility])

Section 504 of the Rehabilitation Act of 1973

In addition to the ADA, American health-facility design decision-makers need to be familiar with Section 504 of the Rehabilitation Act of 1973, which prohibits discrimination against individuals on the basis of disability (US Department of Human Services, 2006):

> Section 504's prohibitions against discrimination apply to service availability, accessibility, delivery, employment, and the administrative activities and responsibilities of organizations receiving Federal financial assistance. A recipient of Federal financial assistance may not, on the basis of disability:
>
> – Deny qualified individuals the opportunity to participate in or benefit from federally funded programs, services, or other benefits
> – Deny access to programs, services, benefits or opportunities to participate as a result of physical barriers
> – Deny employment opportunities, including hiring, promotion, training, and fringe benefits, for which they are otherwise entitled or qualified . . .
>
> These and other prohibitions against discrimination based on disability can be found in the DHHS Section 504 regulation at 45 CFR Part 84 (US Department of Health and Human Services, 2006).

Designing to Comply with Federal Legislation on Disability Rights

A verbatim description of all of the accessibility guidelines and requirements included in federal legislation, as they pertain to healthcare facilities, is beyond the scope of this book. We advise readers to consult online resources, such as the website of the US Access Board (www .access-board.gov):

> The U.S. Access Board is a federal agency that promotes equality for people with disabilities through leadership in accessible design and the development of accessibility guidelines and standards for the built environment, transportation, communication, medical diagnostic equipment, and information technology.
>
> The Access Board is responsible for developing and updating design guidelines known as the ADA Accessibility Guidelines (ADAAG). These guidelines are used by the Department of Justice (DOJ) and the Department of Transportation (DOT) in setting enforceable standards that the public must follow. As of 2015, both DOJ's and DOT's current ADA Standards are based on the Board's updated ADAAG (2004). As a result, for the most part, these two sets of standards are very similar. However, each contains additional requirements that are specific to the facilities covered by the respective agencies. These additional requirements define the types of facilities covered, set effective dates, and provide additional scoping or technical requirements for those facilities. DOJ's ADA Standards apply to all facilities except public transportation facilities, which are subject to DOT's ADA Standards. The edition of the ADA Standards provided on the Board's website includes DOJ's and DOT's additional provisions (www.access-board.gov).

Readers can access the ADA standards, as well as related graphics and animations, through the Access Board's website: www.access-board.gov/guidelines-and-standards /buildings-and-sites/about-the-ada-standards/guide-to-the-ada-standards

In addition, toll-free telephone assistance at (800) 872–2253 and links to other federal websites (such as Disability.gov; and Regulations.gov) are available on the Access Board website to further elucidate accessibility requirements for particular healthcare facility design projects.

Readers with questions about requirements for healthcare facility design as specified in the ADA, the Patient Protection and Affordable Care Act, or Section 504 of the Rehabilitation Act of 1973 may also wish to consult the US Department of Justice Technical Assistance Manual for Title III (www.ada.gov/taman3.html) or search for the latest available information at www.ada.gov, the Department of Justice website for ADA regulations that apply to state and local governments.

Universal Design

An important emphasis of both Section 504 of the Rehabilitation Act of 1973 and the first Americans with Disabilities Act was on *participation* (US Department of Human Services, 2014). Delivery of goods and services must be made available in an *integrated* setting to the maximum extent appropriate; individuals must have "an equal opportunity to participate in or benefit from the goods and services offered" (Americans with Disabilities Act, ADA Title III Technical Assistance Manual, n.d.).

In the decades since the passage of this legislation, thinking about disability has undergone profound changes. Disability was once regarded as characterizing a subset of people with relatively stable limitations (Fletcher, 2010). As discussed in the introduction to the World Health Organization's *International Classification of Functioning, Disability and Health* (ICF):

> Previously, disability began where health ended; once you were disabled, you were in a separate category. We want to get away from this kind of thinking. We want to make ICF a tool for measuring functioning in society, no matter what the reason for one's impairments. . . This is a radical shift. From emphasizing people's disabilities, we now focus on their level of health. . . ICF thus "mainstreams" the experience of disability and recognizes it as a universal human experience. (World Health Organization, 2002, p. 3. www.who.int /classifications/icf/training/icfbeginnersguide.pdf)

Disability is now widely recognized as a "contextual variable, dynamic over time, and in relation to circumstances" (Fletcher, 2010, p. 365). Universal Design recognizes and responds to the facts of human diversity in age and abilities.

Slowly but surely, the concept of Universal Design is gaining hold globally. Universal Design, also known as *inclusive design, human-centered design*, or *design for all*, is a way of focusing:

> on the user, on the widest range of people operating in the widest range of situations without special or separate design. . . Universal design is human-centered design (of everything) with everyone in mind. (Fletcher, 2010, p. 363)

> Disability is a gradient on which every person functions at different levels due to personal and environmental factors. (Brault, 2012, p. 1)

Experience with accessible and barrier-free policies in a number of developed nations led to the realization that "design could do more than reduce barriers. It could enhance everyone's experience" (Fletcher, 2010, p. 364). Design that enables people with disabilities rarely inconveniences and usually helps everyone. As one architectural journal put it:

> Automatic doors relieve everyone of manual effort; grab bars in showers protect everyone from falls; telephone volume controls help everyone hear better in a noisy environment; and talking exit signs aid everyone's evacuation of a building. (Fisher, 1985, p. 123)

Design principles now go beyond the removal of barriers to ensuring, enabling, and supporting environments that facilitate both capacity and performance. Universal Design seeks "user-friendly and elegant solutions . . . to improve the environment for as many people as possible" (Herssens and Heylighen, 2007). Research and innovation are required to meet the challenge of designing across the full spectrum of functional issues in the full range of environments: physical, communication, information, policy, and social.

And as the Institute for Human Centered Design's Executive Director, Valerie Fletcher, notes:

> Many interior designers, especially young interior designers, have little direct knowledge of functional limitations and the ways in which design can either impede or enhance daily life and choice. (Fletcher, 2010, p. 364)

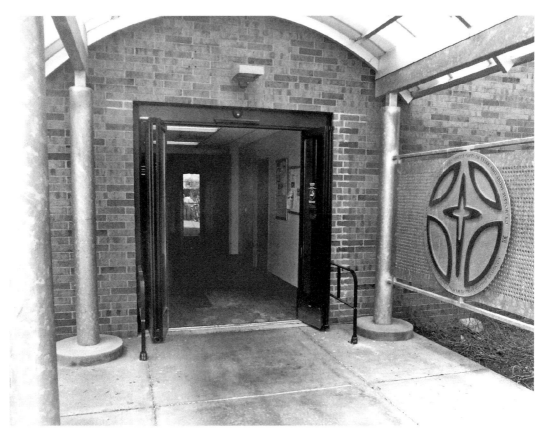

This hospital entrance provides a smooth, accessible transition between indoors and outdoors. Motion-sensitive automatic door openers eliminate the need to push open heavy doors.

Photo credit: Courtesy of St. Joseph Mercy Ann Arbor

Central to achieving the purposes of Universal Design, therefore, is the engagement of "user/experts"—such as wheelchair users, people with low vision, parents of toddlers, caregivers, or older people experiencing the functional changes associated with aging—whose natural experience gives them particular insight into the functionality and accessibility of designed environments (Fletcher, 2010; Ostroff, 1997).

Design principles and guidelines have been developed to assist design decision-makers in creating environments that respond to the wide range of abilities in cognition, vision, hearing, speech, and physical functions (Iezzoni and O'Day, 2006; NCODH and NCSU Center for Universal Design, 2007; Story, Mueller, and Mace, 1998).

The seven principles of Universal Design (see Boxes 9.2 and 9.3) were developed by a working group of environmental design researchers, architects, product designers, and engineers funded by the National Institute on Disability and Rehabilitation Research and the US Department of Education (Connell et al., 1997; NCODH and NCSU Center for Universal Design, 2007).

BOX 9.2. PRINCIPLES OF UNIVERSAL DESIGN AND ASSOCIATED GUIDELINES

Principle 1. Equitable Use

The design is useful and marketable to people with diverse abilities.

Guidelines:

1a. Provide the same means of use for all users: identical whenever possible; equivalent when not.

1b. Avoid segregating or stigmatizing any users.

1c. Provisions for privacy, security, and safety should be equally available to all users.

1d. Make the design appealing to all users.

Principle 2. Flexibility in Use

The design accommodates a wide range of individual preferences and abilities.

Guidelines:

2a. Provide choice in methods of use.

2b. Accommodate right- or left-handed access and use.

2c. Facilitate the user's accuracy and precision.

2d. Provide adaptability to the user's pace.

Principle 3. Simple and Intuitive Use

Use of the design is easy to understand, regardless of the user's experience, knowledge, language skills, or current concentration level.

Guidelines:

3a. Eliminate unnecessary complexity.

3b. Be consistent with user expectations and intuition.

3c. Accommodate a wide range of literacy and language skills.

3d. Arrange information consistent with its importance.

3e. Provide effective prompting and feedback during and after task completion.

Principle 4. Perceptible Information

The design communicates necessary information effectively to the user, regardless of ambient conditions or the user's sensory abilities.

Guidelines:

4a. Use different modes (pictorial, verbal, tactile) for redundant presentation of essential information.

4b. Provide adequate contrast between essential information and its surroundings.

4c. Maximize "legibility" of essential information.

4d. Differentiate elements in ways that can be described (i.e., make it easy to give instructions or directions).

4e. Provide compatibility with a variety of techniques or devices used by people with sensory limitations.

Principle 5. Tolerance for Error

The design minimizes hazards and the adverse consequences of accidental or unintended actions.

Guidelines:

5a. Arrange elements to minimize hazards and errors: most used elements, most accessible; hazardous elements eliminated, isolated, or shielded.

5b. Provide warnings of hazards and errors.

5c. Provide fail safe features.

5d. Discourage unconscious action in tasks that require vigilance.

Principle 6. Low Physical Effort

The design can be used efficiently and comfortably and with a minimum of fatigue.

Guidelines:

6a. Allow user to maintain a neutral body position.

6b. Use reasonable operating forces.

6c. Minimize repetitive actions.

6d. Minimize sustained physical effort.

Principle 7. Size and Space for Approach and Use

Appropriate size and space is provided for approach, reach, manipulation, and use regardless of user's body size, posture, or mobility.

Guidelines:

7a. Provide a clear line of sight to important elements for any seated or standing user.

7b. Make reach to all components comfortable for any seated or standing user.

7c. Accommodate variations in hand and grip size.

7d. Provide adequate space for the use of assistive devices or personal assistance.

Please note that the Principles of Universal Design address only universally usable design, while the practice of design involves more than consideration for usability. Designers must also incorporate other considerations such as economic, engineering, cultural, gender, and environmental concerns in their design processes. These Principles offer designers guidance to better integrate features that meet the needs of as many users as possible.

BOX 9.3. UNIVERSAL DESIGN RESOURCES

The Institute for Human Centered Design (Boston) recommends the following resources related to Universal Design. See their website for a full list:

http://www.humancentereddesign.org/universal-design/universal-design-resources

Barker, P., Barrick, J., and Wilson, R. *Building Sight: A Handbook of Building and Interior Design Solutions to Include the Needs of Visually Impaired People.* New York: AFB Press, 1995.

Clarkson, J., Coleman, R., Keates, S., and Lebbon, C., editors. *Inclusive Design: Design for the Whole Population.* London: Springer, 2003.

Clarkson, J., and Keates, S. *Countering Design Exclusion: An Introduction to Inclusive Design.* London: Springer, 2003.

Coleman, R. *Living Longer: The New Context for Design.* London: Design Council, 2001.

Covington, G., and Hannah, B. *Access by Design.* New York: Wiley, 1997.

Lebovich, W. *Designing for Dignity: Accessible Environments for People with Disabilities.* New York: Wiley, 1993.

Leibrock, C. A. *Beautiful Barrier Free: A Visual Guide to Accessibility.* New York: Wiley, 1992.

Leibrock, C. A., and Harris, D. D. *Design Details for Health: Making the Most of Interior Design's Healing Potential.* New York: Wiley, 1999.

Leibrock, C. A., and Terry, J. E. *Beautiful Universal Design: A Visual Guide (2nd ed.)* New York: Wiley, 1999.

Lifchez, R. *Rethinking Architecture: Design Students and Physically Disabled People.* Berkeley: University of California Press, 1986.

Mueller, J. L. *Case Studies on Universal Design.* Raleigh: North Carolina State University, Center for Universal Design, 1998.

New York Mayor's Office for People with Disabilities (MOPD), City of New York, and the Center for Inclusive Design and Environmental Access (IDEA), School of Architecture and Planning, University at Buffalo, State University of New York. 2001. *Universal Design New York.* Free publication by MPOD. www.nyc.gov.

Norman, D. A. *The Design of Everyday Things.* New York: Basic Books, 2013.

Pirkl, J., and Pulos, A. J. *Transgenerational Design: Products for an Aging Population.* New York: Wiley, 1997.

Preiser, W. F. E., and Smith, K. H. *Universal Design Handbook* (2nd ed.) New York: McGraw Hill Professional, 2011.

Story, M. F., Mueller, J. L., and Mace, R. L. *The Universal Design File: Designing for People of all Ages and Abilities.* Raleigh: North Carolina State University, Center for Universal Design, 1998.

Design Considerations for Patients and Visitors with Mobility Disabilities

In addition to following all current ADA requirements and guidelines, healthcare-facility decision-makers should consider the following guidelines in order to meet the needs of users with mobility disabilities:

- Install automatic doors with controls at a height reachable by people in wheelchairs and out of the way of the door swing (Iezzoni and O'Day, 2006; Insights into, 2004; Jones and Tamari, 1997).

- Provide smooth, level surfaces at doorways; be sure weather matting (both temporary and permanent) and thresholds do not interfere with wheelchair use or are loose and become trip hazards (Iezzoni and O'Day, 2006; Insights into, 2004; Jones and Tamari, 1997; NCODH and NCSU Center for Universal Design, 2007).

- Provide continuous handrails on both sides along circulation routes.

- Provide resting areas with seats along lengthy corridors.

- Provide a reception desk with a portion of the surface low enough to welcome people in wheelchairs and another portion high enough for people who have difficulty bending.

- Be sure tables, reception and information desks, and counters for filling out paperwork allow for the use of chairs with arms, so people with mobility limitations and joint problems can sit and rise independently.

- Be sure tables, desks, and counters for filling out paperwork have ample space underneath to accommodate wheelchair users. Because of the wide variety of wheelchairs, a flexible, adjustable table may be more accommodating than one with a fixed height (Iezzoni and O'Day, 2006; Jones and Tamari, 1997; NCODH and NCSU Center for Universal Design, 2007).

- Install grab bars in bathrooms in a way that accommodates wheelchair users and people with disabilities on their left or right sides. Ensure that personal assistants can move grab bars out of the way (Edlich et al., 1998; Jones and Tamari, 1997; Tetlow, 1995).

- Place soap, hand dryers, dispensers, changing stations, and mirrors so wheelchair users can easily use them (Iezzoni and O'Day, 2006; Jones and Tamari, 1997; NCODH and NCSU Center for Universal Design, 2007).

- Provide good contrast between fixtures, flooring, and walls.

- Avoid glare and shadows when designing and selecting lighting.

- Avoid putting floor drains in accessible routes.

Guidelines for Accessible Exam and Treatment Rooms

With regard to the design of examination rooms for people with mobility disabilities, it is important to provide:

- An accessible route to and through the room (US Department of Justice, 2010 [Access to Medical], p. 5).
- An entry door with adequate clear width, maneuvering clearance, and accessible hardware (US Department of Justice, 2010 [Access to Medical], p. 5).
- Appropriate models and placement of accessible examination equipment (US Department of Justice, 2010 [Access to Medical], p. 5).
- Adequate clear floor space inside the room for side transfers and use of lift equipment (US Department of Justice, 2010 [Access to Medical], p. 5).

Entry Doors

- An accessible doorway must have a minimum clear opening width of 32 inches (~81.3 centimeters) when the door is opened to 90 degrees (US Department of Justice, 2010 [Access to Medical], p. 5).
- The maximum force for pushing or pulling open a door (interior hinged doors) shall be 5 pounds (ADA Accessibility Guidelines (ADAAG) as amended through September 2002, 4.13.11).
- Maneuvering clearances on both sides of the door must also comply with the ADA standards (US Department of Justice, 2010 [Access to Medical], p. 5).
- The door hardware must not require tight grasping, tight pinching, or twisting of the wrist in order to use it (US Department of Justice, 2010 [Access to Medical], p. 5).
- The hallway outside of the door and the space inside the door should be kept free of boxes, chairs, or equipment, so that they do not interfere with the maneuvering clearance or accessible route (US Department of Justice, 2010 [Access to Medical], p. 5).

Clear Floor and Turning Space inside Examination Rooms

- In order for accessible equipment to be usable by a person who uses a wheelchair or other mobility device, that person must be able to approach the exam table and any other elements of the room to which patients have access (US Department of Justice, 2010 [Access to Medical], p. 5).
- The exam table must have sufficient clear floor space next to it so that an individual using a wheelchair can approach the side of the table for transfer onto it. The minimum amount of space required is 30 by 48 inches (~76.2 by 121.9 centimeters). Clear floor space is needed along at least one side of an adjustable height examination table (US Department of Justice, 2010 [Access to Medical], pp. 5–6).

Features of an Accessible Examination Room

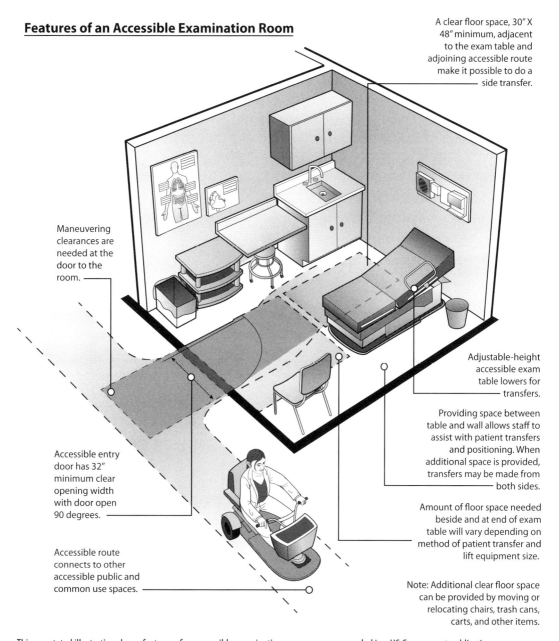

A clear floor space, 30" X 48" minimum, adjacent to the exam table and adjoining accessible route make it possible to do a side transfer.

Maneuvering clearances are needed at the door to the room.

Accessible entry door has 32" minimum clear opening width with door open 90 degrees.

Accessible route connects to other accessible public and common use spaces.

Adjustable-height accessible exam table lowers for transfers.

Providing space between table and wall allows staff to assist with patient transfers and positioning. When additional space is provided, transfers may be made from both sides.

Amount of floor space needed beside and at end of exam table will vary depending on method of patient transfer and lift equipment size.

Note: Additional clear floor space can be provided by moving or relocating chairs, trash cans, carts, and other items.

This annotated illustration shows features of an accessible examination room, as recommended in a US Government publication.

Adapted from: Access to Medical Care for Individuals with Mobility Disabilities. US. Department of Justice, Civil Rights Division, and the Department of Health and Human Services, Civil Rights Division, 2010. www.ada.gov/medcare_mobility_ta/medcare_ta.pdf

– Because some individuals can only transfer from the right or left side, providing clear floor space on both sides of the table allows one accessible table to serve both right- and left-side transfers. Another way to accommodate transfers to either side of exam tables, particularly when more than one accessible examination room is available, is to provide a reverse furniture layout in another accessible examination room (US Department of Justice, 2010 [Access to Medical], p. 6).

- The room should also have enough turning space for an individual using a wheelchair to make a 180-degree turn, using a clear space of 60 inches (~1.5 meters) in diameter or a 60 by 60 inch (~1.5 meter by 1.5 meter) T-shaped space. Movable chairs and other objects, such as wastebaskets, should be moved aside if necessary to provide sufficient clear floor space for maneuvering and turning (US Department of Justice, 2010 [Access to Medical], p. 6).

- When a portable patient lift or stretcher is to be used, additional clear floor space will be needed to maneuver the lift or stretcher. Ceiling-mounted lifts, on the other hand, do not require the additional maneuvering clear floor space because these lifts are mounted over-head (US Department of Justice, 2010 [Access to Medical], p. 6).

Guidelines for Accessible Medical Equipment

Health facilities should be equipped with medical equipment that is accessible to people with mobility disabilities:

> Such equipment includes adjustable-height exam tables and chairs, wheelchair-accessible scales, adjustable-height radiologic equipment, portable floor and overhead track lifts, and gurneys and stretchers (US Department of Justice, 2010 [Access to Medical], p. 8).

As described previously, the US Access Board has developed accessibility standards for medical diagnostic equipment under the "Patient Protection and Affordable Care Act" (United States Access Board [Proposed Accessibility], 2012).

In addition to these standards, consider the following guidelines:

- Provide an adjustable-height table that allows patient transfer from a wheelchair (Iezzoni and O'Day, 2006; NCODH and NCSU Center for Universal Design, 2007; Schott et al., 2002; US Department of Justice, 2010 [Access to Medical]).

- Provide a handle or support rail for stability during a transfer and during the examination (Iezzoni and O'Day, 2006; Schott et al., 2002; US Department of Justice, 2010 [Access to Medical]).

- Provide equipment such as a transfer board or patient lift Iezzoni and O'Day, 2006; Schott et al., 2002; (US Department of Justice, 2010 [Access to Medical]).

- Provide different types of exam tables for different purposes (US Department of Justice, 2010 [Access to Medical]).

- Provide tilt, adjustability, headrests, footrests, and armrests (US Department of Justice, 2010 [Access to Medical]).

- Provide mammography equipment that can accommodate a wheelchair user (Connell et al., 1997; Schott et al., 2002; US Department of Justice, 2010 [Access to Medical]).

- Provide scales that can weigh people sitting in wheelchairs or people who have difficulty standing (NCODH and NCSU Center for Universal Design, 2007; Iezzoni and O'Day, 2006; Schott et al., 2002; US Department of Justice, 2010 [Access to Medical]).

Design Considerations for Patients and Visitors with Hearing Disabilities

In 2008 there were an estimated 35 million Americans with hearing disabilities, with the total projected to rise to over 40 million by 2025 (35 million Americans, 2013). Yet the vast majority of people who are hard of hearing do not use hearing aids or cochlear implants (American Speech-Language-Hearing Association, 2008; Chien and Lin, 2012; Lin, 2012). Among the 26.7 million US adults ages 50 years or older with clinically significant hearing loss, for example, fewer than 15 percent use hearing aids (Chien and Lin, 2012; Lin, 2012). To onlookers, hearing loss can remain an invisible disability.

The critical factor is not the measurable amount of hearing loss, but rather the limitations on verbal communication skills that result (Wyatt, 1983). This is of particular concern in a healthcare setting, where people with hearing disabilities often do not inform healthcare providers of their hearing loss, instead simply catching what information they can. The communication skills so important to human interaction are often severely limited for people with hearing disabilities, and the hearing population is generally uninformed about how to communicate with people who have hearing disabilities (Carpman et al., 1984 [unpub. No. 30]). Through both policy and design, healthcare-facility staff should provide the support that will make communication possible.

The widest possible range of methods must be made available. These may include sign language, specialized software and hardware systems, closed-circuit television systems, vibrating pagers, texting, handwritten notes, supplemental hearing devices, and others. New assistive technologies are always being developed, yet even older technologies, such as the TTY, may still be valuable for patients who need to communicate with loved ones and/or are less adept with newer systems. TTYs may still be federally mandated under some conditions (ADA Questions, 2015; Gips, personal communication, June 16, 2015).

There are no firm statistics on the number of people with hearing limitations who use sign language; for example, researchers at Gallaudet University have found estimates ranging from 100,000 to more than 15 million for American Sign Language (ASL) (Mitchell et al., 2006). The data range suggests that in the United States ASL is anywhere from the fourth to the tenth most-used language and is gaining because of use by non-verbal young people with autism. Sign language interpreters should be available within the healthcare facility or on call. Staff should know how to arrange remote interpreting via video relay systems, which use a computer, high-speed internet, video camera, and speaker to enable immediate access to interpretation services (American Sign Language Interpreter Network, 2015; Gips, personal communication, June 16, 2015). These systems are also valuable in meeting requirements under the 1964 Civil Rights Act for limited English proficient (LEP) patients and visitors (Chen, Youdelman, and Brooks, 2007; US Department of Health and Human Services, 1980).

Because almost no one with *acquired* hearing loss uses sign language, other methods of communication must also be available. Versatile and sophisticated software or hardware technologies can be used for remote interpreting and real-time print communication such as texting and instant messaging, as well as facilitating face-to-face communication (Interpretype Communications, 2015). This technology is also valuable for situations in which people, deaf or hearing, are concerned about privacy. In addition, an optional language translation feature can aid some LEP users.

T-coil hearing-loop induction systems, which transmit amplified sounds directly to hearing aids by means of a thin wire around the perimeter of a room, are inexpensive, broadly scalable, and accessible (Tierney, 2011). Such assistive listening devices are mandated by the ADA in public spaces where audible communication is necessary. The benefits of the technology, however, are little known, and these systems have rarely been installed (Lin, 2012).

Patients should have the option to use e-mail or texting to set up appointments and receive reminders and clinical information. They should also be able to learn about the healthcare facility online (Access to health services, 2014; Iezzoni and O'Day, 2006).

In accordance with ADA regulations and the philosophy and recommendations of the World Health Organization, people with hearing disabilities should be integrated to the maximum extent possible into the mainstream of healthcare-facility services. However, options and technologies have become so complex and sophisticated that healthcare organizations will typically find it necessary to have an identified staff member with this expertise (Americans with Disabilities Act, ADA Title III Technical Assistance Manual, n.d.; Iezzoni and O'Day, 2006; National Association of the Deaf, 2016; US Department of Human Services, 2014; US Department of Justice, 2014).

Facility design elements, such as lighting, sound attenuation, and availability of visual cues, are important factors in supporting communication with patients and visitors who have hearing limitations. Not all people with hearing limitations are totally deaf. For those who depend on hearing aids, it is important that background noise levels be reduced to a minimum and that certain frequencies of sound be controlled (Iezzoni and O'Day, 2006; Milner, 1981; Pipedown International, 2014; Royal National Institute for Deaf People, 2014). As with the reduction of background noise on patient floors, everyone benefits from attention to ambient sound levels in waiting areas, lobbies, and exam rooms. Addressing obtrusive noise makers, such as background music, beeping, TVs, and HVAC systems, will ease communication and make a healthcare facility more inviting.

Because people with hearing disabilities rely heavily on their sense of sight, it is crucial to develop environments that enhance visual cues. This includes providing as much natural light as possible while also addressing glare, avoiding back-lighting, and locating light sources so that shadows are not thrown on staff interpreting or giving information (Iezzoni and O'Day, 2006). It is essential to provide easily understood signage, as well as other written or graphic wayfinding information (Iezzoni and O'Day, 2006). And because users with hearing limitations may not be able to hear fire alarms or other warning signals, decision-makers should consider employing flashing lights, variable-intensity fans, and other warning devices (Iezzoni and O'Day, 2006; Leibrock, 1990; Milner, 1981).

In association with the ASL Deaf Studies Department at Gallaudet University, the Deaf-Space Project has developed a catalog of more than 150 elements of the built environment of particular importance to the deaf community. These address space and proximity, sensory reach, mobility and proximity, light and color, and acoustics. The DeafSpace website stresses that "common to all of these categories are the ideas of community building, visual language, the promotion of personal safety and well-being" (DeafSpace Concepts, 2014; What Is Deaf-Space, 2014).

Lighting systems can be useful in a number of situations, such as knock sensors that flash a light to alert patients that someone is at the door (Iezzoni and O'Day, 2006). Colored lights can be used to signal when patients should take certain actions while getting X-rays, CT scans, and so on (Iezzoni and O'Day, 2006). Cell phones, light signals, number displays, or vibrating pagers can be used in waiting areas to indicate to patients that it is their turn (Iezzoni and O'Day, 2006; Mulley and Ng, 1995; Ubido, Huntington, and Warburton, 2002).

Assigning patients who are totally deaf or who have severe hearing disabilities to rooms near the activity hub of an inpatient unit may be another way healthcare-facility staff can meet these users' needs for information. Rooms near the nursing station tend to be noisy places for hearing patients, but they may provide profoundly deaf patients with a better opportunity to interact with staff members—something essential for providing them with the information and social contact they would otherwise miss. In view of the problems associated with ambient noise, however, such room assignments must be made with care, on a case-by-case basis.

Design Considerations for Patients and Visitors Who Are Blind or Have Low-Vision

Users who are blind or have low-vision may have difficulty finding their way around and negotiating obstacles. With limited sight or no sight at all, patients and visitors are unable to use traditional signs and other wayfinding aids. However, through the use of raised letters, Braille, significantly contrasting colors, audible signals, audible signage systems, and tactile guides, such as textured strips, wayfinding ease can be increased (Harkness and Groom, 1976; Proud, 1989; Rashtian, 2007; Wayfinding: Tactile Signage Leads the Way, 2004; Zimring and Templer, 1983–84). Digital devices may offer audible wayfinding guidance. Providing this range of cues is important, because only 20–25 percent of the blind population in the United States uses Braille (Berkowitz et al., 1979; Goldish, 1967).

Obstacles limit the mobility of blind and low-vision users and put them in potential danger. Pathways obstructed by furniture, equipment, posts, or protrusions from the wall, such as water fountains, are safety hazards. Stairways, roadways, and other structures should be marked by tactile warning signals, such as grooves or strips (Genensky, 1981; Harkness and Groom, 1976; NCODH and NSCU, 2007; Proud, 1989; Rashtian, 2007; Zimring and Templer, 1983–84).

Tactile signage can be effective in leading blind and low-vision people out of a building in case of fire or other emergency requiring evacuation. A study in the United Kingdom tested the effectiveness of different types of emergency lighting and wayfinding systems in a smoke-filled environment (Wayfinding, 2004). One was a tactile wall system consisting of a strip along the walls at rail height. Rather than Braille, this system used shapes (for example, wedges and bumps) to indicate which direction to walk and when to turn to follow exit routes. The study found that this tactile wall system gave the most confidence to low-vision and blind people and increased evacuation speeds by more than 40 percent over conventional overhead emergency lighting. An alternative to the full wall system is the use of similar tactile cues at doors, corners, and other decision-points (Wayfinding, 2004).

In buildings dedicated to people who are blind and low-vision, thoughtfully designed circulation areas can be especially helpful. Hard surfaces should be avoided on floors, ceilings, and hallway walls, because these reflect and redirect sounds that can act as important spatial location cues. Such hard surfaces can cause a sound, such as conversation, to appear to be on one side of the corridor when it is really on the other.

Corridors that intersect at right angles are the easiest for most users to negotiate; oblique or acute angles are more difficult to perceive and remember (Iezzoni and O'Day, 2006). Right angles, however, reduce sight lines and cause problems when people approaching cannot see each other. Right angles are also less easy than gentle curves or straight lines for people to

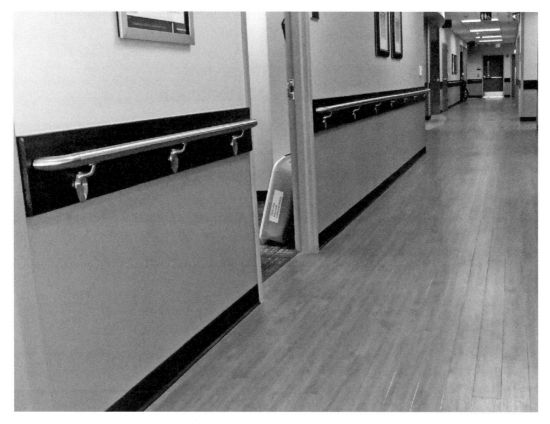

The transition between the base of the wall and the edge of the floor needs to be easy to distinguish, especially for people with vision disabilities. The dark band used here makes the edge of the floor easy to recognize.

Photo credit: Courtesy of St. Joseph Mercy Chelsea

negotiate when using mobility devices. Design decision-makers must assess the actual conditions when selecting a layout. One response to these conflicting needs is the use of glazed panels or lower walls at corners, so that blind or low-vision users can navigate easily, while people with hearing disabilities have a visual cue of someone approaching (Super, personal communication, April 4, 2014).

Stairs can be treacherous places for blind and low-vision users. Ramp and stair width and tread height need to be consistent. Railings should begin before the ramp or first step and run continuously, flattening out along landings and rising or descending again with the next flight on both sides of the stair or ramp.

Elevators with audible warnings are essential for blind and low-vision users. Knowing whether the car is going up or down, which button has been pushed, and what floor has been reached helps them avoid confusion, false starts, asking for help, and backtracking.

People with low vision often cannot distinguish subtle variations in color. In order to minimize potential difficulties and dangers, the items they need to recognize should offer significant contrast with the background or with adjacent items. For instance, the colors of clinic registration counters should contrast with the color of the paper forms used, toilet seats should contrast with the floor, and showers or tubs should contrast with the floors and walls around them (Bright and Cook, 2010; Proud, 1989).

Consider these guidelines:

- In addition to following ADA signage guidelines (including raised lettering and Braille on certain types of permanent signs), provide wayfinding and other graphic signs that are as legible as possible to people who are blind or have low vision, using high contrast between text and background and text large enough to be legible from a distance.

- In addition to signs, consider other means for communicating key information to people who are blind or have low vision, including audible signals, audible signage systems, and tactile guides such as textured strips (Harkness and Groom, 1976; Proud, 1989; Rashtian, 2007; Wayfinding, 2004; Zimring and Templer, 1983–84).

- Train staff to work with patients and visitors who are blind or have low vision and consider how to best use technology (such as audible wayfinding guidance) to communicate key information.

- Make sure interior pathways are not obstructed by furniture, equipment, posts, or protrusions from the wall (such as water fountains) (Genensky, 1981; Harkness and Groom, 1976; NCODH and NSCU, 2007; Proud, 1989; Rashtian, 2007; Zimring and Templer, 1983–1984).

- Make sure potential hazards such as stairways and roadways are marked by tactile warning signals, such as grooves or strips (Genensky, 1981; Harkness and Groom, 1976; NCODH and NSCU, 2007; Proud, 1989; Rashtian, 2007; Zimring and Templer, 1983–84).

- In buildings dedicated to users who are blind or have low vision, avoid using hard surfaces on floors, ceilings, and walls of hallways because these surfaces reflect and redirect sounds that can act as important spatial location cues.

- Design ramp and stair width and tread height to be consistent. Begin railings before the ramp or first step and run them continuously, flattening out along landings and rising or descending again with the next flight on both sides of the stair or ramp.

- Include audible warnings in elevators, if possible, so people who are blind or have low-vision can rely on audible cues.

- Consider the importance of significant color contrast between objects and backgrounds. For instance, the colors of clinic registration counters should contrast with the color of the paper forms used, toilet seats should contrast with the floor, and showers or tubs should contrast with the floors and walls around them (Bright and Cook, 2010; Proud, 1989).

Design Considerations for Older Patients and Visitors

It is essential that healthcare facilities be designed to meet the needs of older patients and visitors. In 2010, there were an estimated 40.2 million people in the United States who were age 65 or older, constituting 13 percent of the US population (US Census, 2010). Nearly 10,000 Americans will turn 65 each day through 2030 (Pew Research Center, 2010). Older people are more prone to chronic conditions and are more frequently hospitalized than are younger people.

Older consumers have particular requirements as a result of the physiological, social, emotional, and psychological changes associated with aging. Although a great deal of research has investigated the environmental requirements of the aging population, most of it has focused on housing or long-term-care facilities (especially nursing homes) and facilities for people with dementia, rather than on healthcare facilities. Design decision-makers need to extrapolate from this related research to the needs of older patients and visitors in inpatient and outpatient healthcare settings. Nevertheless, the design-related needs of older patients and visitors clearly deserve further research attention.

Physiological and Psycho-Social Changes

Physiological changes—usually diminished abilities—are characteristic of the normal aging process. Changes in the various systems of the body usually result in reductions in mobility, balance, strength, stamina, visual acuity, hearing, tactile sensitivity, and thermal sensitivity (American Institute of Architects Foundation, 1986; Developments in Aging, 1986; Koncelik, 1982). Older people normally experience losses in all of these areas rather than having one single disability. It is the combination of physiological changes that often leads to a general sense of vulnerability (American Institute of Architects Foundation, 1986). More specifically, physiological changes may include any or all of the following:

Vision

The lens of the eye thickens, resulting in loss of acuity, narrowing of the visual field, slowed accommodation to temporal or spatial changes in illumination, sensitivity to glare, and some loss of color differentiation (Iezzoni and O'Day, 2006; Lawton, 1979). Three times as much task lighting may be necessary for an older person to perceive and discriminate small detail than would be required for a younger person (Koncelik, 1976). In addition, older people may have difficulty looking up, resulting in problems in reading some wayfinding signs (Iezzoni and O'Day, 2006). Use of bifocal or trifocal lenses can lead to perceived blurring or double images and can have serious safety implications for stair use (Drader, 1982).

Hearing

Hearing becomes less acute, especially in the higher frequency range on which speech and other signals (such as bells and sirens) depend for their clarity. Auditory distortion may result, and older people may be less able to filter out extraneous sounds, as in discerning one voice from a background of competing sounds or voices (Abend and Chen, 1985; American Institute of Architects Foundation, 1986; Drader, 1982; Iezzoni and O'Day, 2006; Koncelik, 1982; Lawton, 1979).

Tactile and Thermal Sensitivity

Due to declines in sensitivity to pain and temperature, older people may be less aware of dangerous changes in temperature and, at the same time, be less able to tolerate such changes. There is increased susceptibility to hypothermia, the lowering of body temperature to potentially fatal levels. If older people are aware of temperature changes, as most are, they are likely to prefer more warmth in winter, to be less able to endure heat in summer, and to be particularly uncomfortable in drafts. Older people may also experience a sensation of insufficient air circulation in buildings with sealed windows (American Institute of Architects Foundation, 1986).

Mobility

Older people may move slowly, and have reduced strength and stamina, stooped posture, difficulty walking and turning, and stiff joints. Loss of balance and dizzy spells may result as side effects from certain medications or neuropathies (American Institute of Architects Foundation, 1986; Drader, 1982).

Memory and Learning

Aging does not impair intelligence per se, but the speed with which information is processed, stored, summoned, and expressed may decline (American Institute of Architects Foundation, 1986). Older people may experience short-term memory deficits, longer times required to learn new information, the need for more repetitions, and longer times required to process sensory information (Drader, 1982). In addition, older people may have increased difficulty creating mental images of unfamiliar settings, which can lead to wayfinding problems (American Institute of Architects Foundation, 1986).

Older people experience a number of psychological and social changes as well as physiological ones, and environmental design needs to be supportive of these changes, too. Older patients and visitors may be experiencing bereavement, social isolation, feelings of uselessness, or an inability to cope with rapidly changing environmental circumstances, such as a move from their home of many years. Social and psychological needs include being able to choose when to be private and when to be social; having access to information; maintaining a sense of control, identity, and independence; and feeling personally safe and secure (Facilities for the Elderly in Canada, 1984).

Design-related Issues for Older Patients and Visitors

A well-designed environment can help mitigate the difficulties older patients and visitors experience by providing physical assistance, psychological support, and behavior cues (American Institute of Architects Foundation, 1986). It is likely that older patients, more often than their younger counterparts, will be at least temporary wheelchair users and that, when hospitalized, they will have longer lengths of stay. This, in addition to older patients' vulnerability, makes the functional nature of facility design and of all the objects within it even more important. However, the physical environment needs to achieve a delicate balance between being supportive of physiological and psychosocial needs and providing a healthy degree of challenge (Koncelik, 1982).

The following principles, adapted for health facilities, have been suggested as a guide for providing well-designed, caring environments for older users.

Safety

Safety should be addressed during the early stages of design. Factors contributing to a lack of patient and visitor safety are often handled too late in the design process. Safety features should not only guard against the possibility of accidental injury but also afford patients and visitors a sense of confidence that they can negotiate spaces themselves (Facilities for the Elderly in Canada, 1984). Slipping and falling, blacking out in unobserved areas, bumping into furnishings with sharp edges, tripping over unseen low obstructions, and other dangers are real hazards faced by many older users. It is important to consider providing effective lighting, rounded corners and edges on all furnishings, carefully designed (even recessed) bed rails, and walls with sufficient surface texture to help prevent hands from slipping (Koncelik, 1982).

Independence

In the face of increasing physical difficulties after many years spent as competent adults, older people tend to highly value their independence and appreciate design features and policies that support their competence. An environment conducive to continued independence is also important for those experiencing dementia or Alzheimer's disease (Koncelik, 1982).

Access

Whether patients and visitors use wheelchairs or are ambulatory—perhaps with the aid of other mobility devices such as canes or walkers—it is essential that features of the healthcare facility's physical environment enable them to have independent access. Sidewalks should be smooth in texture, free of steep slopes, and wide enough to allow two people in wheelchairs to pass comfortably. Outdoor seating areas should be designed so that people in wheelchairs can sit with others or transfer comfortably to a bench. Transitions between exterior and interior spaces should be free of steps and steep ramps. In addition to having wheelchair-accessible routes on the inside, older users should be able to reach and manipulate switches, call buttons, the telephone, and the like (Koncelik, 1982; Lawton, 1979).

Management of Sound and Light

It is not enough to simply provide sufficient quantities of sound and light, because the deterioration of hearing and vision of most older people requires some specialized adjustment of these environmental features. Sound and light must be carefully designed and managed in order to support older patients and visitors in their everyday needs (Iezzoni and O'Day, 2006; Koncelik, 1982).

Control Over Social Contact

Whenever possible, older patients and visitors should have control over the types of social situations in which they participate. They should be able to choose when to have contact with others and when to be alone and to have access to visual and acoustical privacy, as they choose (Koncelik, 1982).

Design Guidelines Regarding Older Patients and Visitors

Some design guidelines that have appeared in the literature on aging and environments can be adapted for use in healthcare settings. Most of these guidelines pertain to environmental features that appear throughout a healthcare facility rather than being unique to a specific area. The guidelines also distinguish between environmental areas or features designed to be used exclusively by older patients, such as a geriatric hospital unit, and those features used by patients and visitors of all ages. Many of these guidelines have been recommended by researchers to improve the quality of healthcare for people with disabilities (Iezzoni and O'Day, 2006).

Safety Systems

Safety systems refer to emergency warning devices such as fire alarms, as well as ways of reducing potential dangers within everyday situations, as the following guidelines suggest:

- Determine a minimum radius for the edges of all hard surfaces and protrusions that might cause injuries in spaces that will be used by older patients and visitors. The more a corner or edge is rounded, the broader the impact area and the more dispersed the force of a blow (Koncelik, 1976).

- Make sure that visual warning devices such as exit signs are backed up with tactile signage and a middle-frequency auditory signal, to enhance the ability of older people to locate the exit (American Institute of Architects Foundation, 1986; Iezzoni and O'Day, 2006; Koncelik, 1982; Wayfinding, 2004; Winters, 1989).

- Post signs for accessible escape routes at wheelchair height so users can easily see them. In the event of a fire, the vision problems of older people may be increased, because many signs are placed high on walls or are suspended from ceilings and may be obscured by smoke (American Institute of Architects Foundation, 1986; Iezzoni and O'Day, 2006; Koncelik, 1982; Winters, 1989).

- Provide fire-detection alarms with extra-loud buzzers, since losses in the ability to smell can impair an older person's ability to detect fires (Winters, 1989).

Sound

Changes in the hearing abilities of many older people make it much more difficult for them to distinguish among simultaneous sounds. The environment needs to be designed so that certain sounds—especially conversation—can be clearly heard. For example:

- When possible, reduce ambient background sounds in open public spaces by using sound-attenuating materials for walls, floors, and ceilings. When possible and appropriate, make use of wall hangings, screens, banners, or acoustic panels (Iezzoni and O'Day, 2006; Koncelik, 1982).

- Avoid background music or loud televisions, which can make the whole environment seem uniform and increase the difficulty of distinguishing one place from another (Iezzoni and O'Day, 2006; Koncelik, 1982).

Lighting

Lighting decisions in healthcare facilities used by older patients and visitors should consider: sensitivity to glare, increased adaptation time when moving between darkness and light, and contrast. Glare caused by unshielded artificial lighting, reflections on glass, and direct sunlight can be a major problem, because it can be visually overwhelming and temporarily distract older patients and visitors, diminishing their awareness of the immediate physical environment, as well as their attention span and short-term memory (American Institute of Architects Foundation, 1986; L. H. Hiatt, 1991; Iezzoni and O'Day, 2006; Koncelik, 1982). Entering a bright room from a low-lit corridor can be dangerous for older patients, because it will take some time for them to adapt to the brightness (Iezzoni and O'Day, 2006; Winters, 1989). Even for a period of time after adaptation, there is likely to be insufficient discrimination of fine details or objects, resulting in the potential for injury (Iezzoni and O'Day, 2006; Koncelik, 1976). (See also chapters 4 and 7.) Contrast between walls and floor is essential for space legibility.

Some additional guidelines include:

- Take advantage of natural light where possible.

- Avoid placing windows, mirrors, and other bright or reflective surfaces at the ends of corridors (American Institute of Architects Foundation, 1986).

• Avoid abrupt changes in illumination levels (Iezzoni and O'Day, 2006). For instance, use low-level night lighting in patient rooms and reduce the level of nighttime corridor lighting (American Institute of Architects Foundation, 1986; Drader, 1982).

• Use indirect lighting whenever possible (American Institute of Architects Foundation, 1986).

• Consider using carpeting in corridors to reduce both glare and noise (Koncelik, 1976).

• Consider lighting the first few stairs in a series, because this is where many falls occur (Facilities for the Elderly in Canada, 1984).

• Select warm-toned lighting, if possible. Cool fluorescents not only are unflattering but also emphasize the blue-green tones most difficult for older people to perceive (Iezzoni and O'Day, 2006; Koncelik, 1976).

• Shield all light sources so that bare bulbs are not exposed (Facilities for the Elderly in Canada, 1984; Koncelik, 1976).

• Reduce glare by fitting all windows and large glass panels with some means of light reduction, such as non-reflective glass, frosted adhesive film, shades, blinds, or drapes (Facilities for the Elderly in Canada, 1984; Koncelik, 1976).

• Provide nuanced lighting with dimmers in bedrooms and lounge areas, with supplementary adjustable task lighting where close work or reading will occur (Fong, 2006; L. H. Hiatt, 1991; Super, personal communication, April 4, 2014).

• Monitor fluorescent bulbs to avoid visual vibration. This can produce agitation in older patients (Hiatt, 1991).

Color

In addition to thickening, the lens of the aging eye gradually changes color. Instead of being clear, it becomes yellowish brown, slightly altering the older person's perception of certain colors. Colors of similar intensity or brightness are more difficult to differentiate than contrasting colors, especially when viewed under constant lighting conditions or against similarly textured or reflective surfaces (L. H. Hiatt, 1991). Different pastels, very dark colors, and combinations of blues and greens can be especially difficult to distinguish between their color groups (American Institute of Architects Foundation, 1986). Pure tones or primary colors are likely to be easiest for older users to recognize and name, whereas off-whites and pale grays may appear drab (L. G. Hiatt, 1981).

In environments for older users, color can be used to organize a series of rooms so they appear to be grouped in some way. Color can signify change, suggest outlines or emphasize contours, signal an alert, or work as a background surface on which a focal object can be easily distinguished. It can also camouflage certain spaces or areas (L. G. Hiatt, 1981).

Color coding is not likely to be an effective wayfinding aid in environments used by older people. As one gerontologist noted, color coding is a relatively abstract idea, and with a decline in memory, older people may not be able to rely on those portions of memory that support abstract reasoning. Because recognition memory is often intact, orientation may be better served by objects, signs, and action (L. G. Hiatt, 1981). (See also chapter 4.)

Some guidelines pertaining to the use of color in health facilities used by older patients and visitors include:

- Consider color in conjunction with lighting. Dim lighting may wash out some colors, whereas direct or bright lighting may intensify others (L. G. Hiatt, 1981).

- Consider color in conjunction with texture. Smooth textures can make colors appear lighter, and uneven surfaces make most colors appear darker (L. G. Hiatt, 1981).

- Emphasize changes in planes—such as the intersections of walls and floors or the treads and risers of stairs—with highly contrasting colors (American Institute of Architects Foundation, 1986; Behar, n.d. [unpub.]; Lawton, 1979).

- Avoid the use of patterns, which can be confusing to older users. Broad stripes on a floor can appear to be steps, stripes on a wall can appear to be bars, and wavy patterns can appear to be in motion, causing unsteadiness. If patterns are to be used at all, it may be more effective to use them along one wall only, like a mural, rather than using them repetitively (L. G. Hiatt, 1981; Iezzoni and O'Day, 2006).

- Use contrasting colors on design components in order to make them stand out for older patients and visitors. Such components might include bathroom fixtures, grab bars, doors, door frames, latches, knobs, and switches (Drader, 1982).

Texture

Because so many older users experience losses of both vision and hearing, texture used in design can be quite effective. In addition to Braille and raised letters, other textural elements can be used. Some of these are handrail markers (notches or grooves cut into the handrail to identify location), and changes in the textural surfaces of walls. Textures need to be different enough that users do not become confused by them (Koncelik, 1982). In addition:

- Consider the use of texture to identify different locations within the healthcare facility.

- Avoid surfaces that are so reflective that they cause glare.

- Avoid wall surfaces that are so abrasive that they will injure those who rub up against them. (Koncelik, 1976)

Hardware

Gerontologists explain that architectural hardware plays two important roles in facility design. It can facilitate or impede use by people with disabilities, and it can convey a symbolic

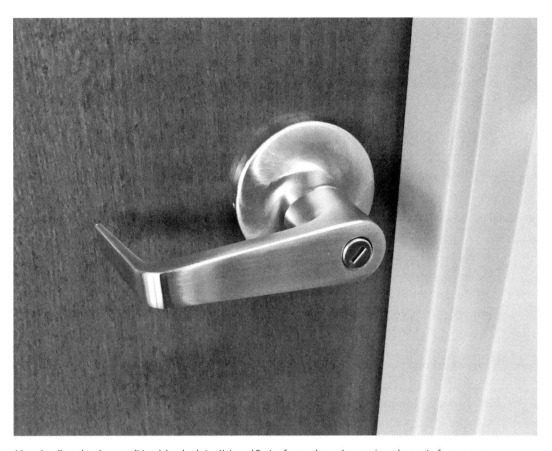

A lever handle, rather than a traditional door knob, is a Universal Design feature that makes opening a door easier for everyone.
Photo credit: Courtesy of St. Joseph Mercy Chelsea

message, usually false, of personal incompetence to users "long before their infirmities reach a point where they [actually] inhibit environmental use" (Koncelik, 1982). Supportive design features, such as hardware, can help facilitate use and feelings of competence on the part of all users.

- Provide door hardware, such as levers and push-type handles that can be operated with one hand and that do not require twisting, turning, or excessive strength (American Institute of Architects Foundation, 1986; Developments in Aging, 1986; Iezzoni and O'Day, 2006; Jones and Tamari, 1997; Leibrock, 1990; US Access Board, ADAAG 2002, 4.13.9).

- Provide door closers that require a maximum of 5 pounds of opening force. (US Access Board, ADAAG 2002, 4.13.11).

Flooring

Flooring materials can prevent older patients and visitors from having to cope with glare or potentially dangerous situations. (See chapter 4.) Guidelines on choosing floor coverings for older users include:

*   Whenever possible, provide low-pile carpeting with a low-contrast pattern rather than hard flooring, because of carpeting's significant glare reduction and safety advantages (Koncelik, 1976).

*   Select stain-resistant carpet with an added guard to prevent bacterial growth and resulting odors (Behar, n.d. [unpub.]).

*   Select a resilient carpet for ease of wheelchair handling, with a pile height of less than ½ inch (~1.27 centimeters) and an uncut or tip sheer in high-density pile (Behar, n.d. [unpub.]; Iezzoni and O'Day, 2006; Jones and Tamari, 1987).

*   Where carpeting is not used, provide flooring that is resilient, non-glare, easy to clean, and nonslip even when wet (Iezzoni and O'Day, 2006; Jones and Tamari, 1997; Koncelik, 1982; Lawton, 1979). Vinyl flooring is generally preferable to ceramic tiles because it is softer and has higher friction ratings (Iezzoni and O'Day, 2006).

*   Make the front edge of each stair tread easily identifiable (Hunt and Ross, 1989).

*   Create contrast between adjoining treads and risers by using color or lighting (Hunt and Ross, 1989).

*   Avoid locating carpet seams on stair treads (Hunt and Ross, 1989).

*   To provide contrast between floor and wall surfaces, use a contrasting color band around the edge of all floor surfaces, except at the entrance to a stairway, ramp, or doorway (Hunt and Ross, 1989).

*   Continue the color of the stair up over the tread of the top step to serve as a warning to those approaching the stair (Hunt and Ross, 1989).

*   Be aware of potential safety problems, such as loose seams, curled edges, and uneven carpet levels (Hunt and Ross, 1989; Iezzoni and O'Day, 2006).

*   Provide handrails that are easily distinguishable from wall surfaces (Hunt and Ross, 1989).

*   Avoid use of carpeting with banding or borders because these may look like objects to older patients and visitors (L. H. Hiatt, 1991; Iezzoni and O'Day, 2006).

Seating

Selecting seating for use by older people in healthcare facilities is especially important, because they often sit for extended periods of time and may have poor circulation. Important considerations include the ease of sitting down on the chair, comfort and support while sitting, and the ease of rising (American Institute of Architects Foundation, 1986). (See chapters 5, 7, and 8 and Research Box 9.4.)

RESEARCH BOX 9.4 GETTING INTO AND OUT OF THE RIGHT SEAT

Many older people have difficulty getting into and out of chairs (Alexander, Schultz, and Warwick, 1991; Finlay et al., 1983; Goetschel, 1987; McGilloway, 1980; Wheeler et al., 1985). Because weakness and disability are eventually experienced by most older people, comfort and the ability to use one's own strength to sit and rise is important, both physically and psychologically. In fact, one study found that older people and those with arthritis rated ease in rising as the most important factor in choosing an "easy chair" (Finlay et al., 1983).

Researchers have studied chair design relative to the biomechanics of rising from a seated position. A central finding is that older adults and some people with disabilities use different strategies for rising from a chair than do younger adults and people without disabilities.

In one study comparing young adults (ages 19–31) with older adults (ages 63–92), with and without apparent difficulty rising from a chair, researchers found that the latter have greater difficulty attaining postural stability (Alexander, Schultz, and Warwick, 1991). To compensate, they tend to rotate their thighs and trunks and flex their legs more than do younger adults. In doing so, they take up to over a half-second longer to lift themselves from the seat, depending on their health and the degree to which they use their hands as an aid.

The process of rising from a chair produces more motion and force on the hips and knees than does walking and, in some cases, than does climbing stairs (Rodosky, Andriacchi, and Andersson, 1989). Thus, although a seat height ~1–2 inches (~2.5–5.1 centimeters) below the knee joint is the most comfortable for sitting, greatest ease in standing up is achieved by a higher chair that minimizes the amount of joint flexion and thrust needed. For people with pathologic conditions of the hip or knee and for those who change between sitting and standing frequently, a chair height that allows a knee angle of up to about 115 degrees may be needed (roughly 18 inches (~45.7 centimeters) high, depending on the individual).

Similarly, higher armrests make for greater leverage in rising. One study of 92 residents in three homes for seniors in England (74 percent women, mean age 81.9 years) found that although 52 percent could not rise without help from standard chairs that had armrests ~6–7 inches (~15.2–17.8 centimeters) above the loaded seat height, 85 percent were able to rise from a chair when the armrests were set at ~9½–10 inches (~24.1–25.4 centimeters) and the occupied seat height was ~17 inches (~43.2 centimeters) (Burdett et al., 1985). The authors also note a critical interaction between seat and armrest heights: there was no benefit when the arm height was optimal and the seat height was low, and vice versa.

Optimizing seat and arm heights for functional chair use would mark an advance in seating design, especially for those large numbers of people who have difficulty rising. Nonetheless, such steps must be coordinated with other elements of chair design: use of firm cushions, elimination of the crossbar located under the front of the seat that blocks leg motion, and backrest angle tilted sufficiently to offer seated comfort but not so much as to become an impediment to rising.

Older people need to be able to center themselves in front of the chair, move their heels underneath it, and sit down rather than fall down. Chair arms aid this process greatly. A clear space under the front of the chair provides an area for placing the heels. When the front of the chair arms is in the same vertical plane as the front edge of the seat, less strength is required for sitting down. Seat height should be just below knee height, and the seat angle should be no more than 4 degrees. A chair seat should never be so high that it lifts the person's feet off the floor, because this can cause damaging interruption of blood flow to the lower legs and feet. Of course, people come in different sizes, so it is difficult to specify an ideal seat height. However, a height that seems to work well for most people is ~17 inches (~43.2 centimeters) (American Institute of Architects Foundation, 1986; Koncelik, 1982).

Seats that are too hard can be uncomfortable and can contribute to or exacerbate skin conditions such as skin ulcers. One way to test a seat's firmness is to press a fist into the center of the seat, gradually increasing the pressure, until one's full weight is on the fist. If the fist

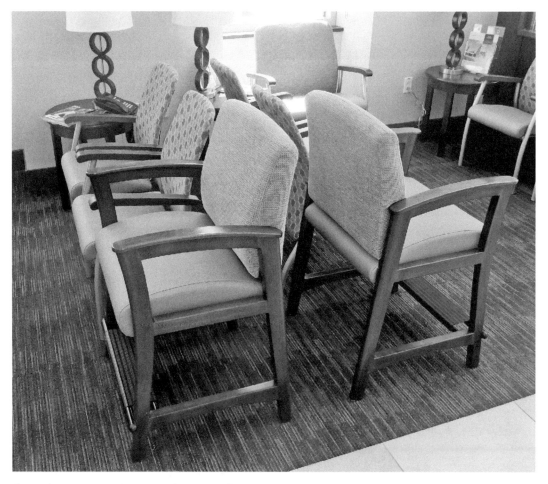

Chairs in this emergency waiting area provide armrests and open space beneath the seats to support visitors as they rise. The two chairs in the foreground provide comfortable seating for people requiring chairs that are larger or higher than usual.

Photo credit: Courtesy of St. Joseph Mercy Chelsea

is stopped by a board or spring, then the seat is probably too hard to accommodate an older person for an extended period of time (American Institute of Architects Foundation, 1986).

Skin ulcers can also be caused by moisture against the skin. Some gerontologists recommend that regardless of the potential for incontinence, nonabsorbent upholstery should be avoided (Koncelik, 1976).

Rising is made easier by the same design features that facilitate sitting down. A chair's arms can help older people pull themselves to the front of the seat. Then they can place their heels under their center of gravity and push up and out, if the front of the chair's arms is in the same vertical plane as the front of the seat (American Institute of Architects Foundation, 1986).

Chair selection guidelines for older patients and visitors include the following:

• Provide a clear space under the front of the chair so that the user's heels can be placed underneath (American Institute of Architects Foundation, 1986).

• Select chairs in which the front edge of the chair arms is in the same vertical plane as, or extends slightly beyond, the front edge of the seat (American Institute of Architects Foundation, 1986).

• Select chairs with arms that can be gripped.

• Make sure the seat angle is no more than 4 degrees (American Institute of Architects Foundation, 1986).

• Avoid seats that are so firm that they may cause skin ulcers (American Institute of Architects Foundation, 1986).

• Avoid non-absorbent upholstery (American Institute of Architects Foundation, 1986; Koncelik, 1976).

• Avoid seat coverings that are rough or slippery (Ellis, 1988).

• Because older adults are somewhat shorter than average, select seating with a height from the floor to the seat's front edge of no more than ~17 inches (~43.2 centimeters) (American Institute of Architects Foundation, 1986; Koncelik, 1982).

• Provide seating designed to accommodate people who are obese in the same style as seating provided for the general population.

• Avoid seating in which the legs are splayed beyond the area of the seat, because the legs can be a tripping hazard.

• Avoid seating where the seat is too deep.

Heating, Ventilation, and Air Conditioning

The following guidelines suggest ways in which the thermal environment needs to be regulated in order to accommodate changes in thermal sensitivity likely to be experienced by older patients and visitors (American Institute of Architects Foundation, 1986):

• Select heating systems capable of maintaining a temperature of 75 degrees Fahrenheit.

- Select cooling systems capable of maintaining a temperature of 78 degrees Fahrenheit.
- Select air-handling systems designed to avoid noise and the creation of drafty areas.

Wayfinding

Although older people may have a good understanding of familiar complex environments, some may have difficulty creating mental images of unfamiliar areas. Finding their way through an unfamiliar complex environment may be stressful (American Institute of Architects Foundation, 1986). Architectural and interior designs that emphasize unique, recognizable, and memorable features and areas help older (and also younger) users who may become confused trying to differentiate among many seemingly repetitive elements (Koncelik, 1982). (See chapter 4.) It is useful to provide information in a hierarchy from general to specific (the closer one is to the destination, the more specific the information). Such a system is common in many public facilities, like airports, and prevents visitors from being overwhelmed with too much unnecessary information (Huelat, 2007). Consider these guidelines:

- Create memorable landmarks throughout the facility, using natural light, color, artwork, unique architectural features, plants, and other design elements (Huelat, 2007; Koncelik, 1982).
- Provide high contrast between the text and background used on signs and between the sign background and the wall color. In areas used predominantly by older patients and visitors, use white symbols on a dark background (Koncelik, 1982).
- Avoid designing signs with reflective surfaces (American Institute of Foundation, 1986, Koncelik, 1982).
- Avoid locating signs opposite windows, so light does not reflect off the sign's surface into viewers' eyes (American Institute of Architects Foundation, 1986; Koncelik, 1982).
- Pay particular attention to letter size on signs and notices that will be read by older patients and visitors. Lettering on directional and identification signs should be a minimum of $1^9/_{16}$ inches (~4 centimeters) high. Notices to older patients and visitors should be printed in large type (Drader, 1982; Koncelik, 1976).
- In places used predominantly by older patients and visitors, consider repeating directional sign messages more frequently than usual (Drader, 1982).

Circulation

Some pedestrian routes involving long distances, obstructions within corridors, or level changes that are difficult to see, can pose difficulties to older users. Design that attends to older users' needs can result in a safer and more pleasant healthcare experience. (See also chapter 4 and Research Box 9.5.) Some guidelines include:

- Minimize distances between frequently used destinations (Drader, 1982).
- Provide rest areas along corridors used regularly by older patients and visitors (Drader, 1982).

- Provide ample storage areas so carts and other large pieces of medical equipment do not need to be stored in hallways and do not act as obstructions to older users (Drader, 1982).

- Avoid protrusions that older patients or visitors might bump into (Drader, 1982).

- Design lighting at entrance and exit areas to allow for older users' slower adaptation rates to dark and light (Drader, 1982).

- Mark glass walls and doors in order to make their presence obvious to older users (Drader, 1982).

- Consider using contrasting colors to accentuate entrances, exits, merging of corridors, steps, handrails, approaches to elevators, ramps, and other changes in level or flooring surfaces (Drader, 1982; Leibrock, 1990).

- Consider using audible signals to indicate when it is safe to enter or exit an elevator (Jones and Tamari, 1997; Koncelik, 1982).

- Consider using a double handrail and kickplate combination in hallways to provide support for older ambulatory users and wheelchair users. Mount one handrail at ~32 inches (~81.3 centimeters) and the other at ~26 inches (~66 centimeters) (Koncelik, 1976).

RESEARCH BOX 9.5 ENABLING OLDER PATIENTS AND VISITORS TO USE STAIRS

Although accident surveillance studies indicate that older people have fewer stair mishaps per capita than those in other age categories, researchers have found that older people have more accidents per amount of use and suffer injuries of greater severity. One hypothesis is that older people avoid using stairs whenever possible, but when they must use stairs, they tend to have more accidents than do younger people. Older people may face even more serious outcomes than accounted for in standard mortality records, given that many die of pneumonia or other problems that stem from stairway accidents but are not directly attributed to them. According to a review by the US National Bureau of Standards, most serious injuries caused by stair accidents occur in descent (Archea, 1985). Overstepping a tread leads to "slips" off the nosing with one foot while the leg on the opposite side collapses under the body. Lower-back sprains and fractured hips and lower legs are common outcomes of such mishaps.

One researcher examined the role of diminished vision in stairway accidents among seniors. He found that, taken together, poor illumination and missing the last step or group of steps through mistaken perception of the bottom accounted for about 40 percent of falls (Sheldon, 1960).

In another study, younger subjects wore special glasses in order to simulate the typical effects of aging eyes. The result was that they had considerable difficulty distinguishing tread and wall boundaries where floral patterns or certain color combinations were used, such as blue/green or more intense red/green (Pastalan, 1982).

(continued)

Inpatient Rooms

When older people are hospitalized, the patient room becomes their home for a time. Because older patients are often more vulnerable than other patients, a supportive environment is especially important. (See also chapter 7.)

Guidelines for beds:

• Select beds that can be lowered to a height of ~20 inches (~51 centimeters) from the floor to the top of the bedding. This height may allow patients to dress and get into and out of bed independently, to position themselves for comfortable conversation with a seated visitor, and to accomplish a wheelchair transfer (Koncelik, 1982).

• Select bedrails that are completely retractable in order to avoid injuries to patients that stem from falling and striking the bedrails (Koncelik, 1982).

• Select beds with rounded corners and edges in order to prevent injuries (Koncelik, 1976).

Guidelines for furnishings:

• Select sturdy furnishings that can help steady a shaky ambulatory patient (Koncelik, 1976, 1982).

• Avoid tables or bedside stands with white or shiny surfaces that cause glare (Koncelik, 1976).

- Select televisions mounted on the wall, rather than arm-mounted televisions that tend to wobble.

- Make sure remote control devices are easy to understand and manipulate, and have large, legibly identified buttons.

   Guidelines for telephones:

- Consider selecting inpatient room telephones having letters and numerals that contrast with the background. Buttons should be larger than the standard size, if possible (Koncelik, 1976).

- Consider providing telephone speaker devices that assist hearing aid users and eliminate interference from ambient noise (Drader, 1982).

   Guidelines for display areas:

- Make provisions for some display of personal items, such as family photographs.

- Allow space to display notes, calendars, signs, and other mechanisms that can help orient older patients to time, place, and activity (Koncelik, 1976).

Inpatient Bathrooms

As one gerontologist noted, "As people age, the bathroom becomes a place of danger" (Koncelik, 1982). Loss of strength and mobility, perceptual difficulties, changes in the performance of tasks, and the privacy typically expected in bathroom use all lead to dangers for older patients. For instance, exposed hot water pipes can cause serious leg burns for wheelchair users, patients can slip and fall when entering or leaving the tub or shower, and toilet grab rails that are incorrectly placed are of little help to a patient in getting on or off the toilet (Koncelik, 1982). Design features can help make the inpatient bathroom a safer place. (See also chapter 7.)

   Guidelines for toilets:

- Install grab bars on both sides of the toilet in a way that accommodates people needing support to lower and raise themselves, people in wheelchairs, and people with disabilities on their left or right sides (Edlich et al., 1998; Jones and Tamari, 1997, Tetlow, 1995).

- Be sure grab bars are placed close enough to be useful (American Institute of Architects Foundation, 1986; Koncelik, 1976).

   Guidelines for sinks:

- Make sure all water pipes are inaccessible and hot water feed pipes are wrapped in order to prevent leg burns (Edlich et al., 1998; Jones and Tamari, 1997; Koncelik, 1982).

- To make it easy for older patients in wheelchairs to use the sink, consider various alternatives for mounting faucets and water controls, such as side mountings, in addition to the traditional back mounting (Iezzoni and O'Day, 2006; Jones and Tamari, 1997; Koncelik, 1976).

- Clearly mark water controls to indicate hot and cold (Koncelik, 1976).

- Select oversized, textured control knobs to enable older patients to identify and grasp them easily (Koncelik, 1976).

- Consider level-handle faucets.

Other bathroom design guidelines:

- Use light bulbs that simulate natural light over bathroom mirrors (American Institute of Architects Foundation, 1986).

- Design towel racks to be extremely sturdy, so that they can support a patient's weight if necessary.

- Consider using brightly colored grab bars (Leibrock, 1990).

Therapeutic Uses of Music

Therapeutic uses of music have been extensively discussed elsewhere in this book. (See chapters 6 and 7.) In addition, research and experience in nursing homes and similar care facilities demonstrates specific benefits of music for people with Alzheimer's, dementia, and related cognitive and physical challenges (Gerdner, 1997, 1999, 2000, 2005; Gerdner and Schoenfelder, 2010; Ragneskog et al., 2001; Sung and Chang, 2005; Sung, Chang, and Abbey, 2006; Sung, Chang, and Lee, 2010). Such benefits are likely transferable to other healthcare settings.

One nonprofit organization, Music & Memory, has explored the use of personalized music to tap into deep memories, bring participants back into contact with their surroundings, and renew social functioning (Music & Memory, 2015). The program is elegant and economical, requiring only headphones and a digital device such as a small iPod containing a playlist that has meaning for the individual. Results have been consistent and remarkable: when they listen to familiar music, people with dementia and related cognitive limitations are visibly happier and more social, they communicate and listen more effectively, and exhibit fewer behavior-management issues.

Design Considerations for Obese Patients

Obesity is on the rise in the United States. According to the Centers for Disease Control and Prevention, 69 percent of the adult population is overweight, and 35.1 percent of these adults are obese (Centers for Disease Control and Prevention, 2015). The weight of bariatric (obese) patients can range from 250 to 1,200 pounds (Harrell and Miller, 2004).

Many hospitals have experienced an increase in the number of severely obese patients seeking treatment for a wide range of medical conditions. Weight varies significantly from one geographic location to another. Therefore, the Health Guidelines Revision Committee of the Facility Guidelines Institute (FGI) recommends that healthcare organizations make their own determinations about the predicted percentage of their patient population expected to be obese. This will affect decisions about paths of egress, as well as fixtures, furniture, and equipment. The FGI plans to develop minimum requirements for accommodating patients of all weights in the 2018 edition of the FGI Guidelines (Facilities Guidelines Institute, 2014).

The rising trend in obesity led to the development of the Bariatric Room Design Advisory Board (BRDAB), a group of bariatric surgeons, nurses, medical equipment designers, and healthcare architects dedicated to the development of industry standards for the design of facilities and equipment for severely obese patients. Their research, as well as the experience of other designers, has led to a number of design recommendations (Harrell and Miller, 2004; Pelczarski, 2007; Thrall, 2005). The BRDAB suggests choosing design features (for example, furniture, toilets, beds, equipment) that can accommodate patients weighing 1,000 pounds (Harrell and Miller, 2004).

Guidelines for Inpatient Rooms for Obese Patients

- Provide a door width of 60 inches (~1.5 meters) so that medical equipment for severely obese patients can fit through the door (Harrell and Miller, 2004).

- Provide a room with a minimum clear floor area of 200 square feet (~18.6 square meters) and preferably 210 square feet (~19.5 square meters), 14 by 15 feet, (~4.3 by 4.6 meters) and that allows 5 feet (~1.5 meters) of clearance around the patient's bed (Facility Guidelines Institute, 2010; Harrell and Miller, 2004; Pelczarski, 2007; Thrall, 2005).

- Consider purchasing bariatric beds that have built-in scales and can be converted to a chair position (Harrell and Miller, 2004; Pelczarski, 2007).

- Allow patients to control the temperature and lighting in the room (Harrell and Miller, 2004).

- Provide a bathroom that is at least 45 square feet (~4.2 square meters) and has doorways that are 60 inches (~1.5 meters) wide (Harrell and Miller, 2004).

- Install floor-mounted toilets and sinks rather than wall-mounted fixtures, unless contraindicated by requirements for accessible design (Facility Guidelines Institute, 2010; Pelczarski, 2007; Thrall, 2005).

- Install toilets and sinks capable of withstanding downward static force of 1,000 pounds (Facility Guidelines Institute, 2010).

- Locate the toilet 24 inches (~61 centimeters) away from the wall (Thrall, 2005).

- Consider installing a bidet, because obese patients may have difficulty cleansing themselves after toileting (Harrell and Miller, 2004).

- Provide reinforced grab bars around toilets and in showers (Harrell and Miller, 2004; Pelczarski, 2007; Thrall, 2005).

- Locate grab bars and toilet paper dispensers in a place where bariatric patients can easily reach them (Harrell and Miller, 2004).

- Provide a mounted handheld nozzle in the shower in a place where caregivers can easily reach it (Harrell and Miller, 2004; Thrall, 2005).

- Provide a shower seat (Harrell and Miller, 2004).

- Be sure the size of the shower allows room for two caregivers to assist the patient (Harrell and Miller, 2004).

Guidelines for Furniture and Medical Equipment for Obese Patients

- In waiting areas, cafeterias, and registration areas, provide some furniture, such as love-seats, that can accommodate bariatric patients and that coordinate with the rest of the furniture (Harrell and Miller, 2004; Pelczarski, 2007; Thrall, 2005).

- Offer seating with and without arms (Harrell and Miller, 2004).

- Provide lift equipment that can be used to transfer obese patients to and from bed. Include built-in mechanical lifts in all newly constructed bariatric-nursing-unit rooms and in 10 percent of the rooms in renovation projects (Harrell and Miller, 2004, Pelczarski, 2007; Thrall, 2005).

- Provide bariatric wheelchairs and bariatric operating room tables (Pelczarski, 2007).

- Provide a scale that measures bariatric patients, accommodates wheelchairs, and respects the privacy of the patient (Harrell and Miller, 2004; Pelczarski, 2007; Thrall, 2005).

- Purchase diagnostic imaging systems that can accommodate bariatric patients (Pelczarski, 2007).

- Purchase extra-large blood pressure cuffs (Pelczarski, 2007).

- Consider installing elevators or lifts where there are floor ramps or inclines so staff do not have to push obese patients up and down the ramps (Thrall, 2005).

- Provide elevators or lifts with a weight capacity that can handle a bariatric patient, bed, transport staff, and specialized equipment (Pelczarski, 2007).

Summary

- Experiencing disability at some stage of life, whether for short or long term, is a universal human experience. Equal accessibility and usability of healthcare facilities is medically important and required by federal law, including the Americans with Disabilities Act. Goods and services must be made available in an *integrated* setting to the maximum extent appropriate. Because disability is now recognized as a contextual variable, dynamic over time, and in relation to circumstances, the principles of Universal Design provide essential guidance in designing built environments that go beyond the removal of barriers to support both capacity and performance in all users.

- Mobility disabilities, whether visible or invisible, permanent or temporary, require facilities that provide smooth and level footing, clear floor and turning space for wheelchairs, supports such as handrails and grab bars, hardware that requires minimal effort to manipulate, and accessible furniture and medical equipment, including exam tables and chairs. Facility design, including lighting, sound attenuation, and the availability of visual cues, must support communication for users who are deaf or who have hearing limitations, and various means of communication must be available, such as sign language interpreters, T-coil hearing-loop induction systems, TTYs, vibrating pagers, knock sensors; email and texting. Wayfinding signs must be as legible as possible to users who are blind or low-vision. Additional means for communicating key information must be provided, including audible signals, audible signage systems, and tactile guides such as textured strips, along with significant color contrast between objects and backgrounds.

○   The normal aging process characteristically involves reductions in mobility, balance, strength, stamina, vision, hearing, and tactile and thermal sensitivity. This combination of physiological changes often leads to a general sense of vulnerability. A well-designed environment can provide physical assistance, psychological support, and behavior cues while still offering older patients a healthy degree of challenge and independence. Safety features are essential, such as well-chosen flooring materials, rounded corners and edges on furnishings, effective lighting, and emergency warning and signage systems. Sound and lighting must be carefully designed and managed in order to support the needs of older patients and visitors. Color and texture can be used to provide valuable orientation cues. Seating must be chosen to accommodate the specific needs of older people.

○   The dramatic rise in obesity in the United States over recent decades means that healthcare facilities must be prepared to serve severely overweight patients and visitors. Some furniture, beds, toilets, and medical equipment, such as wheelchairs, scales, exam tables, blood pressure cuffs, and diagnostic imaging equipment, should be selected to accommodate people weighing up to 1,000 pounds. Room size and layout must be designed accordingly. Seating with and without arms should be provided in waiting areas, cafeterias, and registration areas to accommodate bariatric patients.

DISCUSSION QUESTIONS

1. What is the ADA? Where can one find information about its provisions?
2. What are the central ideas behind the concept of Universal Design? What are the Principles of Universal Design?
3. What are some key requirements for the design and furnishing of accessible exam and treatment rooms?
4. What aspects of facility design support communication for patients and visitors with hearing disabilities?
5. What design features of circulation areas are important to patients and visitors who are blind or have low vision?
6. What features of lighting design are of particular importance to older patients and visitors?
7. What are some design requirements for seating used by older patients and visitors?
8. What are some design requirements for bariatric inpatient rooms and bathrooms?

Design Review Questions

Federal Legislation on Disability Rights

Americans with Disabilities Act

☐ Will the design team review the latest ADA design guidelines for health facilities?

☐ Will all health facility design decisions reflect ADA guidelines and requirements?

☐ Will multi-story buildings housing medical offices provide at least one accessible route or elevator serving each floor? (United States Access Board [Scoping §206.2.3])

☐ Will 10 percent of patient and visitor parking spaces be accessible and compliant with Section 502 parking requirements when they serve hospital outpatient facilities? (United States Access Board [Scoping §208.2.1])

☐ Will 20 percent of patient and visitor parking spaces be accessible and compliant with Section 502 parking requirements when they serve rehabilitation facilities specializing in treating conditions that affect mobility and outpatient physical therapy facilities? (United States Access Board [Scoping §208.2.2])

☐ Will accessible passenger loading zones be available at medical-care and long-term-care facilities? (United States Access Board, [Scoping §209.3])

☐ Will accessible inpatient rooms be dispersed across patient units? (United States Access Board [Scoping §§223–223.2.1], Advisory §223.1.1)

☐ For facilities specializing in treating conditions affecting mobility, will all inpatient rooms provide mobility features complying with Section 805? (United States Access Board [Scoping §223–223.2.1] [Scoping §§805–805.4])

☐ For facilities not specializing in treating conditions affecting mobility, will at least 10 percent of inpatient rooms and resident sleeping rooms and no fewer than one inpatient room and resident sleeping room provide turning space and clear floor space on each side of the bed? Will at least one accessible toilet, lavatory, and tub/shower be provided? (United States Access Board [Scoping §223.2.1], [Scoping §§805–805.4])

Patient Protection and the Affordable Care Act

☐ Will the design team review the Patient Protection and Affordable Care Act for its relevance to health facility design decisions?

☐ Will health facility design decisions reflect requirements of the Patient Protection and Affordable Care Act?

Design That Cares: Planning Health Facilities for Patients and Visitors, third edition, by Janet R. Carpman and Myron A. Grant. ©2016 by Jossey-Bass.

Section 504 of the Rehabilitation Act

☐ Will the design team review Section 504 of the Rehabilitation Act of 1973 for its relevance to health facility design decisions?

☐ Will health facility design decisions reflect Section 504 requirements?

Universal Design

☐ Do health facility design decision-makers understand the principles of Universal Design? (Connell et al., 1997; NCODH and NCSU Center for Universal Design, 2007).

☐ Will health facility design decisions be made with Universal Design principles in mind?

Design Considerations for Patients and Visitors with Mobility Disabilities

☐ Will automatic doors be installed with controls at a height accessible to people in wheelchairs and out of the way of the door swing? (Iezzoni and O'Day, 2006; Insights into, 2004; Jones and Tamari, 1997)

☐ Will smooth, level surfaces be provided at doorways? Will weather matting (both temporary and permanent) and thresholds not interfere with wheelchair use? Will weather matting be fitted flat, so as not to constitute a trip hazard? (Iezzoni and O'Day, 2006; Insights into, 2004; Jones and Tamari, 1997 NCODH and NCSU Center for Universal Design, 2007)

☐ Will continuous handrails be provided on both sides of the corridor along circulation routes?

☐ Will resting areas with seats be provided along lengthy corridors?

☐ Will reception desks provide a portion of the surface low enough to accommodate people in wheelchairs and another portion high enough for people who have difficulty bending?

☐ Will tables, desks, and counters for filling out paperwork allow for the use of chairs with arms, so people with mobility limitations and joint problems can sit and rise independently? (Iezzoni and O'Day, 2006; Jones and Tamari, 1997; NCODH and NCSU Center for Universal Design, 2007)

☐ Will tables, desks, and counters for filling out paperwork provide ample space underneath to accommodate people in wheelchairs? (Iezzoni and O'Day, 2006; Jones and Tamari, 1997; NCODH and NCSU Center for Universal Design, 2007)

Design That Cares: Planning Health Facilities for Patients and Visitors, third edition, by Janet R. Carpman and Myron A. Grant. ©2016 by Jossey-Bass.

☐ Will grab bars in bathrooms be installed in a way that accommodates both people using wheel-chairs and people with disabilities on their left or right side? Will personal assistants be able to move grab bars out of the way? (Edlich et al., 1998; Jones and Tamari, 1997; Tetlow, 1995)

☐ Will soap, hand dryers, paper towel dispensers, changing stations, and mirrors be placed so people in wheelchairs can easily use them? (Iezzoni and O'Day, 2006; Jones and Tamari, 1997; NCODH and NCSU Center for Universal Design, 2007)

☐ Will there be good color contrast between fixtures and flooring and walls?

☐ Will lighting be designed so as to avoid glare and shadows?

☐ Will floor drains not be located along accessible routes?

Guidelines for Accessible Exam and Treatment Rooms

☐ In examination rooms for people with mobility disabilities, will an accessible route be provided to and through the room? (US Department of Justice, 2010 [Access to Medical], p. 5)

☐ Will there be an entry door with adequate, clear width, maneuvering clearance, and accessible hardware? (US Department of Justice, 2010 [Access to Medical], p. 5)

☐ Will appropriate models of accessible examination equipment be used and will they be placed appropriately? (US Department of Justice, 2010 [Access to Medical], p. 5)

☐ Will adequate, clear floor space be provided inside the room for side transfers and use of lift equipment? (US Department of Justice, 2010 [Access to Medical], p. 5)

Entry Doors

☐ Will accessible doorways have a minimum clear opening width of 32 inches (~81.3 centimeters) when the door is opened to 90 degrees? (US Department of Justice, 2010 [Access to Medical], p. 5)

☐ Will the maximum forces for pushing or pulling open a door (interior hinged doors) be 5 pounds? (ADA Accessibility Guidelines (ADAAG) as amended through September 2002, 4.13.11)

☐ Will maneuvering clearances on both sides of the door comply with ADA Standards? (US Department of Justice, 2010 [Access to Medical], p. 5)

☐ Will door hardware not require tight grasping, tight pinching, or twisting of the wrist in order to use it? (US Department of Justice, 2010 [Access to Medical], p. 5)

☐ Will hallways outside of the door and the space inside the door be kept free of boxes, chairs, or equipment, so that they do not interfere with the maneuvering clearance or accessible route? (US Department of Justice, 2010 [Access to Medical], p. 5)

Design That Cares: Planning Health Facilities for Patients and Visitors, third edition, by Janet R. Carpman and Myron A. Grant. ©2016 by Jossey-Bass.

Clear Floor and Turning Space inside Examination Rooms

• In order for accessible equipment to be usable by a person who uses a wheelchair or other mobility device, will that person be able to approach the exam table and any other elements of the room to which patients have access? (US Department of Justice, 2010 [Access to Medical], p. 5)

• Will the exam table have sufficient clear floor space next to it so that an individual using a wheelchair can approach the side of the table for transfer onto it? The minimum amount of space required is 30 by 48 inches (~0.7 by 1.2 meters). Will there be clear floor space along at least one side of an adjustable height examination table? (US Department of Justice, 2010 [Access to Medical], pp. 5–6)

• Because some individuals can only transfer from the right or left side, will clear floor space on both sides of the table be provided so one accessible table can serve both right- and left-side transfers? When more than one accessible examination room is available, will a reverse furniture layout be provided in another accessible examination room? (US Department of Justice, 2010 [Access to Medical], p. 6)

• Will the room provide enough turning space for an individual using a wheelchair to make a 180-degree turn, using a clear space of 60 inches (~1.5 meters) in diameter or a 60 by 60 inch (~1.5 by 1.5 meter) T-shaped space? Will movable chairs and other objects, such as wastebaskets, be moved aside if necessary to provide sufficient clear floor space for maneuvering and turning? (US Department of Justice, 2010 [Access to Medical], p. 6)

• When a portable patient lift or stretcher is to be used, will additional clear floor space be provided to maneuver the lift or stretcher? (US Department of Justice, 2010 [Access to Medical], p. 6)

Guidelines for Accessible Medical Equipment

☐ Will an adjustable-height table be provided that allows patient transfer from a wheelchair? (NCODH and NCSU Center for Universal Design, 2007; Iezzoni and O'Day, 2006; Schott et al., 2002; US Department of Justice, 2010 [Access to Medical])

☐ Will a handle or support rail be provided for stability during a transfer and during the examination? (Iezzoni and O'Day, 2006; Schott et al., 2002; US Department of Justice, 2010 [Access to Medical])

☐ Will equipment such as a transfer board or patient lift be provided? (Iezzoni and O'Day, 2006; Schott et al., 2002; US Department of Justice, 2010 [Access to Medical])

☐ Will different types of exam tables be provided for different purposes? (US Department of Justice, 2010 [Access to Medical])

☐ Will tilt, adjustability, headrests, footrests, and armrests be provided? (US Department of Justice, 2010 [Access to Medical])

☐ Will mammography equipment be provided that can accommodate a wheelchair user? (Connell et al., 1997; Schott et al., 2002; US Department of Justice, 2010 [Access to Medical])

☐ Will scales be provided that can weigh people sitting in wheelchairs or people who have difficulty standing? (Iezzoni and O'Day, 2006; NCODH and NCSU Center for Universal Design, 2007; Schott et al., 2002; US Department of Justice, 2010 [Access to Medical])

Design Considerations for Patients and Visitors with Hearing Disabilities

☐ Will there be a policy of asking all patients if they have difficulty hearing? (Wyatt, 1983)

☐ Will sign language interpreters be available within the facility or on call? (American Sign Language Interpreter Network, 2015; Gips, personal communication, June 16, 2015)

☐ Will various methods of communication be available to patients and visitors with hearing disabilities, including sign language, specialized software/hardware systems, closed-circuit television systems, vibrating pagers, texting, handwritten notes, supplemental hearing devices, or other means? (Interpretype Communications, LTD, 2015)

☐ Will there be a way to install T-coil hearing-loop induction systems around the perimeter of rooms? (Lin, 2012; Tierney, 2011)

☐ Will patients have the option of using use email or texting to set up appointments and receive reminders and clinical information? (Access to health services, 2014; Iezzoni and O'Day, 2006)

☐ Will natural lighting be used as much as possible? (Iezzoni and O'Day, 2006)

☐ Will patient and visitor information, including wayfinding directions, be available in writing? (Iezzoni and O'Day, 2006)

☐ Will fire alarms or other warning signals be available as flashing lights, variable-intensity fans, and other non-sound-based devices? (Iezzoni and O'Day, 2006; Leibrock, 1990; Milner, 1981)

☐ Will various light-based or other nonverbal devices be used to communicate with patients and visitors with hearing disabilities? These may include knock sensors; colored lights that signal when patients should take certain actions while getting X-rays, CT scans, and so on; and cell phones, light signals, number displays, or vibrating pagers used in waiting areas. (Iezzoni and O'Day, 2006; Mulley and Ng, 1995; Ubido, Huntington, and Warburton, 2002)

Design Considerations for Patients and Visitors Who Are Blind or Have Low-Vision

☐ In addition to following ADA signage guidelines (including raised lettering and Braille on certain types of signs), will wayfinding signs be as legible as possible to people with vision disabilities? Will sufficient contrast be provided between text and background? Will text be large enough to be legible from a distance?

☐ Will additional means be considered for communicating key information to people with vision disabilities, including audible signals, audible signage systems, and tactile guides such as textured strips? (Harkness and Groom, 1976; Proud, 1989; Rashtian, 2007; Wayfinding, 2004; Zimring and Templer, 1983–84)

☐ Will staff be trained to work with patients and visitors with vision disabilities and to use technology (such as audible wayfinding guidance), as appropriate, to communicate key information?

☐ Will interior pathways be unobstructed by furniture, equipment, posts, or protrusions from the wall (such as water fountains)? (Genensky, 1981; Harkness and Groom, 1976; NCODH and NSCU, 2007; Proud, 1989; Rashtian, 2007; Zimring and Templer, 1983–84)

☐ Will potential hazards—such as stairways and roadways—be marked by tactile warning signals, such as grooves or strips? (Genensky, 1981; Harkness and Groom, 1976; NCODH and NSCU, 2007; Proud, 1989; Rashtian, 2007; Zimring and Templer, 1983–84)

☐ In facilities dedicated to users who are blind or have low-vision, will hard surfaces be avoided on floors, ceilings, and walls?

☐ Will ramp and stair widths and tread heights be consistent?

☐ Will stair railings begin before the ramp or first step and run continuously, flattening out along landings and rising or descending again with the next flight on both sides of the stair or ramp?

☐ Will elevators contain audible warnings, so people with vision disabilities can rely on sound cues?

☐ Will sufficient color contrast be provided between objects and backgrounds? Will the colors of clinic registration counters contrast with the color of the paper forms used? Will toilet seats contrast with the floor, and showers or tubs contrast with the floors and walls around them? (Bright and Cook, 2010; Proud, 1989)

Design That Cares: Planning Health Facilities for Patients and Visitors, third edition, by Janet R. Carpman and Myron A. Grant. ©2016 by Jossey-Bass.

Design Considerations for Older Patients and Visitors

Design Guidelines Regarding Older Patients and Visitors
Safety Systems

☐ Will a minimum radius be determined for the edges of all hard surfaces and protrusions that might cause injuries in spaces that will be used by older patients and visitors? (Koncelik, 1976)

☐ Will visual warning devices such as exit signs be backed up with tactile signage and a middle-frequency auditory signal, to enhance the ability of older people to locate the exit? (American Institute of Architects Foundation, 1986; Iezzoni and O'Day, 2006; Koncelik, 1982; Wayfinding, 2004; Winters, 1989)

☐ Will signs for accessible escape routes be posted at wheelchair height so users can easily see them? (American Institute of Architects Foundation, 1986; Iezzoni and O'Day, 2006; Koncelik, 1982; Winters, 1989)

☐ Will fire-detection alarms be provided with extra-loud buzzers, since losses in the ability to smell can impair an older person's ability to detect fires? (Winters, 1989)

Sound

☐ When possible, will ambient background sounds in open public spaces be reduced by using sound-attenuating materials for walls, floors, and ceilings? When possible and appropriate, will wall hangings, screens, banners, or acoustic panels be used? (Iezzoni and O'Day, 2006; Koncelik, 1982)

☐ Will background music or loud televisions be avoided? (Iezzoni and O'Day, 2006; Koncelik, 1982)

Lighting

☐ Will natural light be provided wherever possible?

☐ Will windows, mirrors, and other bright or reflective surfaces not be placed at the ends of corridors? (American Institute of Architects Foundation, 1986)

☐ Will abrupt changes in illumination levels be avoided? (American Institute of Architects Foundation, 1986; Drader, 1982; Iezzoni and O'Day, 2006;)

☐ Will indirect lighting be used whenever possible? (American Institute of Architects Foundation, 1986)

☐ Will carpeting be considered for use in corridors in order to reduce glare and noise? (Koncelik, 1976)

☐ Will lighting be provided at the first few stairs in a series, because this is where many falls occur? (Facilities for the Elderly in Canada, 1984)

☐ Will warm-toned lighting be selected? (Iezzoni and O'Day, 2006; Koncelik, 1976)

☐ Will light sources be shielded? (Facilities for the Elderly in Canada, 1984; Koncelik, 1976)

☐ Will glare be reduced by fitting all windows and large glass panels with some means of light reduction, such as non-reflective glass, frosted adhesive film, shades, blinds, or drapes? (Facilities for the Elderly in Canada, 1984; Koncelik, 1976)

☐ Will nuanced lighting with dimmers be provided in bedrooms and lounge areas, with supplementary adjustable task lighting? (Fong, 2006; L. H. Hiatt, 1991; Super, personal communication, April 4, 2014)

☐ Will fluorescent lights be monitored in order to avoid visual vibration? (L. H. Hiatt, 1991)

Color

☐ Will color be planned in conjunction with lighting? (L. G. Hiatt, 1981)

☐ Will color be planned in conjunction with texture? (L. G. Hiatt, 1981)

☐ Will changes in planes (floor to wall, tread to riser) be emphasized with highly contrasting colors? (American Institute of Architects Foundation, 1986; Behar, n.d. [unpub.]; Lawton, 1979)

☐ Will patterns be avoided or used with knowledge and caution in spaces that will be used by older patients and visitors? (L. G. Hiatt, 1981; Iezzoni and O'Day, 2006)

☐ Will contrasting colors be used on design components such as bathroom fixtures, grab bars, doors, door frames, latches, knobs, and switches? (Drader, 1982)

Texture

☐ Will texture be used to help identify different locations within the healthcare facility? (Koncelik, 1982)

☐ Will reflective and shiny surfaces not be specified, especially on floors and bathroom fixtures? (Koncelik, 1976)

☐ Will abrasive wall surfaces not be specified? (Koncelik, 1976)

Hardware

☐ Will door hardware be provided, such as levers and push-type handles that can be operated with one hand and that do not require twisting, turning, or excessive strength?

Design That Cares: Planning Health Facilities for Patients and Visitors, third edition, by Janet R. Carpman and Myron A. Grant. ©2016 by Jossey-Bass.

(American Institute of Architects Foundation, 1986; , Developments in Aging, 1986; Iezzoni and O'Day, 2006; Jones and Tamari, 1997; Leibrock, 1990; US Access Board, ADAAG 2002, 4.13.9)

☐ Will door closers be provided that require a maximum of 5 pounds of opening force? (US Access Board, ADAAG 2002, 4.13.11)

Flooring

☐ Whenever possible, will low-pile carpeting with a low-contrast pattern be provided rather than hard flooring, because of carpeting's significant glare reduction and safety advantages? (Koncelik, 1976)

☐ Will stain-resistant carpet be selected, with an added guard to prevent bacterial growth and resulting odors? (Behar, n.d. [unpub.])

☐ Will resilient carpet be selected for ease of wheelchair handling, with a pile height of less than ½ inch (~1.27 centimeters) and an uncut or tip sheer in high-density pile? (Behar, n.d. [unpub.]; Iezzoni and O'Day, 2006; Jones and Tamari, 1987)

☐ Where carpeting is not used, will flooring be provided that is resilient, non-glare, easy to clean, and nonslip even when wet? (Iezzoni and O'Day, 2006; Jones and Tamari, 1997; Koncelik, 1982; Lawton, 1979)

☐ Will vinyl flooring be used in place of ceramic tiles because it is softer and has higher friction ratings? (Iezzoni and O'Day, 2006)

☐ Will the front edges of stair treads be easily identifiable? (Hunt and Ross, 1989)

☐ Will color or lighting create contrast between adjoining stair treads and risers? (Hunt and Ross, 1989)

☐ Will carpet seams be avoided on stair treads? (Hunt and Ross, 1989)

☐ To provide contrast between floor and wall surfaces, will a contrasting color band be used around the edge of all floor surfaces, except at the entrance to a stairway, ramp, or doorway? (Hunt and Ross, 1989)

☐ Will the color of the stair continue up over the tread of the top step to serve as a warning to those approaching the stair? (Hunt and Ross, 1989)

☐ Will potential safety problems be avoided, such as loose seams, curled edges, and uneven carpet levels? (Hunt and Ross, 1989; Iezzoni and O'Day, 2006)

☐ Will handrails be easily distinguishable from wall surfaces? (Hunt and Ross, 1989)

☐ Will carpeting with banding, patterns, or borders be avoided? (L. H. Hiatt, 1991; Iezzoni and O'Day, 2006)

Seating

☐ Will chairs be selected that have a clear space under the front, so the user's heels can be placed underneath? (American Institute of Architects Foundation, 1986)

☐ Will chairs be selected in which the front edge of the chair arms is in the same vertical plane, or extends slightly beyond, the front edge of the seat? (American Institute of Architects Foundation, 1986)

☐ Will chairs be selected with arms that can be gripped?

☐ Will chairs be selected with a seat angle of no more than 4 degrees? (American Institute of Architects Foundation, 1986)

☐ Will seats be avoided that are so firm that they may cause skin ulcers? (American Institute of Architects Foundation, 1986)

☐ Will nonabsorbent upholstery be avoided? (American Institute of Architects Foundation, 1986; Koncelik, 1976)

☐ Will seat coverings be avoided that are rough or slippery? (Ellis, 1988)

☐ Because seniors are somewhat shorter than average, will seating be selected with a height from the floor to the seat's front edge of no more than 17 inches (~43.2 centimeters)? (American Institute of Architects Foundation, 1986; Koncelik, 1982)

☐ Will seating options be provided for obese people that are the same style as the rest of the seating?

☐ Will seating be avoided where the legs are splayed beyond the area of the seat?

☐ Will seating with overly deep seats be avoided?

Heating, Ventilation, and Air Conditioning

☐ Will heating systems be capable of maintaining a temperature of 75 degrees Fahrenheit?

☐ Will cooling systems be capable of maintaining a temperature of 78 degrees Fahrenheit?

☐ Will air-handling systems be selected to avoid noise and the creation of drafty areas?

Wayfinding

☐ Will memorable landmarks be created throughout the facility, using natural light, color, artwork, unique architectural features, plants, and other design elements? (Huelat, 2007; Koncelik, 1982)

☐ Will high contrast be provided between sign text and background and between the sign background and the wall? (Koncelik, 1982)

Design That Cares: Planning Health Facilities for Patients and Visitors, third edition, by Janet R. Carpman and Myron A. Grant. ©2016 by Jossey-Bass.

☐ Will white letters on a dark background be used in areas used predominantly by older patients and visitors? (Koncelik, 1982)

☐ Will signs with reflective surfaces be avoided? (American Institute of Foundation, 1986, Koncelik, 1982)

☐ Will signs not be located opposite windows, to avoid light reflecting off sign surfaces into viewers' eyes? (American Institute of Architects Foundation, 1986; Koncelik, 1982)

☐ Will directional and identification sign letter sizes be at least $1^9/_{16}$ inches (~4 centimeters) high in areas intended for older patients and visitors? (Koncelik, 1976; Drader, 1982)

☐ Will notices directed to older patients and visitors appear in large type? (Koncelik, 1976; Drader, 1982)

☐ Will directional signs be repeated more frequently than usual in places used predominantly by older patients and visitors? (Drader, 1982)

Circulation

☐ Will distances be minimized between frequently-used destinations? (Drader, 1982)

☐ Will rest areas be provided along corridors used regularly by older patients and visitors? (Drader, 1982)

☐ Will ample storage areas be provided so carts and other large pieces of medical equipment do not need to be stored in hallways and do not act as obstructions to older users? (Drader, 1982)

☐ Will protrusions be avoided so that older patients or visitors don't bump into them? (Drader, 1982)

☐ Will lighting at entrance and exit areas allow for older users' slower adaptation rates to dark and light? (Drader, 1982)

☐ Will glass walls and doors be marked to make their presence obvious to older users? (Drader, 1982)

☐ Will contrasting colors be used to accentuate entrances, exits, merging of corridors, steps, approaches to elevators, ramps, and other changes in level or flooring surface? (Drader, 1982; Leibrock, 1990)

☐ Will audible signals be used to indicate when it is safe to enter or exit an elevator? (Jones and Tamari, 1997; Koncelik, 1982)

☐ Will a double handrail–kickplate combination be used in hallways to provide support for older ambulatory users and wheelchair users? If so, will one handrail mounted at

Design That Cares: Planning Health Facilities for Patients and Visitors, third edition, by Janet R. Carpman and Myron A. Grant. ©2016 by Jossey-Bass.

32 inches (~81.3 centimeters) and the other at approximately 26 inches (~66 centimeters)? (Koncelik, 1976)

Inpatient Rooms
Beds

☐ Can beds be lowered to a height of 20 inches (~50.8 centimeters) from the floor to the top of the bedding? (Koncelik, 1982)

☐ Will bedrails be completely retractable in order to avoid injuries resulting from patients falling against them? (Koncelik, 1982)

☐ Will beds with rounded corners and edges be selected in order to prevent injuries? (Koncelik, 1976)

Furnishings

☐ Will sturdy furnishings be provided so shaky ambulatory patients can use them for physical support, if need be? (Koncelik, 1976, 1982)

☐ Will tables or bedside stands not be selected if they have white or shiny surfaces? (Koncelik, 1976)

☐ Will televisions be mounted on the wall, rather than on adjustable arms?

☐ Will remote control devices be easy to understand and manipulate and have large, legible buttons?

Telephones

☐ Will telephones have illuminated letters and numerals that contrast with the background? (Koncelik, 1976)

☐ Will push buttons be larger than standard size? (Koncelik, 1976)

☐ Will telephone speaker devices assist hearing-aid users and eliminate interference from ambient noise? (Drader, 1982)

Display

☐ Will patients be able to display personal items, such as family photographs? (Koncelik, 1976)

☐ Will space be provided for displaying notes, calendars, signs, and other mechanisms that help orient patients to time, place, and activity? (Koncelik, 1976)

Inpatient Bathrooms

Toilets

☐ Will grab bars be installed on both sides of the toilet in a way that accommodates people needing support to lower and raise themselves, people in wheelchairs, and people with disabilities on their left or right sides? (Edlich et al., 1998; Jones and Tamari, 1997, Tetlow, 1995)

☐ Will grab bars be placed close enough to be useful? (American Institute of Architects Foundation, 1986; Koncelik, 1976)

Sinks

☐ Will water pipes be inaccessible and will hot water feed pipes be wrapped in order to prevent leg burns? (Edlich et al., 1998; Jones and Tamari, 1997; Koncelik, 1982)

☐ To make it easy for older patients in wheelchairs to use the sink, will various alternatives for mounting faucets and water controls be considered, such as side mountings, in addition to the traditional back mounting? (Iezzoni and O'Day, 2006; Jones and Tamari, 1997; Koncelik, 1976)

☐ Will water controls be clearly marked to indicate hot and cold? (Koncelik, 1976)

☐ Will oversized, textured faucet knobs or lever handles enable older patients to identify and grasp them easily? (Koncelik, 1976)

☐ Will level-handle faucets be considered?

Other

☐ Will light bulbs that simulate natural light be used over bathroom mirrors? (American Institute of Architects Foundation, 1986)

☐ Will towel racks be sturdy enough to support a patient's weight, if necessary?

☐ Will brightly colored grab bars be considered? (Leibrock, 1990)

Design Considerations for Obese Patients

Guidelines for Inpatient Rooms for Obese Patients

☐ Will the door be 60 inches (~1.5 meters) wide so that medical equipment for severely obese patients can fit through the door? (Harrell and Miller, 2004)

☐ Will the room have a minimum clear floor area of 200 square feet (~18.6 square meters) and preferably 210 square feet (~19.5 square meters [14 by 15 feet, ~4.3 by 4.6 meters]), allowing 5 feet (~1.5 meters) of clearance around the patient's bed? (Facility Guidelines Institute, 2010; Harrell and Miller, 2004; Pelczarski, 2007; Thrall, 2005)

☐ Will the healthcare organization purchase bariatric beds with built-in scales and that can be converted to a chair position? (Harrell and Miller, 2004; Pelczarski, 2007)

☐ Will patients be allowed to control the temperature and lighting in the room? (Harrell and Miller, 2004)

☐ Will the inpatient bathroom for obese patients be at least 45 square feet (~4.2 square meters)? (Harrell and Miller, 2004)

☐ Will floor-mounted toilets and sinks rather than wall-mounted fixtures be specified, unless contraindicated by requirements for accessible design? (Facility Guidelines Institute, 2010; Pelczarski, 2007; Thrall, 2005)

☐ Will toilets and sinks be capable of withstanding downward static force of 1,000 pounds? (Facility Guidelines Institute, 2010)

☐ Will the toilet be placed 24 inches (~60.9 centimeters) away from the wall? (Thrall, 2005)

☐ Will there be a bidet in the bathroom? (Harrell and Miller, 2004)

☐ Will reinforced grab bars be provided around toilets and showers? (Harrell and Miller, 2004; Pelczarski, 2007; Thrall, 2005)

☐ Will grab bars and toilet-tissue dispensers be located in places where bariatric patients can easily reach them? (Harrell and Miller, 2004)

☐ Will a mounted handheld nozzle be provided in the shower in a place where caregivers can easily reach it? (Harrell and Miller, 2004; Thrall, 2005)

☐ Will a shower seat be available? (Harrell and Miller, 2004)

☐ Will the shower allow room for two caregivers to assist the patient? (Harrell and Miller, 2004)

Guidelines for Furniture and Medical Equipment for Obese Patients

☐ In waiting areas, cafeterias, and registration areas, will some furniture be provided, such as loveseats, that can accommodate bariatric patients and that coordinate with the rest of the furniture? (Harrell and Miller, 2004; Pelczarski, 2007; Thrall, 2005)

☐ Will seating be provided both with and without arms? (Harrell and Miller, 2004)

☐ Will lift equipment be provided that can be used to transfer obese patients to and from bed? Will built-in mechanical lifts be provided in all newly constructed bariatric-nursing-unit rooms and in 10 percent of the rooms in renovation projects? (Harrell and Miller, 2004, Pelczarski, 2007; Thrall, 2005)

☐ Will bariatric wheelchairs and bariatric operating-room tables be available? (Pelczarski, 2007)

☐ Will a scale be provided that measures bariatric patients, accommodates wheelchairs, and respects the privacy of the patient? (Harrell and Miller, 2004; Pelczarski, 2007; Thrall, 2005)

☐ Will diagnostic imaging systems accommodate bariatric patients? (Pelczarski, 2007)

☐ Will extra-large blood pressure cuffs be available? (Pelczarski, 2007)

☐ Will elevators or lifts be installed where there are floor ramps or inclines, so staff members do not have to push obese patients along ramps? (Thrall, 2005)

☐ Will elevators or lifts have a weight capacity that can handle a bariatric patient, bed, transport staff, and specialized equipment? (Pelczarski, 2007)

Design That Cares: Planning Health Facilities for Patients and Visitors, third edition, by Janet R. Carpman and Myron A. Grant. ©2016 by Jossey-Bass.

References

Abend, A., and Chen, A. Developing residential design statements for the hearing-impaired elderly. *Environment and Behavior* 17(4):475–500, July 1985.

Access to health services for people with hearing loss. Action on Hearing Loss: RNID. 2014. www .actiononhearingloss.org.uk/.

ADA Questions and Answers for Health Care Providers. Reprinted with permission from the National Association of the Deaf Law and Advocacy Center. 2015. www.wvdhhr.org/wvcdhh/directories /07TOC/ADAQAHealthCarPro.pdf.

Alexander, N. B., Schultz, A. B., and Warwick, D. N. Rising from a chair: Effects of age and functional ability on performance biomechanics. *Journal of Gerontology* 46(3):M91–98, 1991.

American Institute of Architects Foundation. *Design for Aging: An Architect's Guide.* Washington, DC: AIA Press, 1986.

American Sign Language Interpreter Network. Video relay interpreting. 2015. www.aslnetwork.com /services/video-relay-interpreting.

American Speech-Language-Hearing Association, People with Hearing Loss. Incidence and prevalence of hearing loss and hearing aid use in the United States, 2008 ed. www.asha.org/research/reports /hearing/No. sthash.WdzGvpIU.dpuf.

Americans with Disabilities Act, ADA Title III Technical Assistance Manual Covering Public Accommodations and Commercial Facilities, n.d. http://www.ada.gov/taman3.html.

Archea, J., Collins, B., and Stahl, F. *Guidelines for Stair Safety.* Washington, DC: National Bureau of Standards, BSS 120, 1979.

Archea, J. C. Environmental factors associated with stair accidents by the elderly. *Clinics in Geriatric Medicine* 1(3):555–69, August 1985.

Asher, J. K. Toward a safer design for stairs. *Job Safety Health* 5:27–32, 1977.

Behar, S. Attractive products for independence. Unpublished paper. (No further information available)

Berkowitz, M., et al. *Reading with Print Limitations: Executive Summary.* Prepared for the National Library Service for the Blind and Physically Handicapped. New York: American Foundation for the Blind, 1979.

Brault, M. W. Americans with disabilities: 2010. Household economic studies. Current population reports, 70–131. Issued July 2012. PDF page numbers: 1–23. www.census.gov/prod/2012pubs/p70 –131.pdf.

Bright, K., and Cook, G. *The Colour, Light and Contrast Manual.* Chichester, UK: Wiley-Blackwell, 2010.

Brown, K., and Shoemaker, A. Designing facilities around models of care. Original inquiry brief. *Council of International Hospitals.* February 2004.

Burdett, R. G., Habasevich, R., Pisciotta, J., and Simon, S. Biomechanical comparison of rising from two types of chairs. *Physical Therapy* 65(8):1177–83, August 1985.

Carpman, J. R., Grant, M. A., and Norton, C. Needs of the hearing impaired in a hospital setting. Unpublished research report No. 30, Patient and Visitor Participation Project, Office of Hospital Planning, Research and Development, University of Michigan, Ann Arbor, 1984.

Centers for Disease Control and Prevention (CDC). FastStats Disability and Risk Factors, 2015. www .cdc.gov/nchs/fastats/obesity-overweight.htm.

Chen, A. H., Youdelman, M. K., and Brooks, J. The legal framework for language access in healthcare settings: Title VI and beyond. *Journal of General Internal Medicine* 22(suppl 2):362–67, November 2007. Published online October 24, 2007. doi:10.1007/s11606–007–0366–2. www.ncbi.nlm.nih.gov /pmc/articles/PMC2150609/.

Chien, W., and Lin, F. R. Prevalence of hearing aid use among older adults in the United States. *Archives of Internal Medicine* 172(3):292–93, February 13, 2012.

Connell, B. R., Jones, M., Mace, R., Mueller, J., Mullick, A., Ostroff, E., Sanford, J., Steinfeld, E., Story, M., and Vanderheiden, G. The principles of Universal Design, Version 2.0. Raleigh: North Carolina State University, The Center for Universal Design, 1997. www.ncsu.edu/ncsu/design/cud/about_ud /udprinciples.htm.

DeafSpace Concepts. 2014. www.hbhmarchitecture.com/index.php?/ongoing/deaf-space-design-guide/.

Developments in Aging: 1985. Vol. 3. Washington, DC: US Government Printing Office, 1986.

Drader, D. The design of geriatric assessment units: psychosocial considerations. Consulting report, Department of National Health and Welfare, Ottawa, Canada, 1982.

Edlich, R. F., Neal, J. G., Suber, F., Kirby, D., Woods, J. A., Bentram, D., et al. A new barrier-free burn center. *Journal of Burn Care Rehabilitation* 19:390–98, 1998.

Ellis, M. Everyday aids and appliances: Choosing easy chairs for the disabled. *British Medical Journal* 296(6623):701–2, March 1988.

Facilities for the Elderly in Canada: Design and Environmental Considerations. Vol. 1, Geriatric Units in Hospitals. Ottawa, Canada: Department of National Health and Welfare, 1984.

Facility Guidelines Institute. *Guidelines for Design and Construction of Health Care Facilities,* 2010 edition. 2.2–2.16 Bariatric Care Unit. Chicago: American Society for Healthcare Engineering of the American Hospital Association, 2010.

_____. Major additions and revisions. *2014 FGI Guidelines for Hospitals and Outpatient Facilities.* www .fgiguidelines.org/guidelines2014_HOP.php.

Finlay, O. E., Bayles, T. B., Rosen, C., and Milling, J. Effects of chair design, age and cognitive status on mobility. *Age and Ageing* 12:329–35, 1983.

Fisher, T. Enabling the disabled. *Progressive Architecture,* 119–24, July 1985.

Fitch, J., Templer, J., and Corcoran, P. The dimensions of stairs. *Scientific American* 231:82–90, 1974.

Fletcher, V. A global perspective: Universal Design as socially sustainable design. In C. S. Martin and D. A. Guerin, editors. *The State of the Interior Design Profession,* 362–73. New York: Fairchild Books, 2010.

Fletcher, V. Institute for Human Centered Design. www.HumanCenteredDesign.org.

Fong, D. Evidence-based lighting design. *Healthcare Design,* August 31, 2006. www.healthcaredesign -magazine.com/article/evidence-based-lighting-design.

Genensky, S. M. Design sensitivity: The partially sighted. *Building Operating Management* 28(6):50–54, June 1981.

Gerdner, L. A. Effects of individualized versus classical "relaxation" music on the frequency of agitation in elderly persons with Alzheimer's disease and related disorders. *International Psychogeriatrics,* 12(1), 49–65, March 2000.

_____. An individualized music intervention for agitation. *Journal of the American Psychiatric Nurses Association,* 3(6), 177–84, December 1997.

_____. Individualized music intervention protocol. *Journal of Gerontological Nursing*, 25(10), 10–16, October 1999.

_____. Use of individualized music by trained staff and family: translating research into practice. *Journal of Gerontological Nursing*, 31(6), 22–30, June 2005.

Gerdner, L. A., and Schoenfelder, D. P. Evidence-based guideline. Individualized music for elders with dementia. *Journal of Gerontological Nursing*, 36(6), 7–15, June 2010. doi:10.3928/00989134–20100504–01.

Gips, K., New England ADA Center. 2015. http://newenglandada.org.

Goetschel, G. E. A review of the development of an ergonomically balanced chair. *Journal of Manipulative and Physiological Therapeutics* 10(3):65–69, April 1987.

Goldish, L. *Braille in the United States: Its Production, Distribution, and Use.* New York: American Foundation for the Blind, 1967.

Harkness, S. P., and Groom, J. N. *Building without Barriers for the Disabled.* New York: Watson Guptill, 1976.

Harrell, J. W., and Miller, B. Big challenge. *Health Facilities Management*, 17(3):34–7, March 2004.

Hart, C. Institute for Human Centered Design. www.HumanCenteredDesign.org.

Herssens J., and Heylighen, A. Haptic architecture becomes architectural hap. Paper presented in proceeding of Ergonomics for a Future: Annual Congress of the Nordic Ergonomic Society, Lisekil, January 2007. http://nordiskergonomi.org/nes2007/CD_NES_2007/papers/A34_Herssens.pdf.

Hiatt, L. G. The color and use of color in environments for older people. *Nursing Homes* 30(3):18–22, May–June 1981.

Hiatt, L. H. Breakthroughs in long term care design. Proceedings from the Third Symposium on Health Care Interior Design. *Journal of Health Care Design* 3:205–15, 1991.

Huelat, B. Wayfinding: Design for understanding. A position paper for the Environmental Standards Council of the Center for Health Design. October 2007.

Hunt, M., and Ross, L. Stairway carpet design: A simple preconstruction evaluation approach. *Journal of Applied Gerontology* 8(4):481–91, December 1989.

Iezzoni, L. I., and O'Day, B. L. *More Than Ramps: A Guide to Improving Health Care Quality and Access for People with Disabilities.* New York: Oxford University Press, 2006.

Information and Technical Assistance on the Americans with Disabilities Act. n.d. www.ada.gov.

Insights into facility access. *Health Estate* 58(9):61–63, October 2004.

Interpretype Communications. *Deaf or Hard of Hearing Accessibility Solutions/Language Interpreter Products.* 2015. http://interpretype.com.

Jones, K. E., and Tamari, I. E. Making our offices universally accessible: Guidelines for physicians. *Canadian Medical Association Journal* 156:647–56, 1997.

Koncelik, J. A. *Aging and the Product Environment.* Stroudsburg, PA: Hutchinson, & Ross, 1982.

_____. *Designing the Open Nursing Home.* Stroudsburg, PA: Dowden, Hutchinson, & Ross, 1976.

Lawton, M. P. Therapeutic environments for the aged. In D. Canter and S. Canter, editors. *Designing for Therapeutic Environments,* 233–71. New York: Wiley, 1979.

Leibrock, C. A. Design prescriptions for the disabled. Proceedings from the Second Symposium on Health Care Interior Design. *Journal of Health Care Design* 2:153–58, 1990.

Lin, F. R. Hearing loss in older adults: Who's listening? *Journal of the American Medical Association* 307(11):1147–48, March 21, 2012.

McGilloway, F. A. A chair is a chair, or is it? *Nursing Mirror* 151(4):34–35, July 24, 1980.

Milner, M. Breaking through the deafness barrier: Environmental accommodations for hearing impaired people. Unpublished report, Division of Public Services and Design and Construction Department, Washington, DC: Gallaudet College, 1981.

Mitchell, R. E., Young, T. A., Bachleda, B., and Karchmer, M. A. How many people use ASL in the United States? Why estimates need updating. *Sign Language Studies* 6:3, 306–35, Spring 2006. http:// research.gallaudet.edu/Publications/ASL_Users.pdf.

Mulley, G. P., and Ng, K. Y. Problems encountered by hearing-impaired people in hospitals. *Lancet* 345(8965):1640, June 24, 1995.

Music & Memory. 2015. https://musicandmemory.org.

National Association of the Deaf. Americans with Disabilities Act. Accessed March 25, 2016. https:// nad.org/issues/civil-rights/ADA.

National Center for Health Statistics (NCHS), Centers for Disease Control and Prevention, US Department of Health and Human Services. Prevalence of Overweight and Obesity among Adults: United States, 2003–2004. April 2006. www.cdc.gov/nchs/products/pubs/pubd/hestats/overweight /overwght_adult_03.htm.

North Carolina Office on Disability and Health (NCODH) and North Carolina State University (NCSU)'s Center for Universal Design. *Removing Barriers to Health Care: A Guide for Health Professionals,* 2007. www.fpg.unc.edu/~ncodh/pdfs/rbhealthcare.pdf.

Ostroff, E. Mining our natural resources: The user as expert. INNOVATION *The Quarterly Journal of the Industrial Designers Society of America* 16(1):27–30, 1997.

Pastalan, L. Environmental design and adaptation to the visual environment of the elderly. In R. Sekuler, D. Kline, and K. Dismukes, editors. *Aging and Human Visual Function,* 323–33. New York: Alan B. Liss, 1982.

Pelczarski, K. M. Basic concerns in bariatric design. *Healthcare Design* 7(2): 60–64, March 2007.

Pew Research Center. *Baby Boomers Retire.* 2010. www.pewresearch.org/daily-number/baby-boomers -retire.

Pipedown International. *Piped Music: The Facts.* 2014. www.pipedown.info/storage/pdfs/Fact%20sheet %20final%20version3.pdf.

Proud, G. Pattern for navigation. *Health Service Journal* 99(5154):696–97, June 8, 1989.

Ragneskog, H., Asplund, K., Kihlgren, M., and Norberg, A. Individualized music played for agitated patients with dementia: Analysis of video-recorded sessions. *International Journal of Nursing Practice,* 7(3), 146–155, June 2001.

Rashtian, S. Universal Design, architecture and spatial cognition without sight. In J. Nasar and J. Evans-Cowley, editors. *Universal Design and Visitability: From Accessibility to Zoning.* Columbus: Ohio State University, 2007.

Reiling, J., Knutzen, B., Wallen, T., McCullough, S., Miller, R., and Chernos, S. Enhancing the traditional hospital design process: A focus on patient safety. *Joint Commission Journal on Quality and Safety* 30(3):115–24, March 2004.

Rodosky, M. W., Andriacchi, T. P., and Andersson, G.B.J. The influence of chair height on lower limb mechanics during rising. *Journal of Orthopedic Research* 7(2):266–71, 1989.

Royal National Institute for Deaf People. Noise Pollution Clearinghouse. *MUZAK: Music to Whose Ears?* 2014. www.nonoise.org/library/muzak/muzak.htm.

Schott, L. H., Sanford T. C., Hagglund K. J., Gay J. W., and Coatney M. A. Removing service barriers for women with physical disabilities: Promoting accessibility in the gynecologic care setting. *Journal of Midwifery and Women's Health* 47(2): 74–79, March–April 2002. www.ncbi.nlm.nih.gov /pubmed/12019989.

Sheldon, J. On the natural history of falls in old age. *British Medical Journal,* 1960, 1685–90.

Story, M., Mueller, J., and Mace, R. *The Universal Design File: Designing for People of All Ages and Abilities.* Raleigh: North Carolina State University, Center for Universal Design, 1998.

Sung, H. C., and Chang, A. M. Use of preferred music to decrease agitated behaviours in older people with dementia: A review of the literature. *Journal of Clinical Nursing,* 14(9), 1133–40, October 2005.

Sung, H. C., Chang, A. M., and Abbey, J. The effects of preferred music on agitation of older people with dementia in Taiwan. *International Journal of Geriatric Psychiatry,* 21(10), 999–1000, October 2006.

Sung, H. C., Chang, A. M., and Lee, W. L. A preferred music listening intervention to reduce anxiety in older adults with dementia in nursing homes. *Journal of Clinical Nursing* 19(7–8), 1056–64, April 2010. doi: 10.1002/gps.2761.

Super, R. Personal communication, 2013. Institute for Human Centered Design. www.HumanCentered Design.org.

_____. Personal communication, 2014. Institute for Human Centered Design. www.HumanCentered Design.org.

Tetlow, K. Beyond the ADA. *Interiors* 154(10): 76, October 1995.

35 million Americans suffering from hearing loss. hear-it.org. www.hear-it.org/page.dsp?area=858.

Thrall, T. H. Design with dignity. *Hospitals and Health Networks* 79(11): 48–50, 52, November 2005.

Tierney, J. A Hearing aid that cuts out all the clatter. *New York Times* October 23, 2011. www.nytimes .com/2011/10/24/science/24loops.html.

Ubido, J., Huntington, J., and Warburton, D. Inequalities in access to healthcare faced by women who are deaf. *Health and Social Care in the Community* 10: 247–53, July 2002.

US Access Board, ADA Accessibility Guidelines (ADAAG), as amended through September 2002. n.d. www.access-board.gov/guidelines-and-standards/buildings-and-sites/about-the-ada-standards /background/adaag.

_____. ADA Accessibility Guidelines (ADAAG), as amended through September 2002. n.d. www .access-board.gov/guidelines-and-standards/buildings-and-sites/about-the-ada-standards/ada -standards.

_____. Chapter 5: General site and building elements. 502 parking spaces. n.d. www.access-board .gov/guidelines-and-standards/buildings-and-sites/about-the-ada-standards/ada-standards /chapter-5-general-site-and-building-elements.

_____. Proposed accessibility standards for medical diagnostic equipment, February 9, 2012. www .access-board.gov/guidelines-and-standards/health-care/about-this-rulemaking/proposed-standards.

_____. Scoping Requirements, §§223–223.2.1. n.d. www.access-board.gov/guidelines-and-standards /buildings-and-sites/about-the-ada-standards/ada-standards/chapter-2-scoping-requirements.

_____. Scoping Requirements, §§805–805.4. n.d. www.access-board.gov/guidelines-and-standards /buildings-and-sites/about-the-ada-standards/ada-standards/chapter-2-scoping-requirements.

_____. Scoping Requirements, §206.2.3. n.d. www.access-board.gov/guidelines-and-standards /buildings-and-sites/about-the-ada-standards/ada-standards/chapter-2-scoping-requirements.

———. Scoping Requirements, §208.2.1. n.d. www.access-board.gov/guidelines-and-standards /buildings-and-sites/about-the-ada-standards/ada-standards/chapter-2-scoping-requirements.

———. Scoping Requirements, §208.2.2. n.d. www.access-board.gov/guidelines-and-standards /buildings-and-sites/about-the-ada-standards/ada-standards/chapter-2-scoping-requirements.

———. Scoping Requirements, §209.3. n.d. www.access-board.gov/guidelines-and-standards /buildings-and-sites/about-the-ada-standards/ada-standards/chapter-2-scoping-requirements.

———. Scoping Requirements, §223.2.2. n.d. www.access-board.gov/guidelines-and-standards /buildings-and-sites/about-the-ada-standards/ada-standards/chapter-2-scoping-requirements.

US Census Bureau. Americans with Disabilities: 2010. Table 1. www.census.gov/people/disability /publications/sipp2010.html.

US Department of Health and Human Services. 45 Fed. Reg. 82972 (December 17, 1980). (Notice).

US Department of Human Services. Office of Civil Rights. Your rights under Section 504 of the Rehabilitation Act. Fact sheet, June 2006. www.hhs.gov/ocr/civilrights/resources/factsheets/504.pdf.

US Department of Justice, Civil Rights Division, Disability Rights Section. Access to medical care for individuals with mobility disabilities, July 2010. www.ada.gov/medcare_mobility_ta/medcare_ta.pdf.

US Department of Justice, Civil Rights Division, Disability Rights Section. ADA requirements: Effective communication, 2014. http://www.ada.gov.effective-comm.htm.

US Department of Justice. 2010 ADA Standards for accessible design: Medical care facilities. www.ada .gov/2010ADAstandards_index.htm.

Wayfinding: Tactile signage leads the way. *Health Estate Journal* 58(9):74–75, October 2004.

What Is DeafSpace? 2014. www.gallaudet.edu/campus_design/deafspace.html.

Wheeler, J., Woodward, C., Ucovich, R. L., Perry, J., and Walker, J. M. Rising from a chair: influence of age and chair design. *Physical Therapy* 65(1):22–26, January 1985.

Winters, R. Adapting the environment to age-related sensory losses. *Journal of the American Academy of Nurse Practitioners* 1(4):106–11, October–December 1989.

World Health Organization. Towards a common language for functioning, disability, and health (ICF), 2002. www.who.int/classifications/icf/training/icfbeginnersguide.pdf.

Wyatt, H. J. You and your deaf patients. Seminar materials, National Academy of Gallaudet College, Washington, DC, 1983.

Zimring, C. M., and Templer, J. Wayfinding and orientation by the visually impaired. *Journal of Environmental Systems* 13(4):333–52, 1983–84.

CHAPTER 10

SPECIAL PLACES AND SERVICES

Throughout this book, we have discussed typical patient and visitor activities and the places where they occur in many healthcare facilities. This chapter deviates from that path to cover some special places, such as food service areas, spaces for prayer and meditation, consultation and grieving rooms, emergency departments (EDs), rehabilitation units, and patient and visitor information areas. We also consider design issues related to services that can make a big difference to patients and visitors, including overnight accommodations, shops, hair care, fitness centers, and spas. While some of these may not be found in all healthcare facilities, their design features are important to consider wherever they do occur.

Special Places

Food Service Areas

The quality and healthfulness of food, as well as the inviting and pleasant atmosphere of food services, play a large role in patient and visitor satisfaction with healthcare facilities (Resnick et al., 1999; Rose, 1983). People are increasingly concerned about food allergies, nutrition, and calorie counts; they also care about the freshness and sustainability of the foods they eat. The culture shift in healthcare philosophy, from just treating the illness to treating and promoting the well-being of the whole person, has resulted in quality food service being understood as an integral component of patient and family care. Since a variety of cultural and religious groups may be using a facility's food services, management needs to be sensitive to food preferences and dietary customs.

LEARNING OBJECTIVES

- Become familiar with design issues related to food service areas, spaces for prayer and meditation, and consultation and grieving rooms, and how these can support and enhance care for patients and visitors.

- Understand the range of design features of Emergency Departments that provide care and comfort for patients and their companions.

- Learn how design features of inpatient rehabilitation units can support patients and families.

- Become familiar with important design features of patient information areas.

- Become aware of additional services that support and enhance care for patients and≈visitors, such as overnight accommodations, shops, hair care, fitness centers, and spas.

Good food served in attractive surroundings is one important way of demonstrating to patients and visitors that their needs are understood, valued, anticipated, and attended to by healthcare facility decision-makers. A meal prepared to individual tastes can be a bright spot in a patient's day. Ambulatory patients may find drinking coffee with visitors in a cafeteria a pleasant distraction. Visitors attending sick patients, often around the clock, need nutritious food offered in a pleasant environment to help sustain them during the ordeal. And when attractive eating options are available in-house, busy healthcare workers will save time by not having to travel off-campus for meals and breaks (Gatoade, 2010).

Healthcare facilities are meeting these requirements with a range of dining options, from grab-and-go and fast-casual to cook-to-order. Particularly in urban hospitals, cafés or restaurants are being located along the healthcare facility's street frontage, with large windows that offer views of the street scene, admit plenty of natural light, and invite patrons in without having to encounter a "hospital" environment (Brandau, 2014; Gatoade, 2010). Such dining areas may even include uncommon amenities, such as exhibition-cooking stations and wine service. Improved patient and visitor satisfaction has been reflected in increases of as much as

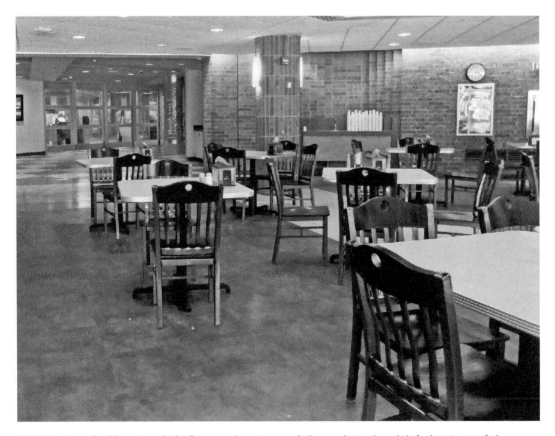

Well-designed, comfortable seating and other features, such as noise control, plants, and artwork, can help food service areas feel welcoming to patients and visitors, as well as staff.

Photo credit: Courtesy of St. Joseph Mercy Ann Arbor

40 percent in food sales, with the accompanying economies-of-scale advantages (Los Angeles Medical Center, 2011).

The importance of quality food service for patient satisfaction has led to dramatic changes in the way patient meals are provided. Many hospitals have adopted personalized tray service, where patients order from restaurant-style menus and meals are cooked and delivered to order. Patients appreciate being able to order as much or as little as they wish to eat. Savings from fewer trays ordered and less food wasted can offset the costs of adapting to this personalized tray-service system, including setting up a call center and tracking system, and hiring staff to take and deliver orders. Since trays must still be delivered in batches, although smaller ones, warming and cooling stations are desirable on inpatient units in hospitals that offer this type of service (Foodservice Changes, 2012; Lee, 2013).

Where a personalized tray-service model is not economically feasible, healthcare organizations can meet patient expectations with a mixture of room service and a traditional tray line, with personalized ordering and set mealtimes. All the food for patients on a given floor unit can be cooked and delivered at one time, with patient orders being taken in batches during less busy times. With this system, it is important to include nutrition rooms on each inpatient unit, for snacks and after-hours nutrition needs (Schilling, 2011).

Although expenditure on food plays a relatively small part in healthcare facility budgets, food costs are steadily rising. While the healthier foods that patients and visitors seek do not always cost more, cost-saving measures must be a part of the design strategy (Lee, 2013). Savings can be had from a kitchen designed for cook/chill, "prepare to inventory" production, rather than hot-bulk, same-day meal production. Energy-efficient equipment—such as Energy Star-rated dishwashers, low-flow spray valves, and high-efficiency fryers with self-cleaning burners—conserves water, fuel, and electricity (Los Angeles Medical Center, 2011). A cool roof that reflects heat and sunlight, state-of-the-art exhaust systems, and the use of natural light whenever possible are other cost-saving and environmentally friendly strategies (Boss, 2012).

Consider these design guidelines for food service areas:

- Provide warming and cooling stations on inpatient units that offer personalized tray service (Foodservice Changes, 2012; Lee, 2013).

- Provide nutrition rooms on inpatient units, for snacks and after-hours nutrition needs (Schilling, 2011).

- Design cafeterias, coffee shops, and other healthcare facility dining spaces to have a relaxing, inviting atmosphere (Henderson, 2015).

- Design healthcare facility dining spaces to be accessible to and usable by everyone.

- Use warm, light colors and a mix of natural light and subdued artificial lighting (Henderson, 2015).

- Use multiple light sources rather than exclusively using standard overhead lighting. Avoid using fluorescent fixtures (Henderson, 2015).

- Consider using artwork and special features, such as electric fireplaces, water walls, murals, and live plants to enhance aesthetics (Gatoade, 2010; Olsen, 2014).

- Provide outside views, if possible (Henderson, 2015).

- Select seating that is comfortable and moveable, with high backs and comfortable upholstery. Provide barriers between seating areas to help ensure visual and acoustical privacy.

- Provide tables of various sizes to accommodate groups of different sizes. Select tables large enough to accommodate cafeteria trays.

- Design ample space for circulation within seating areas for ambulatory patients, visitors, and staff with trays; people with walkers; wheelchair users; people with strollers; patients with rolling IV poles, and others (Henderson, 2015).

- Consider installing update monitors, similar to airport arrival and departure boards that provide information on patient status by means of a personalized code. Alternatively, visitors can be given pagers, similar to the ones used by restaurants (Reizenstein and Grant, 1981 [unpub. No. 4a).

- Consider separating staff dining areas from public dining areas (Henderson, 2015).

- Consider ways to mitigate noise in food service areas, including providing carpeting and sound-absorbing wall and ceiling materials and keeping background noise to a minimum, especially during busy times (Hiatt, 1978).

- Consult with specialists when designing food service circulation areas and areas for food ordering, pick-up, and self-service (Henderson, 2015).

- Provide ample circulation space within food ordering, pick-up, and self-service areas for wheelchair users and users of other mobility devices. Wheelchair users need to be able to easily see food selections (Henderson, 2015).

- Because some people using the food service area may have difficulty with muscle control and spill food easily, provide some dishes with rims. Consider avoiding flimsy throwaway dishes and trays in favor of more stable dishware and trays (Hiatt, 1978).

Sacred Spaces

In recent years the medical profession has been returning to an awareness that healing is a matter of body, mind, and spirit. Spaces designed for prayer and meditation, for reflection, renewal, and reprieve from stressful situations, have taken on new importance and new forms (Peteet, 2013).

Formerly, hospital chapels and meditation rooms tended to be either religiously and denominationally specific, reflecting donor preferences or the affiliation of the healthcare facility, or strictly neutral and generalized, and thus often resembling conference or waiting areas more than sacred spaces (Christian, 2011; Madden, n.d.). Now spaces are designed to welcome all belief systems.

Consider the following design guidelines:

- Rather than installing permanent religious symbols, provide a portable altar, such as a wheeled cart covered by a red cloth, for Roman Catholic mass (James, 2010).

- Provide storage space for religious materials and items, such as hymnals, Bibles, prayer books, prayer rugs, kneeling stools, and sacred texts (Madden, n.d.).

- Provide space for a small piano or organ.

- Provide a generous number of electrical outlets in the altar area in order to accommodate musical instruments, lighting, sound systems, and other equipment.

- Since devotion to nature is common to many faiths, consider creating focal points using stained glass panels or other artwork depicting nature (James, 2010; Madden, n.d.; Texas Children's Hospital, n.d.).

- Include points of the compass since Muslims must face east toward Mecca when they pray, and cardinal directions are important in other beliefs, such as Wicca and Native American faiths (James, 2010).

- Provide moveable furnishings, allowing a variety of configurations (James, 2010).

- Select comfortable chairs (James, 2010).

- Arrange seating to allow visual privacy (James, 2010).

- Provide adjustable lighting levels.

- Insulate the walls and use sound-attenuating materials, such as carpeting, to keep the space quiet.

- Make sure sacred spaces are accessible to and usable by everyone, including people with functional limitations.

Consultation and Grieving Spaces

Consultation and grieving spaces are needed in most healthcare facilities. A family faced with the death of a loved one must have a place to deal with the news in private; a woman who has been raped needs to talk with a social worker in confidence; and patients wrestling with difficult decisions about their treatment need private, quiet places to discuss options with their health-care team. Consultation and grieving need to be accommodated in nearly all patient-care spaces, such as the emergency department, inpatient floors, diagnostic and treatment areas, the surgery area, the labor and delivery area, and intensive care units. When a specific room is not dedicated for this purpose, these activities continue to occur, but they will occur in public—in hallways, waiting areas, or semi-private inpatient rooms—compromising patient and family privacy.

In addition to private grieving and consultation areas, one or more gathering spaces are desirable, where grieving families can be with one another and, perhaps, with other grieving families. These more public spaces can include a kitchenette with a family dining area, digital devices with internet access, a children's area, and laundry facilities (What is inpatient, 2014).

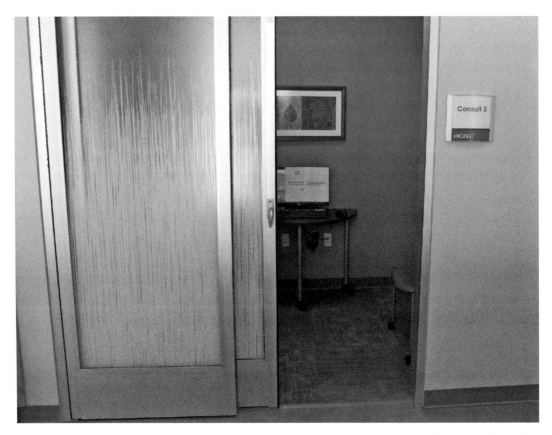

Consultation rooms with closeable doors can provide private places for family members to meet with medical staff in a variety of hospital areas, such as Surgery Waiting and Emergency.
Photo credit: Courtesy of St. Joseph Mercy Ann Arbor

When a healthcare facility includes an inpatient hospice unit, patient rooms must be large enough to allow family members to stay with patients around the clock. Sleeping accommodations for visitors should be provided, such as convertible sleep sofas, and a bathroom where visitors can shower.

Increasingly, healthcare organizations are recognizing and responding to the particular grieving processes that accompany the death of a fetus or baby. Parents in these circumstances should not have to remain in maternity units, where they will encounter families celebrating births (Fry, 2014). Although infant mortality rates have dropped dramatically, one out of every 160 pregnancies in the U.S. ends in stillbirth (March of Dimes, 2015). These deaths are often unexpected, allowing the family no time to prepare. Friends and family may have difficulty acknowledging the grief associated with the death of a fetus or a baby (Brody, 2011; Stillbirth: The facts, 2015). Therefore, it is particularly important for healthcare organizations to validate this grief by providing a private space where families can get to know their babies, at least for a short while. Many of the same design issues apply to the NICU. Since parents are usually the only ones allowed into the NICU, a private room will enable other family members to bond with the baby and seek closure.

All such private spaces should have as soothing and homelike an atmosphere as possible. Furniture should include a sofa, and if possible a double bed, a rocking chair, a sink, and a mini-fridge. A cool cot or other cooling facility is an important feature, since a deceased baby's body deteriorates rapidly if it is not kept cool. Keeping the baby's body cool enables families to be with their babies for longer periods of time, allowing them to mourn on their own schedule (Davies, 2014). Materials should be stored nearby to allow the taking of hand- and footprints.

Consider these guidelines when designing consultation and grieving spaces:

- Locate grieving and consultation rooms so people do not have to walk a long way before they can deal with their situations in private.

- Provide several grieving and consultation rooms in emergency departments, because these are likely to be in high demand.

- Separate postpartum grieving spaces and the NICU from the main maternity area.

- Provide a cool cot or other cooling mechanism in postpartum grieving rooms.

- Design grieving rooms large enough to accommodate numerous family members.

- Provide both visual and acoustical privacy.

- Avoid an institutional ambience by selecting subdued colors, carpeting, and table lamps or other types of indirect or incandescent lighting.

- Use natural light where possible.

- Provide comfortable seating, including chairs and couches.

- Provide coat racks or hooks for personal belongings.

- To avoid unnecessary disturbances, place an adjustable sign on the door to indicate whether or not the room is occupied. (Petersen, 1981)

Emergency Departments

Since the mid-1980s, the volume of emergency-department (ED) visits in the U.S. has increased by almost 3 percent annually, driven by patterns of increased ED usage, general population growth, and escalating numbers of older users (Welch, 2012; Zilm, Crane, and Roche, 2010). By 2006, over 113 million people were treated in hospital-based emergency facilities: one visit for every three people in the country (Zilm, 2007). In most large hospitals, the emergency service now accounts for more than 50 percent of admissions and the emergency entrance has become a second main entrance portal to the hospital (Zilm, 2007).

Patient satisfaction with ED performance has become critical for the reputation of the hospital as a whole, with implications for return patronage, liability, and remuneration (Crane and Noon, 2010; Soremekun, Takayesu, and Bohan, 2011). It has been estimated that three times as many patients create their impressions of a hospital through the ED as through admissions (Exadaktylos and Velmahos, 2008).

By 2005, 69 percent of urban EDs were over capacity (Welch, 2012). Increased demand can contribute to prolonged patient wait times, increased patient complaints, decreased staff satisfaction, decreased physician productivity, and—most worrying—sub-optimal patient outcomes (Bernstein et al., 2009; Exadaktylos and Velmahos, 2008; Magid et al., 2009; Soremekun et al., 2011; Trzeciak and Rivers, 2003; Wiler et al., 2009).

Crowded conditions are only one factor affecting the way EDs operate. Particularly as the baby boom generation reaches and passes retirement age, new demands will be placed on healthcare facilities, as well as on information systems, diagnostic and therapeutic procedures, and personnel (Welch, 2012). Individual EDs have instituted innovations, but many have not yet been validated by formal studies or peer review. Many clinicians are unaware of the available research and information. In selecting optimal organizational models, open dialogue and collaboration are essential among design professionals, architects, consultants, department/ hospital leadership, clinicians, and front-line staff.

In a number of ways, the issues involved in the design of an ED are similar to those of an outpatient diagnostic and treatment area. (See chapter 6.) An important difference, however, is the nature of the situation: many people come to the ED with acute illnesses or serious injuries which may be life-threatening. They are under an unusual amount of stress and may be experiencing considerable pain. The design of the built environment has a significant role to play in achieving good outcomes (Hamilton, 2013). Strategies to assure patient satisfaction and avoid problems—such as patient aggressiveness, leaving without being seen, or leaving before treatment is completed—require particular attention (Kamali et al., 2013).

Finding and Entering the ED

During an emergency, being able to find one's destination is particularly critical. Patients may be traveling to the ED for the first time or visiting it in the middle of the night. Often, when dealing with a stressful situation, neither patients nor their companions have the extra mental energy necessary to navigate confusing traffic patterns during arrival or confusing pedestrian routes once they are inside the facility.

Consider the following guidelines for emergency entrance areas (see also chapter 4):

- Provide a visible, clearly labeled entrance with a covered and convenient patient drop-off/ pick-up area (Carpman Associates, 1984 [unpub.]; A New ED, 2012; New Emergency Entrance, n.d.; Zilm, 2007).

- Make sure exterior signage is legible from a distance during daylight, after dark, and in inclement weather (Carpman Associates, 1984 [unpub.]).

- Make sure the automobile route to the emergency entrance is clearly differentiated from the ambulance route (Carpman Associates, 1984 [unpub.]).

- Provide separate ambulance and walk-in entrances so walk-in patients and visitors don't have views to arriving ambulances (Carpman Associates, 1984 [unpub.]; Department of Health [UK], 2013).

- Provide ambulance parking adjacent to the ambulance entrance, to avoid congestion (Carpman Associates, 1984 [unpub.]; Department of Health [UK], 2013).

- Consider providing a second public entrance for use in high-volume surge conditions and for triage of contaminated patients (Carpman Associates, 1984 [unpub.]; Zilm, 2007).

- Make ED interior signage legible and easy to understand (Carpman Associates, 1984 [unpub.]).

- Provide nearby parking within view of the drop-off entrance, so companions can drop off patients, park, and easily find their way back (Carpman Associates, 1984 [unpub.]).

- Consider providing space for valet parking services (Carpman Associates, 1984 [unpub.]; A New ED, 2012).

- Consider providing a separate entry into the pediatric ED or mark a child-friendly pathway from the adult ED to the pediatric ED (Carpman Associates, 1984 [unpub.]; Department of Health [UK], 2013; Pebble Project, 2014; Pediatric Emergency Department, 2015).

ED Size and Configuration

Despite the ever-growing volume of ED usage nationwide, lower-volume ERs tend to be more efficient and consistently perform better on metrics such as arrival-to-provider time ("door to doc"), length of stay, patients leaving without being seen or before treatment is completed, and ratio of patient complaints (Augustine, 2011; Hutten-Czapski, 2010; Welch et al., 2012). The problem of ED overcrowding, especially for outdated and inefficient facilities, cannot be solved simply by building more and larger facilities (Wheary, 2014).

Under normal conditions, ED patients arrive in predictable cycles, with peak loads three to four times as great as non-peak loads (Welch, Jones, and Allen, 2007). Knowing the census and the arrival curve of an ED allows decision-makers to plan for an effective number of intake spaces; recent estimates give a ratio of 1,400–1,500 annual visits per bed (Welch, 2012; Zilm, 2007).

Natural and manmade disasters have shown that EDs need to be prepared for surges of at least four times normal rates (Zilm, 2007). Accordingly, EDs are turning away from the traditional "ballroom" layout, with 16–18 open exam and treatment bays arranged around a central core of charting and support functions, to designs and operational schemes that offer greater flexibility (Zilm, 2007). The trend is to an ED designed to size up or down in response to demand. A variety of strategies can be employed to achieve this, perhaps different ones at different stages of the 24-hour cycle. Smaller functional units dedicated to patients with similar acuities, with a specific zone for each medical team, can improve communication and clinical care. This design choice also has direct advantages for the team itself: under traditional conditions, ED nurses walk an average of 5.2 miles per shift (Leighty, 2007).

ED Layout Alternatives

Current ED layout alternatives include pods, inner core, doughnut, separate functional units, streaming systems, and fast-track (express care) systems. No doubt there will be other alternatives developed in the future. Whatever the layout, several secure rooms are required, for behavioral care and security-restricted patients, as well as at least one negative-pressure room for at-risk patients (Christmann, 2011).

> *Pods.* A pod arrangement groups clusters of 8–12 exam rooms with a support area and circulation to other pods (Zilm, 2010).

> *Inner Core.* In an inner core concept, staff members work in zones supporting 10–12 exam rooms which patients and visitors access from a perimeter corridor (Zilm, 2010).

> *Doughnut Layout.* In a doughnut layout, staff work areas are located in the center and a perimeter corridor gives access to the patient by family, while protecting staff from cross-traffic (Zilm, 2007).

> *Separate Functional Units.* A larger ED might be divided into several smaller functional units, each an ED-equivalent with the full complement of standard sub-spaces.

> *Streaming Systems.* High-volume EDs are trending toward "streaming" systems, with patients divided according to acuity, and examination and support spaces clustered for specific types of care (Zilm and Lennon, 2003). Higher-acuity patients require larger rooms, with space for stretchers, a resuscitation team, ventilator, EKG machine, and portable X-ray machine all at once, as well as direct sightlines to the staff work station. Lower-acuity patients are often best accommodated in reclining chairs, which take up less space and are often judged more comfortable (Welch, 2012; Wheary, 2014).

> *Fast-Track (Express Care) Systems.* The "fast track" for lower-acuity patients (see "ED Front-End Areas") is proving an attractive option, although rarely employed for the full 24 hours even in the largest hospitals (Welch, 2012). Such fast-track or "express care" may take place in a dedicated section of the ED, with its own exam rooms and/or chair-centric space and an exit path away from more seriously ill patients (Allison and Kunz, 2011; Chandler Hospital Emergency Department, 2014).

Accommodating Disasters

Few current EDs were constructed with sufficient space and facilities to cope with high-risk events such as infectious pandemics or the probable four-fold surge from a natural or man-made disaster. Not all components of the federally funded "ER One" prototype will be within the resources of every institution, but any new ED design should consider the following guidelines:

- Provide more than the usual amount of waiting area space, in order to accommodate possible conversion to a treatment area.

- Provide extra-wide corridors, with flexibility so they can be used as triage and emergency treatment spaces.

- Provide larger-than-usual examination rooms with double headwall provisions, in order to accommodate double occupancy, as needed.

- Provide a patient bathroom between every two treatment rooms, in order to minimize exposure to infectious diseases.

- Provide a large storage area for disaster equipment, such as stretchers and disposable protective equipment.

- Provide more than one air isolation room.

- Provide a modified mechanical system, to allow for the quarantine of groups of patients.

- Provide a separate entrance directly into a decontamination area, with room around it to accommodate containment tents and fire and rescue services. (Zilm, 2007)

ED Patient Rooms

Individual rooms are becoming the norm in EDs, providing greater privacy, as well as better isolation capabilities and space for family; a minimum of 120 net square feet (~11.2 square meters) is recommended (Facility Guidelines Institute, 2014 [2.2–3.1.3.6 (2)]). Acuity-adaptable rooms, with standardized size, shape, and headwall, are desirable, in order to eliminate transfers (Pebble Project, 2014). Reducing or eliminating specialized equipment allows for flexibility and efficiency (Zilm et al., 2010).

When possible, patient rooms should have access to daylight and views to nature (Faulkner, 2006). Colors and textures should be used to create a soothing atmosphere and artwork is a desirable feature. Particularly when rooms are designed to accommodate team triage, they must provide space for the full care team and all necessary equipment, including large items such as an EKG machine. It is important to design for the presence of family members in all areas of the ED, including resuscitation (Bradley, Lensky, and Brasel, 2013; Choi and Bosch, 2013; Department of Health [UK], 2013; Emergency Nurses Association, 2005).

ED Information Technology

Many EDs are implementing a fully integrated emergency-department information system (EDIS), with patient tracking, digital charting and order entry, and direct access to patient records from the hospital data repository. ED design must include the latest information technology (IT), with Wi-Fi capability and space for the necessary digital devices—ideally, one for each member of the healthcare team, including social workers and case managers, plus a bank of common-use equipment for transient staff such as respiratory therapists and x-ray technicians (Welch, 2012; Zeit, 2012). There must never be a delay in either medical or clerical work because of a shortage of IT equipment. In addition, all countertops should be large enough to hold keyboards, tablets, and other IT equipment, and the design must accommodate arm- and wall-mounted screens where appropriate (Welch, 2012).

Other ED Spaces

Emergency Departments should contain ample storage space for portable equipment such as an ultrasound machine and mobility equipment such as stretchers, wheelchairs, and crutches. The trauma area must have room for an ice machine (Allison and Kunz, 2011; Department of Health [UK], 2013).

Additional spaces to consider include staff break rooms, ideally with a view to the outside and an attached pantry, and changing rooms with showers (Allison and Kunz, 2011; Department of Health [UK], 2013).

A resuscitation area should be located adjacent to the ambulance entrance and out of view of other patients. There should also be direct access from assessment and treatment rooms. Immediate access is desirable both from the ambulance entrance and from a rooftop helipad, via large trauma elevators (Allison and Kunz, 2011). Ample space must be provided for 360-degree access to the patient, all staff required for care, and accompanying family members, as well as the parking and maneuvering of equipment (Department of Health [UK], 2013).

Consider these ED design guidelines:

- Consult experts, as well as ED physicians, staff, and facility planners, when designing or renovating Emergency Departments, to be sure decision-makers have access to the latest thinking on ED size, configuration, equipment, IT systems, user needs and requirements, and the like (Allison and Kunz, 2011).

- Calculate the number of treatment rooms needed with reference to the ED census (Welch, 2012; Zilm, 2007).

- Design ED areas for maximum flexibility, on the basis of the typical arrival curve (Welch, 2012; Zilm, 2010).

- Design for efficient patient flow and use of ED space from a square-foot-per-treatment perspective (Zilm, 2010).

- Design ED exam and treatment rooms with space for the activities of an entire medical team and all necessary equipment (Facility Guidelines Institute, 2014 [2.2–3.1.3.6 (2)]).

- When rooms will accommodate team triage, provide space for the full care team and all necessary equipment, including large items such as an EKG machine (Department of Health [UK], 2013).

- Provide ample space in resuscitation areas for 360-degree access to the patient, all staff required for care, and accompanying family members, as well as the parking and maneuvering of equipment (Department of Health [UK], 2013).

- In resuscitation areas, define clear zones for patients, the care team, and family members (Bradley et al., 2013; Choi and Bosch, 2013; Department of Health [UK], 2013; Emergency Nurses Association, 2005).

- Locate a resuscitation area adjacent to the ambulance entrance and out of view of other patients (Allison and Kunz, 2011).

- Allow for immediate access to the ED from the ambulance entrance and a rooftop helipad, via large trauma elevators (Allison and Kunz, 2011).

- Consider ED configurations that allow flexibility in relation to patient flow, such as pods, inner core, separate functional units, streaming systems, fast-track systems, doughnut layouts, and others (Allison and Kunz, 2011; Chandler Hospital Emergency Department, 2014; Christmann, 2011; Welch, 2012; Wheary, 2014; Zilm, 2007, 2010; Zilm and Lennon, 2003).

- Design ED work areas for maximum staff interaction and visual connectivity (Zilm, 2010).

- Locate ED work areas, supplies, and medications to minimize staff travel (Zilm, 2010).

- Make sure ED countertops are large enough to hold keyboards, tablets, and other IT equipment (Welch, 2012).

- Ensure that the ED accommodates arm- and wall-mounted screens, where appropriate (Welch, 2012).

- Provide ample storage space for portable equipment such as an ultrasound machine and mobility equipment such as stretchers, wheelchairs, and crutches (Allison and Kunz, 2011; Department of Health [UK], 2013).

- Ensure that the trauma area has room for an ice machine (Allison and Kunz, 2011; Department of Health [UK], 2013).

- Provide staff break rooms, ideally with a view to the outside and an attached pantry, as well as changing rooms and showers (Allison and Kunz, 2011; Department of Health [UK], 2013).

- Consider providing standardized, individual, acuity-adaptable patient ED rooms (Pebble Project, 2014; Zilm et al., 2010).

- Include highly visible hand-wash sinks and alcohol-based hand-rub dispensers in the ED (Pebble Project, 2014).

- Select ED surfaces and finishes to minimize noise and contamination (Pebble Project, 2014).

- When possible, ensure that ED patient rooms have access to natural light and outside views (Faulkner, 2006; Pebble Project, 2014).

- Use artwork, colors, and textures to create a soothing atmosphere (Faulkner, 2006; Pebble Project, 2014).

- Accommodate family members in areas of the ED, including resuscitation (Bradley et al., 2013; Choi and Bosch, 2013; Department of Health [UK], 2013; Emergency Nurses Association, 2005).

- Provide ample corridor and circulation space to allow family access to patients without resulting cross-traffic with ED staff (Zilm, 2007).

- Provide flexibility for future ED growth through internal adaptation or expansion (Zilm, 2010).

ED Front-End Areas

Emergency departments are developing strategies for improving patient flow, or "throughput." Expediting front-end processing—which typically includes initial patient presentation, triage, registration, bed placement, and medical evaluation—can reduce length of stay and improve both ED efficiency and patient satisfaction (Wiler et al., 2009). Choices of an optimal organizational model depend on the demographics of the population served and factors such as acuity and admission rates, as well as the processes used by clinicians. Design decisions are an integral part of the selection process (Designing a "no wait," 2011).

Triage and registration areas have traditionally constituted the first opportunity for emergency walk-in patients to be assessed and receive help. These areas have also been a source of considerable patient dissatisfaction, associated with operational redundancies and lengthy wait times (Subash et al., 2004). One response is the trend toward immediate bedding (the "no-wait ED") in which patients are immediately placed in a treatment room and a care team, often including a physician, "converges on the patient like a pit crew servicing a race car" (Allison and Kunz, 2011; Kamali et al., 2013; Millburg, 2011; Wheary, 2014). Registration takes place at bedside, an immediate medical assessment is made, and a technician takes blood pressure and other vital signs. Interventions are provided at once, not triaged; X-rays and lab work are ordered. While this care model may call for larger treatment rooms, it substantially removes the need for a traditional waiting area—space that can then be used for other purposes—although patients may sometimes be moved afterwards to a discharge holding area, to free up treatment rooms for the next patients (Goralnick, Walls, and Kosowsky, 2013; Millburg, 2011).

In a related care model ("rapid assessment"), after assessment and immediate treatment, patients are moved to another section of the ED for further care, thus maintaining flow through the rapid-assessment area. The goal is "not to let simple cases back up" and to assure efficient use of space (Millburg, 2011; Wheary, 2014).

Another strategy finding wide acceptance is the "fast track," which treats lower-acuity patients more efficiently (Crane and Noon, 2010; Kamali et al., 2013; Rodak, 2012; Travers and Lee, 2006; Welch, 2012). In traditional triage systems, those patients who could be seen and treated quickly often have to wait longest, making EDs in effect "the nation's most expensive waiting rooms." In the fast-track system, advanced practice nurses are able to promptly see and manage some 90 percent of the cases (Allison and Kunz, 2011; DiFazio and Vessey, 2014; Emergency Nurses Association, 2012; Rodak, 2012; Subash et al., 2004). When a physician is part of the fast-track team, research shows that 30–40 percent, and in some cases up to 50 percent, of patients can be discharged directly from triage (Welch and Savitch, 2012; Wiler et al., 2009). In addition, fast-track patients can frequently be treated "vertically," that is, not on beds or stretchers but in chairs or recliners. Differentiating between "vertical patient flow" and "horizontal patient flow" and creating chair-centric layouts in such areas as the fast-track or internal waiting areas allows treatment of more patients per square foot, facilitates flow through the system, and often makes patients, especially seniors, significantly more comfortable (Christmann, 2011; Welch, 2012; Welch and Davidson, 2010; Wheary, 2014; Wilber et al., 2005).

In many intake models that employ a care team, especially one including a physician, activities may include initiating care orders, drawing blood, and starting intravenous lines. A bigger space may therefore be required, with clinical work areas and storage for supplies (Welch, 2012). It is becoming standard practice to perform an EKG on any patient with symptoms "between the nose and the navel." When triage/treatment spaces are not large enough or do not afford enough privacy for an EKG, an adjacent space must be provided, such as a curtained alcove next to the triage pod (Welch, 2012).

Because confidential information is discussed in all of these areas, the spaces should be designed to provide acoustical privacy. In lower-acuity, higher-density areas, a small, adjoining consultation room should be available to patients desiring greater privacy. Signs can be posted prominently with messages such as, "To Our Patients: Conversations in this area are NOT private. Please tell us if you prefer to have any discussion about your healthcare in a more private setting" (Allison and Kunz, 2011). Electronic privacy window screens can be installed in the triage area, to allow nurses to create immediate visual privacy when needed (New Emergency Department, n.d.).

Under Title VI of the 1964 Civil Rights Act, as made explicit in a 1980 notice from the Department of Human Services, limited English proficient (LEP) patients have a legal right to language assistance, although at this writing, the form and extent of such assistance can vary in response to local conditions and relevant state laws (Chen, Youdelman, and Brooks, 2007; US Department of Health and Human Services, 1980). As a minimum condition, the Facility Guidelines Institute recommends at least one connection for telephone access to translation services in the ED registration and triage area (Facility Guidelines Institute, 2014).

One technology that can dramatically streamline the intake process is palmar scanning, similar to ocular scanning, which can be used to generate an immediate identifier for a patient, tied to an ID number. This process offers reliable identification of very ill or unconscious patients, as well as speed (identification in less than 15 seconds), reducing the risk of misidentification or duplication (Welch and Savitch, 2012).

The following are some ED front-end area design guidelines to consider:

- Consult with hospital and ED department leadership, clinicians, front-line staff, and ED experts on strategies, configuration, and space requirements for front-end processes (Carpman Associates, 1984 [unpub.]).
- Design for patient visual and acoustical privacy during ED front-end processes (Carpman Associates, 1984 [unpub.]; Dubbs, 2003).
- In lower-acuity areas, provide consultation rooms, when possible. Inform patients about available areas for private consultation (Allison and Kunz, 2011).
- Consider providing electronic window screens in triage areas (New Emergency Department, n.d.).
- Make assistance available to patients and companions with LEP (limited English-proficiency). Provide at least one connection for telephone access to translation services (Chen et al., 2007; Facility Guidelines Institute, 2014; US Department of Health and Human Services, 1980).

ED Patient Waiting Areas

Despite the trend to no-waiting EDs, patients will inevitably spend some time just waiting. Intake procedures cannot always be started immediately upon walk-in. After triage and registration, many EDs escort patients into a separate patient waiting area where those with non-urgent needs wait under the supervision of a nurse (Rodak, 2012). After treatment but before discharge, patients may have to wait for medications or test results; many hospitals have created an internal disposition area (IDA) for this purpose (Wheary, 2014). Most waiting areas should be designed to accommodate patients on stretchers or those using mobility devices, such as wheelchairs and walkers. Valuable space can often be saved by making an IDA chair-centric and by making available recliner seating, often a preferred option (Wheary, 2014; Wilber et al., 2005).

Waiting time is one of the key drivers of patient satisfaction with an ED (Boudreaux and O'Hea, 2004). Almost 40 percent of patients wait over an hour to see a physician; 25 percent wait over four hours (Welch et al., 2012). Inefficient patient flow and overcrowding are associated with some 2.6 million people annually—2 percent of all ED visits—leaving without being seen by a physician (Welch et al., 2012).

Studies have found, however, that *perceived* wait times are as important as or more important than *actual* wait times (Soremekun, Takayesu, and Bohan, 2011; Yoon and Sonneveld, 2010; Thompson et al., 1996). Additionally, perception of wait time by staff frequently does not match patient perceptions (Yoon and Sonneveld, 2010). Improvements in waiting-area comfort, a soothing atmosphere, caring attitudes from ED staff, and timely provision of information to patients can do much to reduce perceived wait times (Patient Satisfaction, 2010; Strategies for Improving, 2010).

Because patients typically feel vulnerable and powerless and may need emergency assistance, waiting areas should be designed to reassure them that help is available. Signage must explicitly communicate the correct place for treatment and key staff contacts. Flowcharts can be posted to inform patients about how the ED functions and the steps they can anticipate as they progress through treatment. Digital bus-stop-style screens can show live estimated waiting times for the main categories of procedures. Knowing one's place in the queue and projected waiting times has proved helpful in reducing anxiety and providing a sense of control. Where such systems are in place, incidents of patient aggression have been dramatically reduced. Staff members also report a significant reduction in stress, and measures of staff well-being and retention have improved (Hohenadel, 2013).

Waiting areas should look attractive to patients. Seating should be comfortable; recliners and high-rise chairs are desirable options. Windows to a nature view should be provided, if possible. Artwork, colors, and textures offer visual interest and positive distraction. TVs provide distraction, too, but also have drawbacks: program content may not be soothing, and multiple TVs raise noise levels. One successful strategy has been to replace some or all TV content with videos of serene nature images. This not only lowers noise levels directly, but also correlates with fewer incidents of raised voices, one of the signs of stress (Nanda and Hathorn,

2012). Positive distractions can also lead to increased socializing and conversation (Nanda and Hathorn, 2012).

Keep in mind that ED staff members are under stress, too. Many of the design elements that ease patient stress and anxiety are also helpful to caregivers and should also be deployed behind the scenes.

In designing ED patient waiting areas, consider the following:

- Provide good visual access from the ED patient waiting area to a staff area (Carpman Associates, 1984 [unpub.]).

- Provide large, noticeable information on how the ED functions and estimated waiting times. Consider a digital information system (Carpman Associates, 1984 [unpub.]; Hohenadel, 2013).

- Install an easily identified and operated nurse-call mechanism (Carpman Associates, 1984 [unpub.]).

- Provide reclining seats or some other way for patients to lie down (Carpman Associates, 1984 [unpub.]).

- Allow space for patients on stretchers and patients in wheelchairs (Wheary, 2014; Wilber et al., 2005).

- Provide seating high enough for older patients to sit and rise with a minimum of difficulty (Carpman Associates, 1984 [unpub.]).

- Select seating with good back support and padded armrests (Carpman Associates, 1984 [unpub.]).

- Consider providing some high-rise seating (Carpman Associates, 1984 [unpub.]).

- If possible, provide an outside view to nature, as well as artwork, plants, and other items of visual interest (Carpman Associates, 1984 [unpub.]; Nanda and Hathorn, 2012).

- Provide positive distractions such as TVs, tablets loaded with videos, or digital music players (such as iPods) loaded with a variety of music. Provide individual headphones (Nanda and Hathorn, 2012). (See the discussion in chapter 9.)

ED Visitor Waiting Areas

Family and friends who accompany patients to an emergency department may have to wait for hours while tests, examinations, and treatments are completed. Information on the status of a patient and progress through the ED system can ease visitor stress and diminish perceived wait times. A Patient Status Board can give information in the following categories: patient being prepared for procedure, patient in procedure, patient out of procedure, patient in recovery, patient moved to inpatient room, and patient discharged (Rush University Medical Center, n.d.).

Comfort, privacy, and access to amenities are important considerations in visitor waiting areas (see also chapter 5).

In addition, consider these guidelines for ED visitor waiting areas:

• Provide an outside view, if possible, but avoid views of arriving ambulances (Carpman Associates, 1984 [unpub.]; Drury and Rosen, 1977; Petersen, 1981; Welch, 1977).

• Provide visual access between the waiting area and attending staff (Carpman Associates, 1984 [unpub.]; Drury and Rosen, 1977; Petersen, 1981; Welch, 1977).

• Provide signage and digital systems that explain ED processes and give information on patient progress (Carpman Associates, 1984 [unpub.]; Drury and Rosen, 1977; Petersen, 1981; Rush University Medical Center, n.d.; Welch, 1977).

• Locate restrooms, vending machines, and water fountains near visitor waiting areas (Carpman Associates, 1984 [unpub.]; Drury and Rosen, 1977; Petersen, 1981; Welch, 1977).

• Provide a television and a way to limit TV sound to those watching it. If possible, provide a section of the waiting area away from the television (Carpman Associates, 1984 [unpub.]; Drury and Rosen, 1977; Petersen, 1981; Welch, 1977).

• Provide a children's area, separated from but visually connected to the main waiting area (Carpman Associates, 1984 [unpub.]; Drury and Rosen, 1977; Petersen, 1981; Welch, 1977).

Senior Emergency Departments

The typical ED environment, set up "to be good at treating trauma and to treat it quickly," may not be well suited to the healthcare needs of older patients, who tend to have multiple health problems, require more time and attention than younger patients, be more frail, and be more prone to anxiety and confusion (Kelly et al., 2011; Salvi et al., 2007; Shapiro, 2009). To serve this rapidly growing sector of the population, some healthcare organizations have created separate senior EDs. A senior ED not only provides the care needed in a quieter, more supportive atmosphere, but also frees up beds in the regular ED.

Here are some design guidelines to consider for senior EDs:

• Separate treatment bays in the senior ED by walls, rather than by curtains (Shapiro, 2009).

• Provide handrails in strategically-located places (Shapiro, 2009).

• Provide effective, soft lighting (Shapiro, 2009).

• Provide non-reflective, nonslip flooring (Shapiro, 2009).

• Select wall colors with aging eyes in mind. Contrasting trim helps patients see where one area stops and another begins (Shapiro, 2009).

• Provide mattresses designed to help prevent the skin breakdown that can lead to bedsores (Baker, 2009).

• Make a blanket warmer available (Baker, 2009).

- Provide TVs with headsets, clocks with large numerals, and telephones and remote controls with large buttons.

- Consider offering patients choices about listening to music using headphones and digital devices, such as iPods. (See the discussion in chapter 9.)

Pediatric Emergency Departments

Pediatric emergency departments should be experienced by children and parents as non-threatening and soothing in order to counter the stressful reasons for the ED visit. A number of design features can help:

- Provide a separate entrance to the Pediatric ED. If a separate entrance is not possible, provide a well-marked, child-friendly pathway from the adult ED to the Pediatric ED.

- Make sure children in the Pediatric ED can't be seen by patients and visitors waiting in the Adult ED (Department of Health [UK], 2013).

- Consider providing two waiting areas in the Pediatric ED: one for sick children and one for well children (Department of Health [UK], 2013).

- Select color schemes and furnishings that will be appealing to children who range in age from babies to young teens (Christmann, 2011; Pediatric Emergency Department, 2015).

- Consider providing play tables, toys, and digital play stations (Christmann, 2011; Pediatric Emergency Department, 2015).

- Consider providing a big-screen TV, with headphones (Christmann, 2011; Pediatric Emergency Department, 2015).

- Design restrooms that can be used by children and adults. Consider using touch-free toilets (Pediatric Emergency Department, 2015).

- Provide Wi-Fi access and digital devices and headphones that can be borrowed by parents in order to access information, music, movies, and children's games.

Rehabilitation Units

Patients who have suffered orthopedic trauma, paralysis, amputations, strokes, or other catastrophic medical events may need acute-care inpatient rehabilitation as they recover from and adapt to their injuries or illnesses. Such rehabilitative care requires a large and ongoing amount of interdisciplinary coordination among caregivers and scrupulous attention to the details of the built environment. Consultation and communication in the design of the unit is particularly important, not only between the clinical and the architectural teams, but also by involving community stakeholders, furniture and equipment specialists, interior designers, IT specialists, and the like (Kennedy, 2010).

The entire unit—patient rooms, treatment areas, and communal rooms—should be located on one level, with no stairs and minimal use of ramps. Where ramps cannot be avoided, slopes should be no more than 1:20 (Infrastructure Unit Support Systems, 2014). This both enhances independence for patients using wheelchairs or mobility devices, such as crutches or walkers, but also allows patients who are still bedridden to be brought to the gym and other treatment areas. In addition, it facilitates evacuation in case of emergency (Infrastructure Unit Support Systems, 2014). Wherever possible, the rehabilitation unit should be located at grade level with outdoor recreation areas nearby.

Inpatient rehabilitation rooms should have private bathrooms. Bedside controls will be needed to manipulate lights, window shades, and nurse-call buttons. Specifying the latest bed designs and overhead lift systems can protect caregivers from injury by reducing or eliminating the need to lift and reposition patients (Kennedy, 2010). Bed-sensor technology, integrated with the nurse-call system, minimizes the need for restraints, while reducing the danger of patient falls (Kennedy, 2010). Including video surveillance capability in some rooms increases the safety of patients subject to confusion due to stroke or other brain injury (Gwen Neilsen Anderson Rehabilitation Center Facilities, n.d.). And as family support is a vital element in the entire rehabilitation process, rooms should be furnished with recliners, sleep sofas, or the like.

Decor should be as welcoming and homelike as possible. Attractive communal spaces encourage socializing, which can have great therapeutic benefits. Patients may not believe the message that "things will get better" when they hear it from therapists, nurses, and other caregivers, but when other patients deliver it, it carries more conviction (Infrastructure Unit Support Systems, 2014; New State of the Art, n.d.).

Dining and recreation rooms should accommodate a minimum of 60 percent of the inpatient population, along with caregivers and staff. To allow ample turning and maneuvering space for wheelchairs, total floor area should be calculated on the basis of two square meters per patient (Infrastructure Unit Support Systems, 2014).

The therapy gym needs both a large open area and smaller, private treatment areas. These can be achieved in many cases by curtaining off sections of the larger space. Separate treatment rooms, large enough for patient, therapist, and a family member or other caregiver, should also be available, not only for enhanced privacy, but also for times when patients require isolation. Some patients, such as children or those with head injuries, may be noisy, so acoustical privacy should also be provided (Infrastructure Unit Support Systems, 2014).

The main gym area will need various plinths, with accompanying ramps, to make therapeutic exercise equipment fully accessible. The upholstered edges of the plinths must be reinforced, to prevent fraying from repeated knocks and abrasions (Infrastructure Unit Support Systems, 2014). State-of-the-art therapeutic equipment should be provided. Overhead body-weight suspension systems offer patients additional safety when practicing walking and using treadmills, parallel bars, and the like (Infrastructure Unit Support Systems, 2014; Inpatient Rehabilitation Unit, 2015). The ceiling must be high enough and reinforced to accommodate these and other types of equipment, as well as ball-throwing activities. Oxygen and suction equipment should be at hand, as well as an emergency call system, accessible from wheelchair height (Infrastructure Unit Support Systems, 2014). Since therapy will take place both in and out of wheelchairs, space to store these should be provided near the gym entrance (Infrastructure Unit Support Systems, 2014). Space should also be provided for family members to observe patient treatment, both for present support and because they may need to assist in the therapy when the patient is discharged.

The rehabilitation unit also needs to include *nonaccessible* training spaces for patients to practice household activities, also known as activities of daily living (ADL) (Gwen Neilsen Anderson Rehabilitation Center Facilities, n. d.; Inpatient Rehabilitation Unit, 2015; New State of the Art, n.d.). A fully equipped training kitchen should include a dining area for patients to practice such skills as bringing dishes from stove to table while using a walker. A training bathroom should be furnished with the full range of assistive devices, to aid in selecting appropriate features for the patient's home (Inpatient Rehabilitation Unit, 2015). A training laundry is also desirable.

Outdoor recreation spaces and healing gardens can be designed for specific therapeutic purposes, with a variety of walks, gradients, and other features that replicate real-life challenges (State of the art, n.d.). Amenities, such as putting greens, offer patients the opportunity to practice hand–eye coordination.

Locating outpatient and homecare services adjacent to the inpatient facility is desirable, in order to facilitate coordination and continuity of care. Separate entrances for inpatients and outpatients, however, minimize emotional barriers to treatment for patients who have transitioned to a more independent status (Infrastructure Unit Support Systems, 2014).

Design guidelines for rehabilitation units include:

- Locate the inpatient rehabilitation unit on one level, with no stairs and minimal use of ramps (Infrastructure Unit Support Systems, 2014).

- If ramps are unavoidable, make sure the slope is no more than 1:20 (Infrastructure Unit Support Systems, 2014).

- Provide patient rooms with private bathrooms (Kennedy, 2010).

- Make sure patient rooms employ the latest bed design and overhead lift systems (Kennedy, 2010).

- Provide bedside controls for lights, window shades, and the like (Kennedy, 2010).

- Provide bed sensor technology (Kennedy, 2010).

- Consider providing video surveillance capability in some rooms (Gwen Neilsen Anderson Rehabilitation Center Facilities, n.d.).

- Provide sleeping accommodations for family in patient rooms.

- Design communal areas to be large enough to accommodate a minimum of 60 percent of the inpatient population, along with caregivers and staff (Infrastructure Unit Support Systems, 2014).

- Design the therapy gym with both a large open area and private treatment rooms (Infrastructure Unit Support Systems, 2014).

- Equip the gym with plinths and ramps, in order to make therapeutic equipment fully accessible (Infrastructure Unit Support Systems, 2014).

- Consider providing overhead body-weight suspension systems (Infrastructure Unit Support Systems, 2014; Inpatient Rehabilitation Unit, 2015).

- Design the ceiling high enough and reinforce it to accommodate equipment and ball-throwing exercises (Infrastructure Unit Support Systems, 2014).

- Provide oxygen and suction equipment (Infrastructure Unit Support Systems, 2014).

- Provide emergency call buttons, accessible from wheelchair height (Infrastructure Unit Support Systems, 2014).

- Allow space in the gym for visitors to observe patient treatment.

- Provide fully equipped *non-accessible* training spaces, such as a kitchen, dining room, bathroom, and laundry (Gwen Neilsen Anderson Rehabilitation Center Facilities, n.d.; Inpatient Rehabilitation Unit, 2015; New State of the Art, n.d.).

- Locate outpatient and homecare services adjacent to the inpatient facility, to facilitate coordination and continuity of care.

- Provide separate entrances to inpatient and outpatient rehabilitation areas (Infrastructure Unit Support Systems, 2014).

Patient and Visitor Information Areas

Time spent recuperating in a healthcare facility can be boring. The sense of wasting time or spending time unproductively may aggravate already high levels of stress. Patients may appreciate having something to read or an opportunity to learn more about their illnesses. In one study, nearly 60 percent of the visitors surveyed said they would like to use a reading room within the hospital, and over 80 percent said they would like to learn more about a particular illness (Reizenstein et al., 1981 [unpub. No. 4]).

Not only do information areas and libraries appeal to patients and visitors, but research has demonstrated that such resources often improve patient outcomes (Kantz et al., 1998). Health facilities following the Planetree model encourage education and personal growth and view them as integral parts of the healing process (Arneill and Frasca-Beaulieu, 2003; Frampton et al., 2008).

To encourage use, the information area or library should have a quiet and warm ambience, with comfortable, well-lighted places to sit and read, as well as areas for online research. Some facilities offer classrooms where patients and visitors take wellness, nutrition, or exercise classes, or learn more about particular illnesses and treatments (Arneill and Frasca-Beaulieu, 2003).

Information areas should be accessible to and usable by everyone. They should accommodate wheelchairs, walkers, and rolling IV poles. Consequently, ample circulation space should be provided between bookshelves, as well as within reading areas. Books should be displayed so titles are easy to read and easily reached by people with mobility limitations. Signs used within the information area should be legible to people with vision disabilities (Kamisar, 1979). Many users with vision disabilities may need books with large type or other reading aids. The weight of books should also be considered, since heavy books will be hard to handle for some patients (McGee, 1999). (See also chapter 9.)

Library and patient-education areas can be used only when patients and visitors are aware of their existence. In a study at the University of Michigan Medical Center, for example, nearly a third of the patients interviewed did not know that a patient library was available (Reizenstein and Grant, 1981 [unpub. No. 2]). An effective system should be developed for conveying information to patients and visitors about the library/information area and its services. In addition, awareness of the information area will likely be greater when it is located along a major circulation route.

Library carts also provide a helpful service. Stocked with a variety of titles and taken to patients' bedsides by volunteers, these carts provide access to library materials for bedridden patients and enhance awareness about the patient information area.

Consider these guidelines for patient information areas:

- Let patients and visitors know the location of the patient information area (Reizenstein and Grant, 1981 [unpub. No. 2]).

- Locate the information area along a public circulation route, if possible.

- Design the information area to appear inviting and have a quiet, warm ambience (Arneill and Frasca-Beaulieu, 2003).

- Provide comfortable, well-lighted places to sit and read within the information area (Arneill and Frasca-Beaulieu, 2003).

- Make sure the information area is accessible to and useable by everyone. Design it to accommodate people with functional limitations and include circulation space for people in wheelchairs, and those with walkers and rolling IV poles (Kamisar, 1979).

- If the information area includes books, make sure they are within easy reach of people with functional limitations, and that large-print books are available (Kamisar, 1979).

- Use Braille, tactile lettering, and high contrast between sign messages and sign backgrounds in order to make information area signs legible to people with vision limitations (Kamisar, 1979).

- Provide patient and visitor educational materials and internet access.

- Consider having a book cart regularly serve patient-room areas.

Special Services

Hospitals and other large healthcare facilities often become somewhat like small cities, complete with 24-hour-a-day, seven-day-a-week activity. Visitors may eat and sleep in the hospital for days or even weeks. During long hours of waiting, they need emotional and physical supports, as well as positive distractions. Visitors in one study were asked about activities they would participate in if they were at a hospital but unable to be with the patient for a couple of hours. Sixty percent or more said they would enjoy sitting in an outdoor courtyard, walking around the hospital grounds, going to a small mall within the hospital, attending a movie, or using a reading room. The most popular activities seem to involve the least amount of effort on the visitor's part. Visitors want a place nearby to sit, chat, walk, or look around (Reizenstein et al., 1981 [unpub. No. 4]). Such activities perform therapeutic functions for visitors, including relaxation, refreshment, stress release, information, and satisfaction of practical needs. In this section, we discuss some special services for patients and visitors, including overnight accommodations, shops, hair care, fitness centers, and spas.

Overnight Accommodations

Some visitors and outpatients will need to spend the night in or near a healthcare facility. When a family member or friend is very sick and requires a long hospital stay, visitors may want to remain close to the hospital for days or even weeks. Cost is an issue related to overnight accommodations. Family members may travel to the facility from far away and cannot always afford to pay for hotel or motel rooms. Outpatients, who come for daily treatments over a period of weeks, may need nearby, affordable places to stay. As part of a program of family-centered care, healthcare organizations with out-of-town inpatients, outpatients, and visitors should consider providing inexpensive overnight accommodations in close proximity to the facility (Carpman, Grant, and Simmons, 1984; Reizenstein and Grant, 1982 [unpub. No. 13]).

Some alternatives for providing overnight accommodations for visitors include:

- Provide sleeping accommodations in patient rooms using sleep sofas, cots, or folding beds (Carpman et al., 1984; Reizenstein and Grant, 1982 [unpub. No. 13]).

- Consider providing temporary sleeping areas within family lounges by using sleep sofas and room dividers to create separate spaces (Greenwich Hospital, Yale New Haven Health, 2015).

- Accommodate visitors elsewhere inside the healthcare facility, by developing an in-house hotel, or by making available vacant rooms within patient units or in other areas of the facility.

- Consider offering a "host home" program in which visitors and outpatients can be given a place to shower and sleep in the home of someone in the community, either with or without charge (Carpman et al., 1984; Reizenstein and Grant, 1982 [unpub. No. 13]).

- Build, renovate, lease, or otherwise provide some type of lodging facility (apartments, motel, room and bath) for outpatients and visitors.

- Arrange for a discount program with nearby hotels and motels, with transportation provided by shuttle bus (Carpman et al., 1984; Reizenstein and Grant, 1982 [unpub. No. 13]).

- Encourage an outside group, either for-profit or not-for-profit, to build and operate a hotel or hotel-like facility nearby, such as a Ronald McDonald House (Carpman et al., 1984; Reizenstein and Grant, 1982 [unpub. No. 13].

Shops

Research indicates that the number and variety of shops located in a healthcare facility is important to patients, visitors, and healthcare workers and an important driver of customer satisfaction and willingness to recommend the institution to others (Eisingerich and

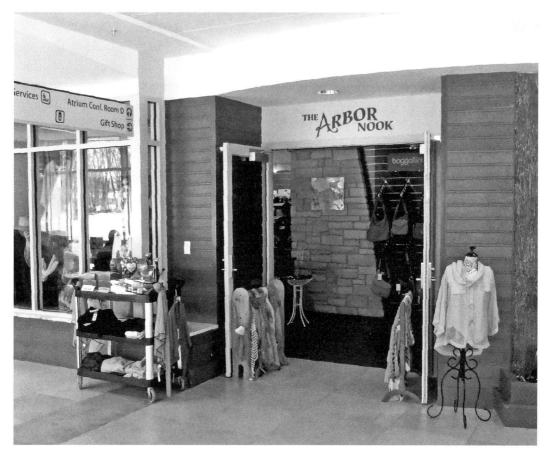

Gift shops and other specialty retail areas within a health facility can be used by patients and visitors for purchasing a variety of niceties and necessities. Shops also provide a setting for browsing, a positive distraction.

Photo credit: Courtesy of St. Joseph Mercy Chelsea

Boehm, 2009). People who pass through a healthcare facility each day have many needs that a well-chosen mix of shops can meet. As well as providing practical services, shops can offer outpatients and visitors some positive distraction during the often lengthy times spent in the facility. Shops offer healthcare workers an activity during breaks from stressful jobs (American Nurse, 2011).

Many healthcare facilities are expanding their retail offerings beyond the familiar gift and flower shops. Patients and visitors appreciate on-site availability of practical items such as toothpaste and toothbrushes, shampoo, makeup, hair accessories, shaving gear, snacks, greeting cards, and stamps, as well as gift items such as flowers, stuffed animals, balloons, games, and jewelry.

In keeping with increased emphasis on treating the whole person, not just the illness, boutiques can offer specialized products and services. An oncology boutique can carry hard-to-find comfort products such as radiation creams, nonmetallic deodorants, wound gels, and rinses (Roper-St. Francis, n.d.). Prostheses and wigs can be purchased and fitted on site while staff coordinate with the registration area for a patient's prescription and insurance information (Cancer center renovation, 2013; Phillips, 2004; Scottsdale Healthcare, 2014). A boutique for pregnant women and new mothers may carry breast pumps and supplies, nursing bras, and infant necessities (Phillips, 2004; Scottsdale Healthcare, 2014). A small grocery is an important convenience for families staying overnight at the healthcare facility or nearby, as well as for busy healthcare workers. Other possibilities include a dry cleaner, bookshop, over-the-counter pharmacy, electronics store, shops focusing on products for healthy living, automatic teller machines (ATMs), and a branch bank or credit union.

With the steady flow of customers, including hospital workers with little free time, such retail operations can prove highly profitable for healthcare organizations (Greene, 2012). A thoughtful array of products and services not available in the immediate neighborhood can also enhance the facility's profile and build links with the surrounding community (Nappi, 2011).

Hair Care

How people feel about their appearance influences their general state of mind, as well as their health. Being a patient does not mean a person ceases to care about personal grooming; in fact, some pampering may go a long way toward increasing a sense of well-being. Beauty salons and barber shops help maintain the morale of long-term patients, help new mothers look their best as they prepare to taken new babies home, and offer a little personal care to caregivers spending long hours in the healthcare facility. When asked about the desirability of providing hair-care services in one large hospital, more than 85 percent of patients and nurses responded positively (Reizenstein and Grant, 1981 [unpub. No. 9]).

Many patients who need hair care services are not able to travel to a barber shop or beauty salon within the hospital. Hair care services, particularly hair washing and cutting, as well as setting, drying, and shaving, need to be brought to the bedsides of these patients.

Fitness Centers

Some healthcare facilities have incorporated health and fitness spaces to attract potential clients and offer a more holistic health and wellness experience. Many facilities contain rehabilitation clinics or fitness spaces, but a growing trend is to plan and build full-service, health club-style fitness centers. Fitness centers can provide services for patients, staff, and the public, regardless of physical ability or age. They reflect the growing emphasis upon "well-care," the preventive aspects of taking care of oneself. They illustrate that the healthcare facility is dedicated to the promotion of well-being and the whole person, in addition to medical treatment (D. McCarthy, 1993; Pallarito, 1994; Spencer, 1998).

Spas

As part of a wellness philosophy that embraces proactive care and the whole person, some healthcare facilities offer in-house spa services to patients, visitors, healthcare workers, and often to the public as well. The "medi-spa," as it is often called, combines medical focus and good clinical practice with complementary therapies (Complementary and Alternative, 2008). Although the mechanism is not thoroughly understood, medical research supports the healing power of touch, including strengthening the immune system (Coan, Schaefer, and Davidson, 2006; Dobson, 2006; Main, 2010).

Physical health is not independent of a person's mental state and mood (Mind-Body, 2008). Just as an environment that creates anxiety may be counterproductive to the healing process, an environment that takes extra measures to offer relaxation and a general sense of well-being may not only encourage people to seek healthcare, but also increase their receptivity to that care (J. McCarthy, 2010).

On maternity wards, where the current medical spa movement began, it was quickly found that daily massage reduced stress, especially among the high-risk population—mothers confined to hospital bedrest for weeks or even months (Osborn, 2005). Stress reduction and self-care prove helpful in a number of cardiovascular and GI conditions and in pain management (Alexander, 2012; Lee, Park, and Kim, 2011). Spas can provide important complementary services for dermatology and plastic surgery and help patients with cosmetic needs arising from medical care, such as surgery or cancer treatment.

A medical spa can become a significant part of a patient's healing process, whether in the spa itself or as part of a bedside-service program. Visitors, too, take advantage of this amenity; a substantial percentage of clients often come from outside the healthcare facility (Osborn, 2005). Healthcare workers benefit, as well. A spa is often seen as a valuable employee perk; some of the most frequent clients may be emergency-department nursing staff, for example (Osborn, 2005).

Developing a medical spa can be complex and costly—notably more costly than any other medical practice—and requires careful planning and consultation (Goldman, Vaiana, and Romley, 2010; Osborn, 2005). Factors to consider include HIPAA compliance, physician involvement, educating hospital staff about spa benefits, a surgical standard of cleanliness, laundry logistics, and size and design of the physical space. The returns, however, can also be high. Amenities like a spa raise the community visibility of a healthcare facility, attract customers, and create new, compatible revenue streams.

Summary

- Offering nutritious food, attending to different food preferences and dietary customs, and providing quality food service demonstrate to patients and visitors that their healthcare facility values good nutrition and its importance in health. Food service areas should be user-friendly: accessible to everyone, attractive, comfortable, and designed to mitigate noise. Facilities for inpatient meals may be designed for traditional tray service, personalized tray service, or some combination of these, according to the policy of the healthcare facility. All food service areas and equipment should be efficient, cost-effective, and environmentally friendly.

- Space for prayer or meditation is important for patients, visitors, and staff members who need time and space for quiet reflection. This type of space can also be used as needed for organized services. The design of "sacred spaces" should be religiously and denominationally neutral, incorporating no permanent religious symbols, but they should not have an institutional appearance. Belief-specific articles and furnishings should be available. Chairs should be comfortable and seating arrangements should be flexible.

- Consultation and grieving spaces are necessary in nearly all patient-care areas, to provide the physical comfort, visual privacy, and acoustical privacy needed for discussing sensitive issues and experiencing emotional situations.

- Emergency departments have particular design and planning requirements and layout options due to the high-volume, high-stress circumstances under which care is sought and offered. Extra attention must be paid to clarity of wayfinding, visual and acoustical privacy, comfort, and access to amenities for patients and companions, including children and seniors. Design must support Emergency Department policies to minimize waiting times, both perceived and actual.

- Acute rehabilitation units should be designed in close collaboration not only with clinical teams, but also with community stakeholders, furniture and equipment specialists, interior designers, IT specialists, and the like. Rehabilitation units should be located on a single level. Patient rooms should be as homelike and welcoming as possible, and incorporate all available safety features. The therapy gym should be equipped with plinths and overhead suspension systems. Common rooms should accommodate a minimum of 60 percent of the inpatient population. The unit should also include a full range of non-accessible spaces useful for patients re-learning activities of daily living (ADL).

○ Many visitors require overnight accommodations, and healthcare organizations can demonstrate their caring mission and enhance their marketing strategy by providing for inexpensive lodging in or close to the facility.

○ Healthcare organizations can offer special services to provide practical necessities, emotional and physical supports, and positive distractions. Various shops can serve the needs of patients, visitors, and healthcare workers; enhance a healthcare facility's profile; build community support; and act as a source of revenue. Hair care services, fitness centers, and "medi-spas," can attract potential clients to a facility and offer a more holistic health and wellness experience.

DISCUSSION QUESTIONS

1. What design elements and other factors are important in making food service areas useful and attractive to patients, visitors, and staff?

2. What factors should be considered in the design of a prayer/meditation room?

3. Why is it important to provide dedicated spaces for consultation and grieving? Where should these be located, and what factors are important in their design?

4. What issues need to be considered in the design of Emergency Departments? What are some options for ED layout and configuration?

5. How can design elements help mitigate the high stress and long wait times patients and visitors often encounter in Emergency Departments?

6. What are some important design considerations in an inpatient rehabilitation unit?

7. What design elements and organizational policies will help make a patient information center attractive, usable, and useful?

8. What are some options for providing overnight accommodations for outpatients and visitors?

9. What are some special services a healthcare facility can provide for patients, visitors, and healthcare workers, and what role can they play in the overall mission of a healthcare facility?

Design Review Questions

Special Places

Food Service Areas

☐ Will warming and cooling stations be provided on inpatient units that offer personalized tray service? (Foodservice Changes, 2012; Lee, 2013)

☐ Will nutrition rooms be provided on inpatient units, for snacks and after-hours nutrition needs? (Schilling, 2011)

☐ Will cafeterias, coffee shops, and other healthcare facility dining spaces be designed to have a relaxing, inviting atmosphere? (Henderson, 2015)

☐ Will the food service area have warm, light colors and a mix of natural light and subdued artificial lighting? (Henderson, 2015)

☐ Will healthcare facility dining spaces be accessible to and usable by everyone?

☐ Will multiple light sources be used, rather than only standard overhead lighting? (Henderson, 2015)

☐ Will fluorescent fixtures be avoided? (Henderson, 2015)

☐ Will artwork and special features, such as electric fireplaces, water walls, murals, and live plants be considered as ways of enhancing aesthetics? (Gatoade, 2010; Olsen, 2014)

☐ Will there be outside views? (Henderson, 2015)

☐ Will seating be comfortable and moveable, with high backs and comfortable upholstery?

☐ Will barriers be provided between seating areas to help ensure visual and acoustical privacy?

☐ Will tables of various sizes be provided in order to accommodate groups of different sizes? Will tables be large enough to accommodate cafeteria trays?

☐ Will there be ample circulation space within seating areas for ambulatory patients, visitors, and staff with trays; people with walkers; wheelchair users; people with strollers; patients with rolling IV poles, and others? (Henderson, 2015)

☐ Will there be update monitors—similar to airport arrival and departure boards—that provide information on patient status by means of a personalized code? Will visitors be given pagers, similar to the ones used by restaurants? (Reizenstein and Grant, 1981 [unpub. No. 4a)

☐ Will separate staff and public dining areas be considered? (Henderson, 2015)

☐ Will there be an effort to mitigate noise in food service areas, including providing carpeting and sound-absorbing wall and ceiling materials and keeping background noise to a minimum? (Hiatt, 1978)

☐ Will decision-makers consult with specialists when designing food service circulation areas and areas for food ordering, pick-up, and self-service? (Henderson, 2015)

☐ Will ample circulation space be provided within food ordering, pick-up, and self-service areas for wheelchair users and users of other mobility devices? Will wheelchair users to be able to easily see food selections? (Henderson, 2015)

☐ Will there be some dishes with rims? Will dishware and trays be stable? (Hiatt, 1978)

Sacred Spaces

☐ Rather than installing permanent religious symbols, will there be a portable altar? (James, 2010)

☐ Will storage space be provided for religious materials and items? (Madden, n.d.)

☐ Will space be provided for a small piano or organ?

☐ Will a generous number of electrical outlets be provided in the altar area in order to accommodate musical instruments, lighting, sound systems, and other equipment?

☐ Since devotion to nature is common to many faiths, will focal points be created using stained glass panels or other artwork depicting nature? (James, 2010; Madden, n.d.; Texas Children's Hospital, n.d.)

☐ Will the points of the compass be included somewhere within the sacred space? (James, 2010)

☐ Will furnishings be moveable, allowing a variety of configurations? (James, 2010)

☐ Will chairs be comfortable? (James, 2010)

☐ Will seating be arranged to allow visual privacy? (James, 2010)

☐ Will lighting levels be adjustable?

☐ Will walls be insulated and will sound-attenuating materials, such as carpeting, be used to keep the space quiet?

☐ Will sacred spaces be accessible to and usable by everyone, including people with functional limitations?

Consultation and Grieving Spaces

☐ Will grieving and consultation rooms be located so people do not have to walk a long way before they can deal with their situations in private? (Petersen, 1981)

☐ Will separate grieving and consultation rooms be provided in emergency departments? (Petersen, 1981)

☐ Will postpartum grieving spaces and the NICU be separated from the main maternity area? (Petersen, 1981)

☐ Will a cool cot or other cooling mechanism be provided in postpartum grieving rooms? (Petersen, 1981)

☐ Will grieving rooms be large enough to accommodate numerous family members? (Petersen, 1981)

☐ Will the design accommodate patients' and visitors' needs for visual and acoustical privacy? (Petersen, 1981)

☐ Will subdued colors, carpeting, and table lamps or other types of indirect or incandescent lighting contribute to a non-institutional ambience? (Petersen, 1981)

☐ Will natural light be used where possible? (Petersen, 1981)

☐ Will comfortable seating be provided, including chairs and couches? (Petersen, 1981)

☐ Will coat racks or hooks be provided for personal belongings? (Petersen, 1981)

☐ Will an adjustable sign on the door indicate whether or not the room is occupied? (Petersen, 1981)

Emergency Departments
Finding and Entering the ED

☐ Will the entrance to the ED be visible and clearly labeled, with a covered and convenient patient drop-off/pick-up area? (Carpman Associates, 1984 [unpub.]; A New ED, 2014; New Emergency Entrance, 2014; Zilm, 2007)

☐ Will exterior signage be legible from a distance during daylight, after dark, and in inclement weather? (Carpman Associates, 1984 [unpub.])

☐ Will the automobile route to the emergency entrance be clearly differentiated from the ambulance route? (Carpman Associates, 1984 [unpub.])

☐ Will separate ambulance and walk-in entrances be provided so walk-in patients and visitors don't have views to arriving ambulances? (Carpman Associates, 1984 [unpub.]; Department of Health [UK], 2013)

☐ Will ambulance parking be provided adjacent to the ambulance entrance? (Carpman Associates, 1984 [unpub.]; Department of Health [UK], 2013)

☐ Will a second public entrance be available for use in high-volume surge conditions and triage of contaminated patients? (Carpman Associates, 1984 [unpub.]; Zilm, 2007)

☐ Will ED interior signage be legible and easy to understand? (Carpman Associates, 1984 [unpub.])

☐ Will nearby visitor parking be located within view of the drop-off entrance, so companions can drop off the patient, park, and easily find the way back? (Carpman Associates, 1984 [unpub.])

☐ Will space for valet parking services be available? (Carpman Associates, 1984 [unpub.])

☐ Will there be a separate entrance into the pediatric ED or a marked, child-friendly pathway from the adult ED to the pediatric ED? (Carpman Associates, 1984 [unpub.]; Department of Health [UK], 2013; Pebble Project, 2014; Pediatric Emergency Department, 2015)

ED Size and Configuration

☐ Will experts be consulted, as well as ED physicians, staff, and facility planners, when designing or renovating Emergency Departments, to be sure decision-makers have access to the latest thinking on ED size, configuration, equipment, IT systems, user needs and requirements, and the like? (Allison and Kunz, 2011)

☐ Will the number of needed treatment rooms be calculated with reference to the ED census? (Welch, 2012; Zilm, 2007)

☐ Will ED areas be designed for maximum flexibility? (Welch, 2012; Zilm, 2010)

☐ Will ED areas be designed for efficient patient flow and use of ED space from a square-foot-per-treatment perspective? (Zilm, 2010)

☐ Will ED exam and treatment rooms be designed with space for the activities of an entire medical team and all necessary equipment? (Facility Guidelines Institute, 2014 [2.2–3.1.3.6 (2)])

☐ When rooms will accommodate team triage, will there be space for the full care team and all necessary equipment, including large items such as an EKG machine? (Department of Health [UK], 2013)

☐ Will there be ample space in resuscitation areas for 360-degree access to the patient, all staff required for care, and accompanying family members, as well as the parking and maneuvering of equipment? (Department of Health [UK], 2013)

☐ In resuscitation areas, will clear zones be defined for patients, the care team, and family members? (Bradley et al., 2013; Choi and Bosch, 2013; Department of Health [UK], 2013; Emergency Nurses Association, 2005)

☐ Will a resuscitation area be provided adjacent to the ambulance entrance and out of view of other patients? (Allison and Kunz, 2011).

☐ Will immediate access to the ED be provided from the ambulance entrance and from a rooftop helipad, via large trauma elevators? (Allison and Kunz, 2011)

☐ Will decision-makers consider ED configurations that allow flexibility in relation to patient flow, such as pods, inner core, separate functional units, streaming systems, fast-track systems, doughnut layouts, and others? (Allison and Kunz, 2011; Chandler Hospital Emergency Department, 2014; Christmann, 2011; Welch, 2012; Wheary, 2014; Zilm, 2007, 2010; Zilm and Lennon, 2003)

☐ Will ED work areas be designed for maximum staff interaction and visual connectivity? (Zilm, 2010).

☐ Will ED work areas, supplies, and medications be located so as to minimize staff travel? (Zilm, 2010).

☐ Will ED countertops be large enough to hold keyboards, tablets, and other IT equipment? (Welch, 2012)

☐ Will the ED accommodate arm- and wall-mounted screens, where appropriate? (Welch, 2012)

☐ Will ample storage space be provided for portable equipment such as an ultrasound machine and mobility equipment such as stretchers, wheelchairs, and crutches? (Allison and Kunz, 2011; Department of Health [UK], 2013).

☐ Will the trauma area accommodate an ice machine? (Allison and Kunz, 2011; Department of Health [UK], 2013)

☐ Will staff break rooms have a view to the outside and an attached pantry, as well as changing rooms and showers? (Allison and Kunz, 2011; Department of Health [UK], 2013)

☐ Will standardized, individual, acuity-adaptable patient ED rooms be considered? (Pebble Project, 2014: Zilm et al., 2010)

☐ Will there be highly visible hand-wash sinks and alcohol-based hand-rub dispensers in the ED? (Pebble Project, 2014)

☐ Will ED surfaces and finishes minimize noise and contamination? (Pebble Project, 2014)

☐ Will ED patient rooms have access to natural light and outside views? (Faulkner, 2006; Pebble Project, 2014)

☐ Will artwork, colors, and textures be used to create a soothing atmosphere? (Faulkner, 2006; Pebble Project, 2014)

☐ Will family members be accommodated in areas of the ED, including resuscitation? (Bradley et al., 2013; Choi and Bosch, 2013; Department of Health [UK], 2013; Emergency Nurses Association, 2005)

☐ Will ample corridor and circulation space allow family access to patients without resulting cross-traffic with ED staff? (Zilm, 2007)

☐ Will flexibility be provided for future ED growth through internal adaptation or expansion? (Zilm, 2010)

Accommodating Disasters

☐ Will more than the usual amount of waiting area space be provided, in order to accommodate possible conversion to a treatment area?

☐ Will flexible, extra-wide corridors be provided so they can be used as triage and emergency treatment spaces?

☐ Will larger-than-usual examination rooms be provided with double headwall provisions, in order to accommodate double occupancy, as needed?

☐ Will a patient bathroom be provided between every two treatment rooms, in order to minimize exposure to infectious diseases?

☐ Will a large storage area be provided for disaster equipment, such as stretchers and disposable protective equipment?

☐ Will more than one air isolation room be provided?

☐ Will a modified mechanical system be provided to allow for the quarantine of groups of patients?

☐ Will a separate entrance be provided, leading directly into a decontamination area, with room around it to accommodate containment tents and fire and rescue services? (Zilm, 2007)

ED Front-End Areas

☐ Will decision-makers consult with hospital and ED department leadership, clinicians, front-line staff, and ED experts on strategies, configuration, and space requirements for front-end processes? (Carpman Associates, 1984 [unpub.])

☐ Will patients have visual and acoustical privacy during ED front-end processes? (Carpman Associates, 1984 [unpub.]; Dubbs, 2003)

☐ Will consultation rooms be provided in lower-acuity areas? Will patients be informed about available areas for private consultation? (Allison and Kunz, 2011)

☐ Will electronic window screens be considered in triage areas? (New Emergency Department, 2014)

☐ Will assistance be available to patients and companions with LEP (limited English-proficiency)? Will access to at least one connection be provided for telephone access to translation services? (Chen et al., 2007; Facility Guidelines Institute, 2014; US Department of Health and Human Services, 1980)

ED Patient Waiting Areas

☐ Will good visual access be provided from the ED patient waiting area to a staff area? (Carpman Associates, 1984 [unpub.])

☐ Will large, noticeable information be provided, describing how the ED functions and show-ing estimated waiting times? Will a digital information system be provided for patients? (Carpman Associates, 1984 [unpub.]; Hohenadel, 2013)

☐ Will an easily identified and operated nurse-call mechanism be provided? (Carpman Asso-ciates, 1984 [unpub.])

☐ Will there be reclining seats or some other way for patients to lie down? (Carpman Asso-ciates, 1984 [unpub.])

☐ Will space be provided for patients on stretchers and patients in wheelchairs? (Wheary, 2014; Wilber et al., 2005).

☐ Will seating be high enough for older patients to sit and rise with a minimum of difficulty? (Carpman Associates, 1984 [unpub.])

☐ Will seating have good back support and padded armrests? (Carpman Associates, 1984 [unpub.])

☐ Will some high-rise seating be provided? (Carpman Associates, 1984 [unpub.])

☐ Will an outside view to nature be provided, as well as artwork, plants, and other items of visual interest? (Carpman Associates, 1984 [unpub.]; Nanda and Hathorn, 2012)

☐ Will positive distractions be provided, such as TV's, tablets loaded with videos, or digital music players (such as iPods) loaded with a variety of music? Will individual headphones be available? (Nanda and Hathorn, 2012)

ED Visitor Waiting Areas

☐ Will an outside view be provided that does not include arriving ambulances? (Carpman Associates, 1984 [unpub.]; Drury and Rosen, 1977; Petersen, 1981; Welch, 1977)

☐ Will visual access be provided between the waiting area and attending staff? (Carpman Associates, 1984 [unpub.]; Drury and Rosen, 1977; Petersen, 1981; Welch, 1977)

☐ Will signage and digital systems explain ED processes and provide information on patient progress? (Carpman Associates, 1984 [unpub.]; Drury and Rosen, 1977; Petersen, 1981; Rush University Medical Center, n.d.; Welch, 1977)

☐ Will visitor waiting areas be located near restrooms, vending machines, and water fountains? (Carpman Associates, 1984 [unpub.]; Drury and Rosen, 1977; Petersen, 1981; Welch, 1977)

☐ Will a television area be provided? Will there be a way to limit television sound for those not watching it? (Carpman Associates, 1984 [unpub.]; Drury and Rosen, 1977; Petersen, 1981; Welch, 1977)

☐ Will a waiting area be provided away from the television? (Carpman Associates, 1984 [un-pub.]; Drury and Rosen, 1977; Petersen, 1981; Welch, 1977)

☐ Will a children's area be provided, separated from but visually connected to the main waiting area? (Carpman Associates, 1984 [unpub.]; Drury and Rosen, 1977; Petersen, 1981; Welch, 1977)

Senior Emergency Departments

☐ Will treatment bays in the senior ED be separated by walls, rather than by curtains? (Shapiro, 2009)

☐ Will handrails be strategically located? (Shapiro, 2009)

☐ Will effective, soft lighting be provided? (Shapiro, 2009)

☐ Will non-reflective, nonslip flooring be provided? (Shapiro, 2009)

☐ Will wall colors be selected with aging eyes in mind? Will contrasting trim help patients see where one area stops and another begins? (Shapiro, 2009)

☐ Will mattresses be provided to help prevent the skin breakdown that can lead to bedsores? (Baker, 2009)

☐ Will a blanket warmer be available? (Baker, 2009)

☐ Will TVs with headsets be provided, as well as clocks with large numerals, and telephones and remote controls with large buttons?

☐ Will patients have choices about listening to music using headphones and digital devices, such as iPods?

Pediatric Emergency Departments

☐ Will a separate entrance be provided to the Pediatric ED? If a separate entrance is not possible, will a well-marked, child-friendly pathway be provided from the adult ED to the Pediatric ED?

☐ Will children in the Pediatric ED not be seen by patients and visitors waiting in the Adult ED? (Department of Health [UK], 2013)

☐ Will two waiting areas be considered in the Pediatric ED: one for sick children and one for well children? (Department of Health [UK], 2013)

☐ Will color schemes and furnishings be appealing to children who range in age from babies to young teens? (Christmann, 2011; Pediatric Emergency Department, 2015)

☐ Will play tables, toys, and digital play stations be provided? (Christmann, 2011; Pediatric Emergency Department, 2015)

☐ Will a big-screen TV with headphones be provided? (Christmann, 2011; Pediatric Emergency Department, 2015)

☐ Will restrooms be usable by children and adults? Will touch-free toilets be considered? (Pediatric Emergency Department, 2015)

☐ Will there be Wi-Fi access? Will digital devices and headphones be available?

Rehabilitation Units

☐ Will the entire unit be located on a single level, with no stairs and minimal use of ramps? (Infrastructure Unit Support Systems, 2014)

☐ If ramps are unavoidable, will the slopes be no more than a ratio of 1:20? (Infrastructure Unit Support Systems, 2014)

☐ Will patient rooms have private bathrooms? (Kennedy, 2010)

☐ Will patient rooms employ the latest bed design and overhead lift systems? (Kennedy, 2010)

☐ Will bedside controls be provided for lights, window shades, and the like? (Kennedy, 2010)

☐ Will bed sensor technology be provided? (Kennedy, 2010)

☐ Will some rooms have video surveillance capability? (Gwen Neilsen Anderson Rehabilitation Center Facilities, n.d.)

☐ Will sleeping accommodations be provided for family in patient rooms?

☐ Will communal areas be large enough to accommodate a minimum of 60 percent of the inpatient population, along with caregivers and staff? (Infrastructure Unit Support Systems, 2014)

☐ Will the therapy gym have both a large open area and private treatment rooms? (Infrastructure Unit Support Systems, 2014)

☐ Will the gym contain plinths and ramps, to make therapeutic equipment fully accessible? (Infrastructure Unit Support Systems, 2014)

☐ Will overhead body-weight suspension systems be provided? (Infrastructure Unit Support Systems, 2014; Inpatient Rehabilitation Unit, 2015)

☐ Will the ceiling be reinforced and high enough to accommodate equipment and ball-throwing exercises? (Infrastructure Unit Support Systems, 2014)

☐ Will oxygen and suction equipment be provided? (Infrastructure Unit Support Systems, 2014)

☐ Will emergency call buttons be provided, accessible from wheelchair height? (Infrastructure Unit Support Systems, 2014)

☐ Will the gym have space for visitors to observe treatment? (Infrastructure Unit Support Systems, 2014)

☐ Will the acute rehabilitation unit contain fully equipped *non-accessible* training spaces, such as a kitchen, dining room, bathroom, and laundry? (Gwen Neilsen Anderson Rehabilitation Center Facilities, n.d.; Inpatient Rehabilitation Unit, 2015; New State of the Art, n.d.)

☐ Will outpatient and homecare services be located adjacent to the inpatient facility, to facilitate coordination and continuity of care? (Infrastructure Unit Support Systems, 2014)

☐ Will inpatient and outpatient areas have separate entrances? (Infrastructure Unit Support Systems, 2014)

Patient and Visitor Information Areas

☐ Will patients and visitors be informed about the location of the patient information area? (Reizenstein and Grant, 1981 [unpub. No. 2])

☐ Will the information area be located along a public circulation route?

☐ Will the information area appear inviting and have a quiet, warm ambience? (Arneill and Frasca-Beaulieu, 2003)

☐ Will comfortable, well-lighted places be provided for patients and visitors to sit and read within the information area? (Arneill and Frasca-Beaulieu, 2003)

☐ Will the information area be accessible to and usable by everyone? Will it accommodate people with functional limitations and include circulation space for people in wheelchairs, and those with walkers and rolling IV poles? (Kamisar, 1979)

☐ If the information area includes books, will they be displayed within easy reach of people with functional limitations? Will large-print books be available? (Kamisar, 1979)

☐ Will signs use Braille, tactile lettering, and high contrast between sign messages and sign backgrounds in order to make information area signs legible to people with vision limitations? (Kamisar, 1979)

☐ Will patient and visitor educational materials and internet access be provided?

☐ Will a book cart be provided?

Special Services

Overnight Accommodations

☐ Will sleeping accommodations be provided in patient rooms using sleep sofas, cots, or folding beds? (Carpman et al., 1984; Reizenstein and Grant, 1982 [unpub. No. 13]).

☐ Will temporary sleeping areas be provided within family lounges by using sleep sofas and room dividers to create separate spaces? (Greenwich Hospital, Yale New Haven Health, 2015)

☐ Will visitors needing to stay overnight sometimes be accommodated in an in-house hotel, in vacant rooms within patient units, or in other areas of the facility?

☐ Will a "host home" program be considered in which visitors and outpatients can be given a place to shower and sleep in the home of someone in the community, either with or without charge? (Carpman et al., 1984; Reizenstein and Grant, 1982 [unpub. No. 13])

☐ Will the healthcare organization plan to build, renovate, lease, or otherwise provide some type of lodging facility (apartments, motel, room and bath) for outpatients and visitors?

☐ Will an outpatient and visitor discount accommodations program be available with nearby hotels and motels, with transportation provided by shuttle bus? (Carpman et al., 1984; Reizenstein and Grant, 1982 [unpub. No. 13])

☐ Will the healthcare organization encourage an outside group, either for-profit or not-for-profit, to build and operate a hotel or hotel-like facility nearby, such as a Ronald McDonald House? (Carpman et al., 1984; Reizenstein and Grant, 1982 [unpub. No. 13])

Shops

☐ Will retail shops be provided within public spaces of the health facility? (Eisingerich and Boehm, 2009; Greene, 2012; Nappi, 2011; Phillips 2004; Roper-St. Francis, n.d.)

Hair Care

☐ Will hair care services be available for ambulatory and bedridden patients? (Reizenstein and Grant, 1981 [unpub. No. 9]

Fitness Centers

☐ Will a fitness center be available in or near the healthcare facility? (D. McCarthy, 1993; Pallarito, 1994; Spencer, 1998)

Spas

☐ Will a spa be available in or near the healthcare facility? (Alexander, 2012; Coan, Schaefer, and Davidson, 2006; Complementary and alternative, 2008; Dobson, 2006; Lee et al., 2011; Main, 2010; J. McCarthy, 2010; Osborn, 2005)

References

Alexander, D. G. Freeing the heart. *Massage Today* 12(01), January 2012. http://massagetoday.com/mpacms/mt/article.php?id=14520.

Allison, P., and Kunz, P. Case study: UK Chandler Hospital Emergency Department. Center for Health Design Research Report. 2011. www.healthdesign.org/sites/default/files/uk_ed_case_study_pmfall-2011.pdf.

American Nurse. Quoted in *The Spokesman-Review* (Spokane, WA). 2011. www.spokesman.com/stories/2011/nov/27/healthy-returns/.

Arneill, B., and Frasca-Beaulieu, K. Healing environments: Architecture and design conducive to health. In S. Frampton, L. Gilpin, and P. Charmel, editors. *Putting Patients First: Designing and Practicing Patient-Centered Care*, 163–90. San Francisco: Jossey-Bass, 2003.

Augustine, J. Boost capacity, slash LWBS rate with POD triage system. *Emergency Department Management* 23(4):40–41, 2011.

Baker, B. Serenity in emergencies: A Silver Spring ER aims to serve older patients. *Washington Post*, January 27, 2009. www.washingtonpost.com/wp-dyn/content/article/2009/01/26/AR2009012601872.html?sid=ST2009012601965.

Baraban, R. A garden that delights. *Food Management,* 196–200, April 1988.

Bernstein, S. L., Aronsky, D., Duseja, R., Epstein, S., Handel, D., et al. The effect of emergency department crowding on clinically oriented outcomes. *Academic Emergency Medicine* 16(1):1–10, January 2009. doi:10.1111/j.1553–2712.2008.00295.x. www.ncbi.nlm.nih.gov/pubmed/19007346

Boss, D. The central kitchen at the Johns Hopkins Hospital in Baltimore. *Food Service Equipment and Supplies*, October 1, 2012. www.fesmag.com/departments/facility-design-project-of-the-month/10231-the-central-kitchen-at-the-johns-hopkins-hospital-in-baltimore.

Boudreaux, E. D., and O'Hea, E. L. Patient satisfaction in the Emergency Department: A review of the literature and implications for practice. *Journal of Emergency Medicine* 26(1):13–26, January 2004.

Bradley, C., Lensky, M., and Brasel, K. Family presence during resuscitation. Fast facts and concepts No. 232. Medical College of Wisconsin End of Life/Palliative Education Resource Center. www.eperc.mcw.edu/EPERC/FastFactsIndex/ff_232.htm.

Brandau, M. Hospitals elevate foodservice with improved restaurants. *Food Service Warehouse.* January 6, 2014. http://nrn.com/onsite/hospitals-elevate-foodservice-improved-restaurants?page=1.

Brody, J. In decline, stillbirths continue to devastate. *New York Times*, August 15, 2011. www.nytimes.com/2011/08/16/health/16brody.html?_r=0.

Cancer center renovation improves patients' quality of life. *Healthcare Facilities Today,* January 3, 2013. www.healthcarefacilitiestoday.com/posts/Cancer-center-renovation-improves-patients-quality-of-life-Renovations—120.

Carpman Associates. St. Joseph Mercy Hospital Emergency Department Behavioral Design Program. Unpublished report. Ann Arbor, MI: Author, 1984.

Carpman, J. R., Grant, M. A., and Simmons, D. A. Overnight accommodations for visitors and outpatients: a nationwide study. *Health Care Strategic Management* 2(6):9–14, June 1984.

Chandler Hospital Emergency Department. 2014. www.ukhealthcare.uky.edu.

Chen, A. H., Youdelman, M. K., and Brooks, J. The legal framework for language access in healthcare settings: Title VI and beyond. *Journal of General Internal Medicine* 22(Supplement 2): 362–67,

November 2007. Published online October 24, 2007. doi:10.1007/s11606–007–0366–2. www.ncbi
.nlm.nih.gov/pmc/articles/PMC2150609/.

Choi, Y.-S., and Bosch, S. J. Environmental affordances: Designing for family presence and involvement
in patient care. *Health Environments Research and Design Journal* 6(4):53–75, September 30, 2013.
https://www.herdjournal.com/article/environmental-affordances-designing-family-presence-and
-involvement-patient-care.

Christian, S. Kaiser unveils meditation room. *Roseville and Granite Bay (CA) Press Tribune*, February 3,
2011. www.thepresstribune.com/article/kaiser-unveils-meditation-room.

Christmann, J. A. CHD research report. *Healthcare Design*, November 22, 2011. www.healthcaredesign
-magazine.com/article/chd-research-report.

Coan, J. A., Schaefer, H. S., and Davidson, R. J. Lending a hand: Social regulation of the neural response to
threat. *Psychological Science* 17(12), 2006. www.investigatinghealthyminds.org/ScientificPublications
/2006/CoanLendingPsychSci.pdf.

Complementary and alternative approaches to health. *NIH MedlinePlus* 3(1):7, Winter 2008.

Crane, J., and Noon, C. Strategies of a "no-wait" ED: How to use operational excellence to achieve superior
patient satisfaction, loyalty and dedication . . . and the truth behind the marketing strategy. *Executive
Insight*, December 13, 2010. http://healthcare-executive-insight.advanceweb.com/Archives/Article
-Archives/Strategies-of-a-No-Wait-ED.aspx.

Davies, D. L. Providing after-death care at home when a baby dies. *Psychology Today*, March 30, 2014.
www.psychologytoday.com/blog/laugh-cry-live/201403/providing-after-death-care-home-when-
baby-dies.

Department of Health [UK]. Health Building Note 15–01: Accident and emergency department. April 2013.
www.gov.uk/government/uploads/system/uploads/attachment_data/file/206267/15_01final3_v3.pdf.

Designing a "no wait" emergency department. The AHA Resource Center. American Hospital
Association Resource Center Blog. 2011. http://aharesourcecenter.wordpress.com/2011/10/21
/designing-a-no-wait-emergency-department/.

DiFazio, R. L., and Vessey, J. Advanced practice registered nurses: Addressing emerging needs in
emergency care. *African Journal of Emergency Medicine* 4(1):43–49, March 2014. doi:10.1016/j
.afjem.2013.04.008 www.afjem.org/article/S2211–419X percent2813 percent2900074–8/references.

Dobson, R. How the power of touch reduces pain and even fights disease. *Independent* October 10,
2006. www.independent.co.uk/life-style/health-and-families/health-news/how-the-power-of-touch
-reduces-pain-and-even-fights-disease-419462.html.

Drury, L. R., and Rosen, P. Multiple use, flexibility key to emergency department planning. *Hospitals*
51(14):201–11, July 16, 1977.

Dubbs, D. Privacy please! *Health Facilities Management* 16(8):20–24, August 2003.

Eisingerich, A. B., and Boehm, L. Hospital visitors ask for more shopping outlets. *Harvard Business Review:
The Magazine,* May 2009. http://hbr.org/2009/05/hospital-visitors-ask-for-more-shopping-outlets/ar/1.

Emergency Nurses Association. Position statement: Advanced practice in emergency nursing. 2012.
www.ena.org/SiteCollectionDocuments/Position percent20Statements/AdvPracticeERNursing.pdf.

_____. Position statement: Family presence at the bedside during invasive procedures and cardiopulmo-
nary resuscitation. Des Plaines, IL: Emergency Nurses Association, 2005. www.ena.org.

Exadaktylos A. K., and Velmahos, G. C. Emergency medicine and acute care surgery: A modern "Hansel
and Gretel" fairytale? *Emergency Medicine Journal* 25(6):321–22, 2008.

Facility Guidelines Institute. Guidelines for Design and Construction of Health Care Facilities, 2014 edition. Emergency Department. Treatment room or area. 2.2–3.1.3.6 (2). Chicago: American Society for Healthcare Engineering of the American Hospital Association, 2014.

Faulkner, J. Creating a no-wait emergency department. *Healthcare Design,* November 1, 2006. www .healthcaredesignmagazine.com/article/creating-no-wait-emergency-department.

Foodservice changes equals satisfied patients. *Foodservice Director,* September 7, 2012. www .foodservicedirector.com/managing-your-business/generating-revenue/articles/foodservice -changes-equals-satisfied-patients.

Frampton, S., Guastello, S., Brady, C., Hale, M., Horowitz, S., Smith, S. B., and Stone, S. *Patient-Centered Care Improvement Guide.* Plaintree, Inc, and Picker Institute, 2008. http://planetree.org/wp-content /uploads/2012/01/Patient-Centered-Care-Improvement-Guide-10–28–09-Final.pdf.

Fry, E. Chilwell couple grieving for stillborn daughter raise £1,000 for charity in six days. *Nottingham Post,* February 6, 2014. www.nottinghampost.com/Couple-grieving-stillborn-daughter-raise-1–000 /story-20566311-detail/story.htmlNo. ixzz30xcGZD2q.

Gatoade, H. Kaiser Permanente's Rejuve(n)ate Café transforms the hospital cafeteria into something truly special. *Healthcare Design* 10(6):40–44, June 2010. www.healthcaredesignmagazine .com/article/kaiser-permanentes-rejuvenate-caf-transforms-hospital-cafeteria-something-truly -special.

Goldman, D. P., Vaiana, M., and Romley, J. A. The emerging importance of patient amenities in hospital care. *New England Journal of Medicine* 363:2185–87, December 2, 2010. doi:10.1056 /NEJMp1009501

Goralnick, E., Walls, R. M., and Kosowsky, J. M. How we revolutionized our emergency department. *Harvard Business Review.* HBR Blog Network, September 26, 2013. http://blogs.hbr.org/2013/09 /how-we-revolutionized-our-emergency-department/.

Greene, J. Intensive wares: Hospitals expand in-house shops for good returns, good will. *Crain's De-troit Business,* March 11, 2012. www.crainsdetroit.com/article/20120311/SUB01/303119987 /intensive-wares-hospitals-expand-in-house-shops-for-good-returns.

Greenwich Hospital, Yale New Haven Health. 2015. www.greenhosp.org/inpatient_oncology_unit.

Gwen Neilsen Anderson Rehabilitation Center Facilities. St. Luke's Magic Valley, Twin Falls ID. n.d. www.stlukesonline.com/magic_valley/specialties_and_services/rehabilitation/inpatient.php.

Hamilton, D. K. Research informed design supports evidence-based ICU medicine. *Health Environments Research and Design Journal,* September 30, 2013.

Henderson, S. How to create a hospital food service environment that encourages rest and relaxation. *Food Service Warehouse,* July 16, 2015. www.foodservicewarehouse.com/education/healthcare-food -service/how-to-create-a-hospital-food-service-environment-that-encourages-rest-and-relaxation /c31070.aspx.

Hiatt, L. G. Architecture for the aged: Design for living. *Inland Architect* 23:6–17, November–December 1978.

Hohenadel, K. Can digital updates on emergency room wait times reduce patient rage? *The Eye,* December 4 2013. www.slate.com/blogs/the_eye/2013/12/04/emergency_room_design_can_digital _updates_reduce_patient_frustration.html.

Hutten-Czapski, P. Rural-urban differences in emergency department wait times. *Canadian Journal of Rural Medicine,* 15(4):153–55, 2010.

Infrastructure Unit Support Systems (IUSS). Health Facility Guides. Adult Physical Rehabilitation [Proposal V.1] 18 March 2014. Department: Health. Republic of South Africa. iussonline.co.za/iuss /wp-content/uploads/2013/10/2014_03_06-IUSS-Adult-Physical-Rehabilitation-proposal1.pdf.

Inpatient Rehabilitation Unit. Cedars-Sinai, Los Angeles, CA. 2015. www.cedars-sinai.edu/Patients /Programs-and-Services/Physical-Medicine-and-Rehabilitation/Treatments-and-Programs /Inpatient-Rehabilitation-Unit.aspx.

James, S. Making hospital chapel welcoming to all faiths. *Bay (CA) Citizen,* October 21, 2010. Reprinted *New York Times,* October 22, 2010. www.nytimes.com/2010/10/22/us/22bcjames.html.

Kamali, M. F., Jain, M., Jain, A. R., and Schneider, S. M. Emergency Department waiting room: Many requests, many insured and many primary care physician referrals. *International Journal of Emergency Medicine* 6:35, 2013. doi:10.1186/1865–1380–6–35. www.intjem.com/content/6/1/35.

Kamisar, H. Signs for the handicapped patron. In D. Pollet and P. Haskel, editors. *Sign Systems for Libraries,* 99–103. New York: R. R. Bowker, 1979.

Kantz, B., Wandel, J., Fladger, A., Folcarelli, P., Burger, S., and Clifford, J. Developing patient and family education services: Innovations for the changing healthcare environment. *Journal of Nursing Administration* 28(2):11–18, February 1998.

Kennedy, C. Rehabilitating rehab: Impact of transdisciplinary collaboration in design and cultural transformation on operational and quality outcomes. Sutter Health: California Pacific Medical Center. 2010. www.cpmc.org/advanced/neurosciences/bulletin/2010–2/rehab_rehab.html.

Lee, J. Changes on the menu. *Modern Healthcare,* April 27, 2013. www.modernhealthcare.com /article/20130427/MAGAZINE/301049827No.

Lee, Y-H., Park, B.N.R., and Kim, S. H. The effects of heat and massage application on autonomic nervous system. *Yonsei Medical Journal* 52(6):982–9, November 2011. doi: 10.3349/ymj.2011.52.6.982

Leighty, J. You called? Hourly rounding cuts call lights. *Nurse.com,* April 2, 2007. news.nurse.com/apps /pbcs.dll/article?AID=2007304020012No. .U1q7J6Jtz-s.

Los Angeles Medical Center cafeteria gets rejuvenated. *Health Care Development,* January 13, 2011. www.healthcaredevelopmentmagazine.com/article/los-angeles-medical-center.html.

Madden, C. Sacred spaces in the hospital setting. St. Louis Children's Hospital. n.d. www.google.com /No. q=hospital+sacred+spaces.

Magid, D. J., et al. The safety of emergency care systems: Results of a survey of clinicians in 65 US emergency departments. *Annals of Emergency Medicine* 53(6):715–23, June 2009. doi:10.1016/j .annemergmed.2008.10.007. www.ncbi.nlm.nih.gov/pubmed/19054592.

Main, E. The best reason to get a massage. *Rodale News,* September 30, 2010. www.rodalenews.com /benefits-massage.

March of Dimes/Loss and Grief/Pregnancy loss/Stillbirth. June 2015. www.marchofdimes.com/loss /stillbirth.aspx.

McCarthy, D. Hospital shapes up its cardiac care continuum with new fitness center. *Health Facilities Management,* 12–13, May 1993.

McCarthy, J. The hospital of the future is more like a hotel. *Mind-Body, Psychology of Spas and Wellbeing,* August 10, 2010. psychologyofwellbeing.com/201008/the-hospital-of-the-future-is-more-like-a-hotel .html.

McGee, P. The patient library service in England. *Health Libraries Review* 16(3):204–207, September 1999.

Millburg, S. No-wait ED doesn't even have a waiting room. *Radiology Daily,* October 21, 2011. www .radiologydaily.com/daily/diagnostic-imaging/no-wait-ed-doesnt-even-have-a-waiting-room/.

Nanda, U., and Hathorn, K. Impact of art on the ED waiting experience. *Heathcare Design,* November 15, 2012. www.healthcaredesignmagazine.com/article/impact-art-ed-waiting-experience.

Nappi, R. As hospitals struggle, gift shops provide spark by making money. *Spokesman-Review,* November 27, 2011. www.spokesman.com/stories/2011/nov/27/healthy-returns/.

A new ED for a new era at Hopkins. 2012. www.hopkinsmedicine.org/emergencymedicine/NEW percent20ED_2012/New_Emergency percent20Department.html.

New emergency department entrance opens. Holy Family Memorial, Manitowoc, WI. n.d. www .hfmhealth.org/Default.aspx?id=1725&sid=1&CWFriendlyUrl=true.

New State of the Art Inpatient Rehabilitation Unit. Faxton St. Luke's, Utica, NY. n.d. http://faxtonstlukes .com/inpatient-rehabilitation.

Olsen, D. St. John's Hospital unveils renovated cafeteria. *State (IL). Journal-Register* May 5, 2014. www .sj-r.com/article/20140505/NEWS/140509678/10298/LIFESTYLE.

Osborn, K. Hospital spas: An unusual union unfolds. *Massage Bodywork,* April/May 2005. www.massage therapy.com/articles/index.php/article_id/910/Hospital-Spas.

Pallarito, K. Hospitals strengthen networks through new fitness facilities. *Modern Healthcare,* 45–46, December 12, 1994.

Patient satisfaction by time spent in the emergency department and comfort of the waiting room. Emergency Department Pulse Report: Patient Perspectives on American Health Care. Press Ganey Associates, 2010. www.osuem.com/education/journalClub/2010_ED_Pulse_Report.pdf

Pebble Project. Chandler Hospital Emergency Department. 2014. www.healthdesign.org/ pebble/partners/university-kentucky-healthcare/chandler-hospital-emergency-department /chandler-hospi

Pediatric Emergency Department (ER). Overview. Stanford Hospitals and Clinics. 2015. www.stanford -childrens.org/en/service/emergency-department

Peteet, T. Sacred spaces in medicine. *State of Formation.* CIRCLE: The Center for Interreligious and Communal Leadership Education, Hebrew College and Andover Newton Theological School, January 8, 2013. www.stateofformation.org/2013/01/sacred-spaces-in-medicine/.

Petersen, R. W. Behavioral criteria: patient and companion needs for reception and waiting areas. Unpublished report. McMinnville, OR: R. W. Petersen and Associates, July 31, 1981.

Phillips, K. Industry trends: Expert says hospitals should tap retail potential. *Nursezone.com.* 2004. http://nursezone.com/Nursing-News-Events/more-features/Industry-Trends-Expert-Says-Hospitals -Should-Tap-Retail-Potential_20792.aspx.

Reizenstein, J. E., and Grant, M. A. Executive summary: Patient hair care and storage. Unpublished research report No. 9. Patient and Visitor Participation Project, Office of Hospital Planning, Research and Development, University of Michigan, Ann Arbor, 1981.

_____. Hospital patient and visitor issues: currently unmet needs and suggested solutions. Unpublished research report No. 4a. Patient and Visitor Participation Project, Office of Hospital Planning, Research and Development, University of Michigan, Ann Arbor, 1981.

_____. Patient activities and schematic design preferences. Unpublished research report No. 2. Patient and Visitor Participation Project, Office of Hospital Planning, Research and Development, University of Michigan, Ann Arbor, 1981.

_____. Visitor preferences for overnight accommodations. Unpublished research report No. 13. Patient and Visitor Participation Project, Office of Hospital Planning, Research and Development, University of Michigan, Ann Arbor, 1982.

Reizenstein, J. E., Grant, M. A., and Vaitkus, M. A. Visitor activities and schematic design preferences. Unpublished research report No. 4. Patient and Visitor Participation Project, Office of Hospital Planning, Research and Development, University of Michigan, Ann Arbor, 1981.

Resnick, M., Gregoire, M., Lafferty, L., and Lipson, S. Marketing can change consumers' perceptions of healthfulness of items served in a worksite cafeteria. *Journal of the American Dietetic Association.* 99(10):1265–67, October 1999.

Rodak, S. 8 Trends in emergency department design. *Becker's Hospital Review*, November 8, 2012. www .beckershospitalreview.com/capacity-management/8-trends-in-emergency-department-design.html.

Roper-St. Francis. The stores. n.d. www.rsfh.com/Patients_and_Visitors/The_Stores.aspx.

Rose, I. C. Marketing new food services. *Hospitals* 57(15):64–66, August 1, 1983.

Rush University Medical Center. Patient and Visitor Services. Smith Lounge–Procedural Waiting Room. n.d. www.rush.edu/rumc/page-1272985403596.html.

Salvi, F., Morichi, V., Grilli, A., Giorgi, R., De Tommaso, G., and Dessì-Fulgheri, P. The elderly in the Emergency Department: A critical review of problems and solutions. *Internal Emergency Medicine* 2(4):292–301, December 2007. www.ncbi.nlm.nih.gov/pubmed/18043874.

Schilling, B. Atlanta's Piedmont Hospital moving away from room service. *Foodservice Director,* October 24, 2011. www.foodservicedirector.com/managing-your-business/controlling-costs/articles /atlantas-piedmont-hospital-moving-away-from-room.

Scottsdale Healthcare. Auxiliary gift shops. 2014. www.shc.org/patients-visitors/gift-shops-boutiques /scottsdale-healthcare-auxiliary-gift-shops-and-boutiques.

Shapiro, J. An emergency room built specially for seniors. *NPR,* February 19, 2009. www.npr.org /templates/story.php?storyId=100823874.

Soremekun, O, A., Takayesu J. K, and Bohan, S. J. Framework for analyzing wait times and other factors that impact patient satisfaction in the emergency department. *Journal of Emergency Medicine* 41(6):686–92, December 2011. doi:10.1016/j.jemermed.2011.01.018. www.ncbi.nlm.nih.gov /pubmed/21440402.

Spencer, J. Go for the gold. *Health Facilities Management* 11(5):24–30, May 1998.

State of the art facilities built to enhance healing. John Muir Health, Contra Costa County, CA. n.d. www .johnmuirhealth.com/services/physical-rehabilitation/inpatient-rehabilitation-unit.html.

Stillbirth: The facts. *Life Challenges,* 2015. www.allaboutlifechallenges.org/stillbirth.htmNo.sthash .L4POnFo4.dpuf.

Strategies for improving satisfaction with wait times. Emergency Department Pulse Report: Patient Perspectives on American Health Care. Press Ganey Associates, 2010. www.osuem.com/education /journalClub/2010_ED_Pulse_Report.pdf.

Subash, F., Dunn, F., McNicholl, B., and Marlow, J. Team triage improves emergency department efficiency. *Emergency Medicine Journal* 21:542–44, 2004 doi:10.1136/emj.2002.003665.

Texas Children's Hospital. n.d. www.texaschildrens.org/AllAbout/VisitingTheHospital/SpiritualCare .aspx.

The Inpatient Rehabilitation Unit. Community Memorial Hospital: The Froedtert and the Medical College of Wisconsin Regional Health Care Network. 2015. www.froedtert.com/community-memorial/rehabilitation/inpatient/unit.

The mind–body connection. *NIH MedlinePlus* 3(1):4, Winter 2008.

Thompson, D. A., Yarnold, P. R., Williams, D. R., and Adams, S. L. Effects of actual waiting time, perceived waiting time, information delivery, and expressive quality on patient satisfaction in the emergency department. *Annals of Emergency Medicine* 28:657–65, December 1996.

Travers, J. P., and Lee, F. C. Avoiding prolonged waiting time during busy periods in the emergency department: Is there a role for the senior emergency physician in triage? *European Journal of Emergency Medicine* 13(6):342–48, December 2006.

Trzeciak, S., and Rivers, E. P. Emergency department overcrowding in the United States: An emerging threat to patient safety and public health. *Journal of Emergency Medicine* 20:402–5, 2003. www.ncbi.nlm.nih.gov/pmc/articles/PMC1726173/pdf/v020p00402.pdf.

US Department of Health and Human Services. 45 Fed. Reg. 82972 (December 17, 1980). (Notice).

Welch, P. Hospital emergency facilities: Translating behavioral issues into design. Report. Cambridge, MA: Harvard University Department of Architecture, 1977.

Welch, S., and Davidson, S. Exploring new intake models for the emergency department. *American Journal of Medical Quality* 25(3):172–80, May–June 2010. doi:10.1177/1062860609360570

Welch, S., and Savitch, L. Exploring strategies to improve emergency department intake. *Journal of Emergency Medicine* 43(1):149–58, July 2012.

Welch, S. J., Augustine, J., Dong, L., Savitz, L., Snow, G., and James, B. C. Volume-related differences in emergency department performance. *Joint Commission Journal on Quality and Patient Safety* 38(9), September 2012. www.edbenchmarking.org/uploads/jcjqps-size-matters-welch-preproofreadiing.pdf.

Welch S. J., Jones S. S., and Allen T. Mapping the 24-hour emergency department cycle to improve patient flow. *Joint Commission Journal on Quality and Patient Safety*, 33(5):247–55, 2007.

Welch, S. J. Using Data to Drive Emergency Department Design. *Health Environments Research & Design Journal*, May 15, 2012. www.herdjournal.com/article/using-data-drive-emergency-department-design-metasynthesis.

What is inpatient hospice care? Frequently asked questions about inpatient hospice. St. Luke's Hospital, Cedar Rapids, IA. 2014. https://www.unitypoint.org/cedarrapids/services-frequently-asked-questions.aspx.

Wheary, J. Rethinking the emergency department. *Healthcare Design*, February 12, 2014. www.healthcaredesignmagazine.com/article/rethinking-emergency-department.

Wilber, S. T., Burger, B., Gerson, L.W., and Blanda, M. Reclining chairs reduce pain from gurneys in older emergency department patients: A randomized controlled trial. *Academic Emergency Medicine* 12(2):119–23, February 2005. www.ncbi.nlm.nih.gov/pubmed/15692131.

Wiler J. L., Gentle C., Halfpenny J. M., Heins A., Mehrotra A., Mikhail M. G., and Fite, D. Optimizing emergency department front-end operations. *Annals of Emergency Medicine* 55(2):142–60, 2009. doi:10.1016/j.annemergmed.2009.05.021

Yoon, J. K, and Sonneveld, M. Anxiety of patients in the waiting room of the emergency department. TEI 10 Fourth International Conference on Tangible, Embedded, and Embodied Interaction, January 25–27, 2010, Cambridge, MA. http://tei-conf.org/10/uploads/Program/p279.pdf.

Zeit, K. D. Two emergency departments, many lessons learned. *Healthcare Design,* November 5, 2012. www.healthcaredesignmagazine.com/article/two-emergency-departments-many-lessons-learned.

Zilm, F. Designing for emergencies. *Health Facilities Management,* November 1, 2010. www.hfmmagazine.com/display/HFM-news-article.dhtml?dcrPath=/templatedata/HF_Common/NewsArticle/data/HFM/Magazine/2010/Nov/1011HFM_FEA_AD.

———. A new era of emergency care: Planning and design consideration. *Journal of Ambulatory Care Management* 30(3):259–63, July–September 2007. doi:10.1097/01.JAC.0000278985.18428.c9. www.zilm.com/New percent20Generation percent20of percent20ED.pdf.

Zilm, F., Crane, J., and Roche, K. T. New directions in emergency service operations and planning. *Journal of Ambulatory Care Management* 33(4):296–306, October–December 2010. www.ncbi.nlm.nih.gov/pubmed/20838109.

Zilm, F., and Lennon, J. New directions in emergency facilities design. *Health Facilities Management* 16(6), June 2003.

CHAPTER 11

USER PARTICIPATION IN HEALTHCARE-FACILITY DESIGN

Commissioning a design and construction project is a bit like buying an expensive new suit. With a suit, you may know the color and style you like, the amount you want to spend, and the size you wear. With a building, you may know functions that must be accommodated, the image to be conveyed, the approximate number of square feet (square meters) desired, the time frame, and the budget. But chances are you would not walk out of the clothing store until the suit had been altered to fit your exact proportions—the waist might need to be taken in, the hips let out a bit, the sleeves lengthened. The same is true of the design of a building. A general set of design parameters, even informed guidelines like the ones presented in this book, must be tailored to each project's specific requirements.

Design guidelines supply information of a general nature: for example, how to arrange cubicles in an admitting area, how to position a window in relation to a patient's bed, and the types of electrical connections needed on a patient-room headwall. However, in order to ensure that these guidelines are relevant to a specific situation—such as an admitting area short on space, an older hospital that cannot afford to change its windows, or a bed design that can abrade electrical plugs—it is necessary to supplement general design guidelines with detailed design-related information gathered from the people—staff, patients, and visitors—who use (and will use) the facility.

Of course, many others will also participate in the process. Designers, including architects, landscape architects, interior designers, and others will make major contributions. Consultants in such areas as Emergency Department design, Food Services, Universal Design, Wayfinding,

LEARNING OBJECTIVES
- Understand the concept of user participation in healthcare-facility design.
- Identify some benefits of user participation.
- Identify user groups who might participate in healthcare-facility design.
- Become familiar with the range of information-gathering mechanisms and techniques related to user participation in design.
- Know the issues related to managing a user participation process.

Materials Management, and others, will contribute to the project as a result of their experience and expertise. Those who manage the organization and maintain the facility will also have significant input into the design in order to make sure it reflects the mission of the organization, its corporate culture, preferences of corporate leaders, as well as the available budget, schedule, regulatory, and other requirements. Philanthropic donors may also weigh in (Sommer, 1983).

What Is User Participation in Design?

User participation refers to a process of systematically gathering information about the design-related needs, expectations, preferences, and experiences of the facility's eventual users and incorporating this information into the design decision-making process. User participation is desirable for any healthcare-facility design project, small scale or large scale, including site planning, architectural design, interior design, and landscape architecture (Brubaker, 1985 [unpub.]).

As far back as the 1970s, the importance of "Participatory Design," as it was then known, was becoming clear (Sanders and Stappers, 2008). Information about consumer needs and preferences, as well as quantitative and qualitative feedback from consumers about products, was recognized as a key to business excellence in producing consumer goods. These criteria now are understood as crucial for service industries such as healthcare, with patients acknowledged as "the ultimate (although not the only) consumers—the *end consumers*—of healthcare services" (Stern et al., 2003).

Evidence-based design emerged as a way of improving functionality by basing design decisions on knowledge about the impact of these decisions on people, costs, and management (Codinhoto et al., 2014). Evidence can provide a solid basis for questioning old standards and promoting innovation. A practice of routinely collecting evidence on the effects of the decisions made and the results achieved can stimulate learning and improve performance (Codinhoto et al., 2014).

Benefits of User Participation

Although orchestrating a participatory design process is complex and time-consuming, it can be beneficial for a number of reasons.

Helps Clarify Design Objectives

With objectives stated and constraints in mind, designers are free to do what they do best: meet these challenges with creative design approaches (Kaplan and Kaplan, 1983). Participation can also help relieve users' anxieties about the otherwise unknown changes ahead (Brill et al., 1985). User participation can encourage realistic expectations, because users can gain a better understanding of the project's financial, regulatory, and physical constraints (Dewulf and van Meel, 2002).

Leads to Better Design Decisions

Without detailed familiarity with what goes on within a given space, design decision-makers may inadvertently fail to accommodate users' needs (Brill et al., 1985; Dewulf and van Meel, 2002; Hall, 1991; Lindamood, 1982; Reizenstein, 1982; Sommer, 1983). Participation can bridge the gap between generally relevant approaches and specifically workable options.

Stimulates Positive Behavior and Attitudes

When people have been involved in a participatory process, they tend to take better care of the resulting design (Kaplan and Kaplan, 1983). They also feel a vested interest in the project, leading perhaps to less staff absenteeism, turnover, theft, or vandalism (Becker, 1977; Brill et al., 1985; Sommer, 1983).

Inspires a Sense of Community

A participatory design process often brings people together to talk about common concerns—something rare in segmented or large organizations. This opportunity for staff—at different levels, in different roles, or in different departments—to work together on an important and challenging task can create at least a temporary sense of teamwork that might otherwise be absent (Sommer, 1983).

Provides Opportunities to Assess Design-Related Organizational Polices

When participants review proposed designs, questions often arise about related policies. For example, the degree to which a clinic waiting area is overcrowded may be a function of scheduling practices, as well as design. Design and policy need to work in concert to achieve organizational objectives (Cleary, 2003).

Acts as a Marketing Strategy

Knowing which design features and amenities are most important to consumers can help healthcare facilities attract patients and visitors. As healthcare organizations become more competitive, references to such design features as parking, comfort, green design, Universal Design, and healing gardens are likely to appear with greater frequency in marketing materials (Falick, 1981). Furthermore, the fact that consumers participated in the design process is a marketable feature in itself (Carpman and Trester, 1986).

User-Experts in the Design Process

Input from users enhances the design process by incorporating a wide variety of knowledge and expertise, making the process not only intrinsically more democratic, but also more productive, resulting in practical solutions.

It is widely recognized that usability is determined not only by the immediate interface between users and design features, but also by how design features fit into the complex organizational environment. Thus documents by themselves cannot be sufficient sources of information. Direct contact with users is also necessary for understanding the *contexts* of use (Kujala, 2003). Designers certainly bring a view of context to the design process, but this will be to some extent, "a guess, a personal view based on personal experiences" (Sleeswijk Visser et al., 2005). Designers may have little experience with healthcare settings. And as one experienced healthcare architect and project designer observes, "We always make a conscious effort to design from the perspectives of the patient, family, and caregivers, but we aren't always fortunate enough to see the space in use" (Zeit, 2013). Moreover, project developers may underestimate the diversity of users over the full spectrum of personal (demographic), task-related, geographic, and social characteristics (Kujala and Kauppinen, 2004).

Research with real users offers "a richer, more dependable view" as the description and selection of representative users evolves (Kujala and Kauppinen, 2004; Sleeswijk Visser et al., 2005). Involving patients, family members, and healthcare staff in the dialogue about healthcare facility environments allows designers and architects "to go beyond their own limited experience with the built environment of a particular healthcare facility" to optimally accommodate users' needs (Stern et al., 2003). After all, "no one can validate flows and prioritize goals like an end-user" (Glushko, 2013).

In addition, designers characteristically have an intensely visual way of knowing and working. This visual expertise is a source of strength, but has its limitations (Franck and Lepori, 2007; Heylighen, Devlieger, and Strickfaden, 2009). The way a space looks is important, as is the way it feels, sounds, smells, and the way one moves through it (Pallasmaa, 2007). Architect Robert Campbell explains that the architect's typical way of working can result in "architecture reduced to two dimensions and one sense, the visual," and can become "increasingly remote from the way lay people describe and prioritize architecture" (Campbell, 2007).

In this context, the lived experience of users—including people with functional limitations—is a valuable resource to ensure multi-sensory values and usability in the built environment. People with functional limitations, for example, are able "through their daily interaction with space . . . to identify and appreciate qualities in buildings and spaces that other people—and designers in particular—are not even aware of" (Heylighen et al., 2009). Recognizing users as "experts of their experience" "strives for user-friendly and elegant solutions and attempts to improve the environment for as many people as possible" (Herssens and Heylighen, 2007; Sleeswijk Visser et al., 2005).

The concept of "users" itself is changing and broadening, giving way in many instances to the idea of "stakeholders": that is, all the people who will be affected by a designed environment, also known as a "system" (Baek et al., 2014). For artifacts and systems to effectively address the needs of the people for whom they are designed, all stakeholders must be integrated into the design process (Schuler, 2014).

The Evolution toward Co-designing

Participation in design can encompass a number of quite different activities, from relatively little or no direct user involvement to a great deal. "Traditionally"—at least since the 1970s and '80s—these have occurred along the following scale of increasing involvement:

- Experienced behavioral consultants might be asked to act as user advocates in the design process.

- Users themselves can participate by conveying information to designers or researchers about their design-related needs and preferences.

- Users might be more involved by reviewing several design concepts and expressing their preferences.

- Users might participate in design more fully still by offering some design ideas themselves. This participation might occur as a natural outgrowth of design review, if the user/reviewer thinks the proposed design does not work well and suggests an alternative. It could also happen during a full-scale simulation in which users manipulate environmental features to best suit their needs (Becker, 1977; Brill et al., 1985).

In recent years, design and design research have been undergoing a transformation (Sanders, 2006). The user-centered approach of informed experts "designing *for users*" is being expanded and sometimes superseded by the idea of co-designing, "designing *with people*" (Glushko, 2013; Sanders and Stappers, 2008). Knowledge useful for a design process can come in many forms: for instance, "knowledge of an end-user about her practice, knowledge of a researcher about some end-users' practices, knowledge of a designer about technology, an end-user's ideas for product improvement, a researcher's hunch about a certain problem, a designer's ambition to create something," and the like (Steen, Kuijt-Evers, and Klok, 2007). Similarly, creativity occurs on several levels, from doing and adapting to making and creating (Sanders and Stappers, 2008). Those with passion and expertise about a subject can, as "experts of their experience," become co-creators in the design process, if they are given effective tools for expressing themselves (Sanders, Brandt, and Binder, 2010; Sanders and Stappers, 2008; Simonsen and Robertson, 2013).

The complexity and scale of design challenges are growing. The best research into past practices and current user preferences cannot provide all the answers to questions about patients and their needs; healthcare staff and their needs, technology and its requirements, managers and their concerns, and the like (Sanders and Stappers, 2008). It is no longer a matter of simply designing a *product* for users. A design movement has arisen that seeks to address "the future experiences of people, communities, and cultures who are now connected and informed in ways that were unimaginable" even a short while ago (Sanders and Stappers, 2008). The design process now must often move to a *purpose* perspective, seeking new techniques and tools (Jensen, 2011; Sleeswijk Visser et al., 2005).

A further challenge to involving users in design is that, in well-learned tasks, much of a user's knowledge becomes tacit: not conscious or easily expressed in words (Kujala, 2003). In addition, while innovation must always aim to solve real problems, some of these may be latent issues that people are not yet aware of, "things you never knew you needed" (Brown, 2014). Strategies are needed that unlock these sources of potential design expertise.

An array of techniques and tools meets these challenges, particularly ones that avoid the high levels of abstraction of traditional design approaches (Sanders et al., 2010; Schuler, 2014; Simonsen and Robertson, 2013). This expansion in thinking is reflected in the language of design: prominent buzzwords include *human-centered design, co-designing, cultural probes, generative design thinking, applied ethnography, contextual inquiry, lead user/ lead consumer approach, and empathetic design*. Overall, the design process has acquired a new outlook: "People who are not educated in design are designing; the line between product and service is no longer clear; the boundaries between the design disciplines are blurring" (Sanders, 2006).

Our aim here is not to single out any one approach for detailed analysis, but rather to lay out general challenges and opportunities at the leading edge of design thinking. Certain themes emerge, however, from an exploration of the literature. Focus is increasingly on "the fuzzy front end" of the design process, formerly called "pre-design": the open-ended exploration of what is to be designed—and sometimes, what should not be designed and manufactured (Sanders and Stappers, 2008). Emphasis is more on experiential concerns than on physical or material ones. A multi-disciplinary approach and communication among *all* the stakeholders are critical (Baek et al., 2014; Jensen, 2011; Steen, Kuijt-Evers, and Klok, 2007). Such conversations need to be more about exploring and exchanging knowledge than about making decisions and reaching closure (Baek et al., 2014). And throughout the design process, there needs to be enough time to allow for multiple iterations of research, design, and analysis.

Examples of User Participation in Healthcare-Facility Design

Some examples may help clarify some participation alternatives. They show that participation can occur throughout the design process and can use a variety of techniques. Some of the following examples occurred in the 1980s as part of the design process for the University of Michigan Medical Center in Ann Arbor, one of the first extensive health-facility user participation projects in the United States. Since then, similar efforts in other hospitals have been made to involve patients and family members in designing new facilities and patient rooms (Johnson, 1999; Spohn, 2007).

Patient Room Mockups Reviewed by Patients, Staff, Designers, and Others

- At Parkland Hospital in Dallas, Texas, mock-ups of key rooms were constructed with a variety of finish options and subjected to routine maintenance by the environmental services staff in order to analyze product performance and select the most effective materials and finishes (Echols, 2014).

- During an early phase of the Parkland Hospital mock-up project, design teams were able to work through an alternative way of installing a trim-free slot light fixture, resulting in significant cost savings (Echols, 2014).

- When detailed decisions needed to be made about the design of the inpatient bathroom at the University of Michigan Medical Center, both staff and recently discharged patients took part in analyzing several full-scale mock-ups. They acted out scenarios (such as a nurse helping a patient into the shower), assessed the degree to which the design of the mock-up worked well, and made suggestions for design changes. The findings from the mock-up studies had a direct impact on the eventual bathroom design (King et al., 1982).

- In the design process for the new Sacred Heart Medical Center at RiverBend in Springfield, Oregon, full-scale plywood mock-ups of patient bathrooms were used. Noting the size difference between a standard bathroom and the ADA-compliant bathroom next door, one team member, a community volunteer, asked, "Why do you have smaller bathrooms? Why aren't they all bigger?" Caregivers had complained for years about the difficulties of getting patients into the bathrooms. Yet as "standard operating procedure," the problem of space had never been addressed. The volunteer's question, however, got hospital leadership thinking, and all patient rooms in the new hospital were designed with larger, ADA-compliant bathrooms, thereby both easing the caregiver workload and eliminating the need for patient transfers (Green, 2008).

- At Parkland Hospital, a typical private patient room was mocked up, complete with furniture and medical equipment, and was used for staff training, as well as for touring by stakeholders and potential donors. It was found, for instance, that the nurse-call button should be separated from the code-blue button, with the nurse-call on the family side of the patient for easier access and the code-blue button on the staff side. Bed outlets were moved off-center to reduce wear and tear on plugs. And the charting station was adjusted so the caregiver could sit facing the patient during charting, in order to facilitate better communication and patient satisfaction (Echols, 2014).

- In the Parkland Hospital mock-up of a labor and delivery room, it was found that, due to narrowness of the room, families had difficulty moving out of the room from the family zone if a delivery complication arose. The room was redesigned to accommodate this change (Echols, 2014).

- A resuscitation room mock-up for Parkland Hospital was found to have more fixed casework than necessary, so all upper cabinets were removed. Countertops needed to be raised in order to accommodate cart storage. In addition, noise levels during scenarios was unacceptably high, so acoustic design was reevaluated (Echols, 2014).

Patient Interviews Using 3D Models

Before decisions were made at the University of Michigan Medical Center about the layout of the acute-care inpatient room, including the location of the bathroom and the relationship of beds to the doorway in a semi-private room, randomly sampled patients were interviewed, using small, three-dimensional models that the patients could hold and manipulate to show the arrangements they preferred. Their preferences, in addition to staff preferences and other considerations, played an important role in decisions about the eventual layout (Reizenstein and Grant, 1981).

Staff Interviews

At the University of Michigan Medical Center, as part of pre-design programming, staff members in each clinical, hospital, and administrative department were interviewed about their requirements for space, equipment, lighting, finishes, and furnishings. This information was recorded and used to guide design.

Staff Prototyping

During preparatory workshops for the new patient tower of the H. Lee Moffitt Cancer Center and Research Institute in Tampa, Florida, nurses co-created a concept for ideal workflow on a patient floor. All the toolkit components were round, to help the nurses think in terms of activities, rather than rooms, at this early stage of the design process. When the team proceeded to co-design the ideal future patient room, a three-dimensional toolkit was used for generative prototyping (Sanders and Stappers, 2008).

Staff Reviews of Department and Furniture Layouts

– Before interior design decisions were made at the University of Michigan Medical Center, working groups comprising key staff members from each department pored over proposed furniture layouts. They tried to envision how each layout would function, debated alternative approaches, and suggested changes. When these suggestions were compatible with other performance criteria, interior designers modified the designs to incorporate users' suggestions.

– Staff participation in the design of the registration and triage area in the Saint Joseph Mercy Hospital (Ypsilanti, Michigan) emergency department led to a different and more workable layout than the one originally proposed (Carpman Associates, 1984 [unpub.]).

– User participation, patient satisfaction surveys, and other quality-improvement initiatives can also introduce needed design changes and improve functioning in existing hospitals. For example, in an effort to respond to needs expressed by family members of hospitalized children, the Children's Hospital of Philadelphia, designed the Connelly Resource Center for Families. The design of the center was largely driven by feedback received from family members. The center provides rooms and facilities for family members to sleep, shower, cook, and wash clothes. The center also includes a library, computers, and a learning center where family members can practice using equipment that their child will need when they return home (Johnson, 1999).

Developing a User Participation Process

Necessary Conditions

A number of conditions are needed in order to achieve maximum benefits from user participation in design:

- A healthcare organization that seeks to promote the well-being and morale of its users and understands the potential benefits of a participatory design process.

- Designers who place a high value on satisfying users' needs and are knowledgeable about and receptive to user participation.

- Users willing to contribute time, effort, and enthusiasm to the participatory process.

- Skilled, experienced participation leaders to guide the process.

- Visual, flexible, easily manipulated information aids and tools to increase the realism of design alternatives. (Sommer, 1983)

Mechanisms for User Participation

User participation in design can occur in a variety of ways. Three frequently used mechanisms are working groups, systematic research, and consultation by outside experts.

Working Groups

User' working groups may meet frequently or infrequently. They might represent a particular occupational group, they might represent users from one department, they might comprise users from several different departments, or they might share some other commonality. A particularly successful strategy is to develop internal expertise through early creation of "think tank" groups that cut across departments, thereby creating thought leaders to promote new ideas and encouraging staff buy-in for proposed changes (Joseph, Bosch, and Frede, 2007).

On a small design project, such as the renovation of an obstetrics and gynecology clinic, one or two working groups may suffice. On a large-scale project, such as the design of a teaching hospital, there may be a need for many working groups: perhaps one for each department, plus some additional groups organized by functional issues such as safety, security, Universal Design, and wayfinding.

These working groups may review relevant studies and reports, visit other facilities, use design tools to generate ideas and develop concepts as co-creators, review the details of proposed design schemes, select from several completed design schemes, and/or try out proposed designs or design features through simulation. Regardless of the ways each group functions, users can collaborate on and respond to different design alternatives and predict what will work for them (Kaplan and Kaplan, 1983; Sanders and Stappers, 2008). By creating understanding of the benefits of innovations, such user participation can result in fostering change, retaining design features that might otherwise have been lost to cost-reduction decisions (Joseph et al., 2007).

The working-group format requires that users and design decision-makers negotiate as they work toward a final design. It is important that all working-group members have an opportunity to contribute and that the process not be dominated by one or two individuals. Otherwise, the design will reflect a unique mode of functioning and could become ineffective if a particular individual leaves the organization. In addition, other working-group members may feel that their own efforts are not valued.

Working groups function most smoothly when they are run by skilled, neutral leaders. Leaders can be responsible for scheduling, setting agendas, procuring necessary documents, and guiding discussions, as well as recording and distributing meeting notes. Because working-group discussions can become heated, the leader's neutrality and group-facilitation skills can maximize the group's productivity.

Systematic Research

Systematic research is another approach to user participation. A large group of users, such as obstetrics and gynecology clinic patients, can be sampled to obtain a reasonably accurate representation of user characteristics and viewpoints. Research techniques might include face-to-face and telephone interviews, online surveys, and simulations such as the evaluation of rough scale models or conceptual drawings (Becker, 1982).

Participation through research may be useful on both small-scale and large-scale projects. It would be a cost-effective and time-effective way for obstetrics and gynecology patients and companions to voice their needs and preferences about a clinic renovation, for example. It would also be a practical way to involve house officers, staff nurses, housekeeping and maintenance staff, clerical staff, and patients and visitors in the design of a new teaching hospital.

User needs and preferences might be tapped in a single study, such as a study of responses to 3D models or drawings showing different layouts for obstetrics and gynecology examination rooms and waiting areas. Or a number of different studies might be needed to optimize user participation in the design of a teaching hospital, such as studies of patients' comfort, nurses' ease of operation of different beds, visitors' preferences about the location of restrooms in relation to waiting areas, and clerical staff's preferences for different office landscape systems.

Although every information-gathering technique has its strengths, there are always corresponding shortcomings. For example, guided interviews with open-ended questions can produce large amounts of data that are rich in detail and yet time-consuming to code or quantify. Selecting more than one technique, however, can often compensate for the shortcomings of each.

Consultants

Information about users' design needs can also be provided by behavioral consultants. This approach may be desirable when a project's success depends on balancing the needs and preferences of multiple user groups, when the schedule and budget do not allow for either direct participation or systematic research, or when users are either unknown or unavailable. Consultants can contribute expert information based on their experience with the design of similar projects, familiarity with relevant design research literature, and/or previous research on and experience with similar facilities. They can act as user advocates, they may have skill at interpreting and reviewing design documents from a behavioral point of view, and they can offer a clear perspective on the design process that insiders might not have (Sommer, 1983).

Techniques for Information-Gathering

Gathering information through user participation can be considered a two-phase process. During the first and preparatory phase, user participation managers need to become as knowledgeable as possible about the relevant design issues. During the second phase, they will gather and analyze users' design-related information about use, needs, and preferences.

For example, consider the design of a private (single-occupancy) inpatient room. First, participation managers will identify relevant codes and regulations. This might be followed by gathering books, articles, and other relevant materials and conducting an online literature review of published studies, unpublished reports, conference presentations, and so on, to discover what is already known about users' design needs and the current state-of-the-art (or ongoing controversies) about meeting these needs. The manager might then review minutes of meetings and other organization records to learn about the history of the design project, discover whether some informal decisions have already been made, and gauge whether or not certain decision-makers favor certain design approaches. The initial learning period could be supplemented by visits to other hospitals for a brief overview of how well their patient rooms appear to function. Finally, the manager might consult with experts. This reconnaissance effort will make it easier and more efficient to plan user participation since key assumptions, preferences, issues, realistic design alternatives, internal political realities, as well as local and national context should all be clear.

In order to gather and analyze information in a way that will provide useful information to design decision-makers and be satisfying to users, realistic design alternatives must be presented in ways users can easily understand and respond to (Kaplan and Kaplan, 1983).

For example, asking nurses or others without architectural training to review a two-dimensional floor plan of a private patient room would not be a useful approach. These nurses would have no alternatives to compare (other than patient rooms where they have worked), they might not be able to make sense of a two-dimensional floor plan, and they might doubt their own expertise on the topic. In this scenario, the nurses might not be able to contribute much of substance and would probably end up feeling frustrated with the exercise.

However, if these same nurses were shown a video or digital images of several three-dimensional arrangements or small, shoebox-sized 3D models, the participation exercise would probably be more successful. They could assess the different design alternatives; they could virtually manipulate the beds, walls, and other features in the images; and they could more easily visualize how different activities would be accommodated. This approach would generate pragmatic design responses and ideas, be more enjoyable, and leave participants feeling satisfied that they had made useful contributions. A group of designers who used this approach in designing hospital rooms for children found that models with moveable parts offered a useful way for participants, particularly children, to provide feedback. Family members and caregivers were also among the participants (Spohn, 2007).

Three-dimensional simulations or games can also be useful and engaging. These simulations allow the viewer to "fly" or "run" through the building and see the space from multiple perspectives. Designers can present the simulations in person or post them online (Dewulf and van Meel, 2002). Computer simulations may facilitate users' abilities to visualize proposed designs; however, their effectiveness in promoting participation satisfying to the user and useful for the designer is not yet well understood.

There are many opportunities for gathering feedback and sharing information online. Online user surveys are easy to develop, send, and analyze. Websites can contain password-protected areas for group communications. And, of course, huge amounts of information can be gathered using various search engines (Dewulf and van Meel, 2002).

Selecting optimal information-gathering techniques for a specific situation is part of the art of managing user participation. One should also consider the expertise available; the schedule; the numbers of users who need to be involved; the relevance, quantity, and quality of information needed; and the budget. Box 11.1 describes some techniques that can provide background information about the design problem at hand (Boisaubin et al., 1985; Brill et al., 1985; Madge, 1965; Michelson, 1975; Reizenstein et al., 1982; Stern, 1979; Webb, 1966; Wohlwill and Weisman, 1981; Zeisel, 2006). (See Box 11.2 for recommended reading.)

BOX 11.1. TECHNIQUES FOR GATHERING BACKGROUND INFORMATION ON FACILITY DESIGN IN RELATION TO USERS

Literature Reviews

Literature reviews are searches for relevant print and online articles, books, reports, conference presentations, codes, standards, and other materials that may have a bearing on the project at hand. Once initial relevant titles are identified, articles need to be located and studied and their bibliographies examined in order to identify further relevant materials.

Review of Project History and Related Archival Documents

Archival records may help explain a project's history and contribute useful insights to the design process. Types of records that may be helpful include print and online position papers; meeting notes; correspondence; reports; design documents; maintenance and repair records; purchase records; health, safety, or medical records; and employee and customer surveys or other feedback (Brill et al.,1985).

Facility Visits

Much can be learned about how new or renovated facilities could work by observing existing environments and behavior in similar organizations. In preparation for a facility visit, design participants need to identify specific environmental features and policies to be investigated. It will be helpful to line up a knowledgeable person (or persons) within the facility being visited to act as a guide. Participants should prepare questions in advance, respond to what they see and hear about during the visit, and learn how to recognize telling "physical traces," evidence that environments may not be working as intended, such as hand-lettered, taped-up signs (Brill et al., 1985; Webb et al., 1966; Zeisel, 2006). Realistic time estimates should be set for the visit: more will be remembered when the facility is toured slowly. The visit should be documented with audio recordings, notes, photos, and videos, depending on what the facility will allow (Zimring, 1994).

BOX 11.2. USER PARTICIPATION IN DESIGN: RECOMMENDED READING

Groat, L., and Wang, D. *Architectural Research Methods.* Hoboken, NJ: Wiley, 2013.

Knight, A., and Ruddock, L., eds. *Advanced Research Methods in the Built Environment.* Oxford, UK: Wiley-Blackwell, 2008.

Kopec, D. *Environmental Psychology for Design* (2nd ed.). New York: Fairchild Books, 2012.

Peña, W., and Parshall, S. *Problem Seeking: An Architectural Programming Primer* (5th ed.). Hoboken, NJ: Wiley, 2012.

Sommer, R. *Personal Space: The Behavioral Basis of Design* (Updated ed.). Bristol, UK: Bosko Books, 2008.

Zeisel, J. *Inquiry by Design: Environment/Behavior/Neuroscience in Architecture, Interiors, Landscape, and Planning.* New York: Norton, 2006.

Zimring, C. *Guide to Conducting Healthcare Facility Visits.* The Center for Health Design, 1994. www.healthdesign.org/sites/default/files/Healthcare%20Facility%20Visits.PDF.

Timing of User Participation

In order to have real impact on the design of healthcare facilities, user participation should occur throughout the design process, from conceptualization through post-occupancy evaluation (also known as "Facility Performance Evaluation" or FPE). (See chapter 1 for a detailed description of phases of the design process.) Recommendations growing out of the participation process must be provided in a timely manner—while design alternatives are being considered—and be geared to key milestone dates in the project schedule. The ways in which participation occurs may vary with the particular stage of design (Frey, 1989; Kaplan and Kaplan, 1983; Kernohan et al., 1992; King, Marans, and Solomon, 1982; Lawrence, 1982; Madge, 1965; Moser and Kalton, 1985; Sanoff, 1977, 2000; Zeisel, 2006).

Users' needs and preferences should be articulated at the earliest stages of a healthcare-facility design project, and be reflected in a mission statement, types and sizes of spaces required, and associated performance criteria (Lickhalter, 1988). Early in the participation effort, users need an overview of the design process for their areas. This mental road map can help clarify where their contributions fit in. Once they have an overview, participants will know when certain types of functional information will be most useful, enabling them to work productively and efficiently (Sommer, 1983).

Once the design process begins, users and/or behavioral consultants can perform periodic design reviews; helping assess the probable performance of the proposed designs, according to a variety of performance criteria. Users can review design progress in person or online by annotating floor plans, providing written comments, attending actual or virtual meetings, and the like. Users may respond to questions, images, scale models, or full-scale mock-ups (Kaplan and Kaplan, 1983; King, Marans, and Solomon, 1982; Reizenstein and Grant, 1982; Sanoff, 1992).

Participation can also occur during the construction phase of a project, when last-minute design changes may occur. If design decisions need to be revisited at this late (and costly) stage, users can weigh-in using all the mechanisms and techniques described above. If participation occurs this late in the process, there need to be mechanisms in place for quickly summarizing user input and revisiting design decisions, as needed.

Post-occupancy evaluation (POE), assessing how new or renovated facilities perform, is another stage of the design process when user participation is valuable. (This is also known as Facility Performance Evaluation—FPE). User participants can contribute to POE planning by helping identify which aspects of the design should be evaluated. They can give feedback on the performance of design features they regularly use and make recommendations for changes in design and related policies (Manasec and Adams, 1987; Ogrodnik, 1985; Preiser, 2002; Reizenstein and Grant, 1982; Zeisel, 2006; Zimring, Rashid, and Kampschroer, 2010; Zimring and Reizenstein, 1980, 1981).

Selecting Participants

Users are *all* the people who come into contact with the physical environment. In healthcare facilities, users include inpatients and outpatients; family members and visitors; medical, nursing, and care staff; allied health professionals; medical, nursing, and allied health students; managers and administrators; staff who provide a range of needed patient care, administrative, clerical, maintenance, information technology, and other services that keep the healthcare facility running; as well as others who use the buildings, including salespeople and delivery workers. All of these users' voices should be reflected and respected in the design process.

When selecting users to participate, consider the type and extent of knowledge they bring, their motivation to participate, their availability, and their ability to represent the views of others (Baek et al., 2008; Brill et al., 1985; Brunnquell, Balik, and Pearson, 1991; Sidhu et al., 2002).

Users can be categorized according to their roles in the facility. For example, the renovation of a department head's office may only require the participation of that physician and an administrator, whereas the renovation of an obstetrics and gynecology clinic may call for the involvement of patients, companions, nurses, clerical staff, physicians, technicians, maintenance staff, housekeeping staff, administrators, and others.

Both the size of the user group and the frequency of facility use should be considered when selecting participants. To continue the example of the obstetrics and gynecology clinic, the nurses on duty every day should each have an opportunity to contribute ideas and review the design's progress, because they will use the renovated clinic frequently. On the one hand, although more than 25,000 patients may visit the clinic each year, a manageable sample of participants could be systematically drawn from this group. Sampling patients, rather than including all of them, is preferable since it would be neither time- nor cost-effective to involve every patient in the design process, and the potential findings are not likely to differ widely within the group. On the other hand, involving only a few patients would probably not result in an accurate representation of the range of experiences, ideas, and opinions (Brunnquell et al., 1991; Walsworth-Bell, 1986).

Political power is another consideration when selecting participants. A rule of thumb is that the more powerful the individuals, the more likely they will participate in the design process anyway. Even so, it is important that these persons be sought out, because they can contribute useful information based on experience and their approval of the design is often necessary. At the same time, it is important to seek out the expertise of less-powerful user groups, such as nurses. They, too, will have important views of how the facility should be designed. Because they are often the people most directly involved in day-to-day operations, their contributions are critical to the long-term success of the project (Dewulf and van Meel, 2002; Hardesty, 1988).

When planning new or renovated facilities, it is not always possible to involve individuals who will still be there when the project is completed. People in working groups may retire or move on to other jobs. In addition, there may be some turnover within working groups over the course of the design process. There is no foolproof solution to this common problem, but it pays to be aware of it before the process begins. One approach is to involve current users with characteristics similar to those of future users. Another option is to refer to research on users in similar types of facilities.

Managing User Participation

User participation in a design project, whether small scale or large scale, requires management, either by in-house staff or consultants. These managers should be familiar with the design needs of healthcare-facility users, ways in which design decisions are made within their organization, the timing of these decisions, and the role of user information in this process. Managers should also be skilled communicators, researchers, advocates, meeting facilitators, interpreters of design graphics, and project managers (Fiedler, 1978).

A manager's biggest challenge is likely to be handling competing design needs and preferences. Users themselves may disagree, users and design decision-makers may disagree, or external constraints such as budgets or codes may make user groups' needs impossible to meet. As a result, user participants must be made aware of the often extensive negotiations that go on among the affected parties and the likelihood that users' recommendations will not always sway design decisions.

Implementing Resulting Recommendations

When users and design decision-makers come together in working groups, users have the opportunity to lobby for their own recommendations. They might argue from personal experience, bring in relevant literature and data, or report the consensus of their colleagues. In addition to a recommendation's objective merits, other factors may play a role in influencing a design decision, such as timing, capital and operating costs, internal politics, values, personality, personal relationships, and organizational norms (Carpman, 1983).

When users participate in design through systematic research, the results of their efforts, including their recommendations, may reach design decision-makers in meetings, presentations, reviews of documents and design graphics, and written reports, as well as in online communications. A detailed study of participation through research in a large-scale design project (the Patient and Visitor Participation Project of the University of Michigan Medical Center) indicated that multiple, face-to-face contacts between users' representatives and design decision-makers were the most effective way of influencing design decisions (Carpman, 1983). On this large-scale project, periodic design reviews were important, and written reports that documented research findings promoted credibility, but neither process was sufficient to ensure utilization. The advantage of face-to-face settings, such as meetings, is that recommendations become better understood through two-way conversations. Troublesome issues can be clarified, and recommendations can be elaborated on and reinforced using visual aids. In addition, alliances can be formed and compromises forged.

Documenting the User Participation Process

It is important to document user participation because it may be the source of many recommendations reflected in the final design. Without such documentation, important information may be lost and some aspects of the design may not function as intended. Users who were not involved in design decision-making may be curious about why certain decisions were made. Documentation also provides a record of design intentions that will be important to understand when the relationship between the facility's design and performance is assessed during post-occupancy evaluation (Facility Performance Evalvation).

Summary

- ○ To ensure that general design guidelines are applicable to a particular project, they must be supplemented with detailed information about design-related needs and preferences of the facility's eventual users and stakeholders, including those who will administer and maintain it. This information should be incorporated into all stages of the design decision-making process. Users can participate in design in various ways: simply conveying information to designers, selecting from various design alternatives, reviewing and commenting on design options (including plans, drawings, models, mock-ups, videos, and the like), and offering design ideas.

- ○ Participation can occur through questionnaires, interviews, working groups, simulations, and other techniques. When such activities are not possible, user participation can be achieved indirectly by conducting literature reviews or by employing behavioral consultants as user advocates.

- ○ User participation has numerous benefits: it clarifies design objectives, leads to better design decisions, stimulates positive behavior and attitudes, inspires a sense of community, provides opportunities to assess design-related organizational policies, and acts as a marketing strategy.

- ○ In recent years, participatory design and design research have been undergoing a transformation. The user-centered approach of informed experts "designing *for users*" is being expanded and sometimes superseded by the idea of co-designing, "designing *with people.*" This shift in thinking is reflected in the language of design: prominent buzzwords include *human-centered design, co-designing, cultural probes, generative design thinking, applied ethnography, contextual inquiry, lead user/lead consumer approach,* and *empathetic design.* Overall, the design process has acquired a new outlook: "People who are not educated in design are designing; the line between product and service is no longer clear; the boundaries between the design disciplines are blurring" (Sanders, 2006).

- ○ Necessary conditions to achieve maximum benefits of user participation in design include:

  - – Healthcare organizations that seek to promote the well-being and morale of their users and understand the benefits of a participatory design process

  - – Designers who value user satisfaction and are knowledgeable about and receptive to user participation

  - – Users willing to contribute time, effort, and enthusiasm to the participatory process

  - – Skilled, experienced participation leaders to guide the process

  - – Visual, flexible, easily manipulated information aids and tools to communicate design alternatives

- ○ The choice of users to involve through participation will depend on the specific project. It is not always possible to involve the individuals who will be future users. Participants should be selected as a function of their knowledge, motivation, availability, and ability to represent the views of others. The most common mechanisms for design participation are working groups, systematic research, and consultation by experts.

○   User participation managers should be familiar with the design needs of healthcare-facility users, how design decisions are made within their organization, and the timing of these decisions. To handle negotiations about competing design needs, participation managers should be skilled communicators, researchers, advocates, meeting facilitators, interpreters of design graphics, and project managers. User participation should be documented to enable assessment of the design and its intended performance.

DISCUSSION QUESTIONS

1. What are some examples of situations in which it would be important to employ user participation over the course of a healthcare-facility design and construction project?

2. What are some benefits of user participation?

3. What conditions are necessary to achieve benefits from user participation?

4. What is "co-design"? How can it contribute to the design process?

5. What are ways in which users can participate directly in a design and construction project?

6. If direct user participation is not feasible, what are other ways to include user information in a design project?

7. What are some criteria for selecting users to participate in the design process?

8. What are some important skills for managers of user participation projects?

References

Baek, E. O., Cagiltay, K., Boling, E., & Frick, T. (2008). User-centered design and development. *Handbook of Research on Educational Communications and Technology* (1):660–68.

Becker, F. D. The evaluation. In W. C. Beck and R. H. Meyer, editors. *The Health Care Environment: The User's Viewpoint*, 231–49. Boca Raton, FL: CRC Press, 1982.

_____. *Housing Messages.* Stroudsburg, PA: Dowden, Hutchinson, & Ross, 1977.

_____. *User Participation, Personalization and Environmental Meaning: Three Field Studies.* Ithaca, NY: Program in Urban and Regional Studies, Cornell University, 1977.

Boisaubin, E. V., Henrikus, D. J., Sanson-Fisher, R. W., and Merrill, J. M. Behavioral mapping to plan a new emergency center. *Journal of Ambulatory Care Management* 8(3):38–43, 1985.

Brill, M., with Margulis, S., Konar, E., and BOSTI. *Using Office Design to Increase Productivity.* Vol. 2. Buffalo, NY: Workplace Design and Productivity, 1985.

Brown, T. Five Tips for experienced designers working to improve healthcare innovation. *UX,* article no. 1317, October 1, 2014. http://uxmag.com/articles/five-tips-for-experience-designers-working-to-improve-healthcare-innovation.

Brubaker, T., ed. Design and construction project manual. Unpublished report, Office of the Replacement Hospital Program, University of Michigan, Ann Arbor, 1985.

Brunnquell, D., Balik, B., and Pearson, T. Appropriate design takes input from all corners. *Health Care Strategic Management,* 16–18, January 1991.

Campbell, R. Experiencing architecture with seven senses, not one. *Architectural Record*, 65–66, November 2007.

Carpman Associates. St. Joseph Mercy Hospital Emergency Department behavioral design program. Unpublished report, Carpman Associates, Ann Arbor, 1984.

Carpman, J. R. Influencing design decisions: An analysis of the impact of the Patient and Visitor Participation Project on the University of Michigan Replacement Hospital Program. PhD diss. University of Michigan, Ann Arbor, 1983. [Available from ProQuest, 789 E. Eisenhower Parkway, Ann Arbor, MI 48108.]

Carpman, J. R., and Trester, K. Marketing implications of consumer-responsive health facility design. In P. Cooper, editor. *Responding to the Challenge: Proceedings of the Sixth Annual Health Services Marketing Symposium*, 55–58. Chicago: American Marketing Association, 1986.

Cleary, P. A hospitalization from hell: A patient's perspective on quality. *Annals of Internal Medicine* 138(1):33–39, January 2003.

Codinhoto, R., Aouad, G., Kagioglou, M., Tzortzopoulos, P., and Cooper, R. Evidence-based design of health-care facilities. *Journal of Health Services Research & Policy* 14:194. doi:10.1258/jhrsp.2009.009094. http://hsr.sagepub.com/content/14/4/194.

Dewulf, G., and van Meel, J. Participation and the role of information and communication technology. *Journal of Corporate Real Estate* 4(3):237–47, 2002.

Echols, L. Mock trial: How mock-ups are beneficial for design. 2014. www.neocon.com/default/assets/File/T261%20Mock%20Trial%20How%20Mock-ups%20are%20Benficial%20for%20Design.pdf.

Falick, J. Humanistic design sells your hospital. *Hospitals* 55(4):68–74, February 16, 1981.

Fiedler, J. *Field Research: A Manual for Logistics and Management of Scientific Studies in Natural Settings.* San Francisco: Jossey-Bass, 1978.

Franck, K. A., and Lepori, B. *Architecture from the Inside Out: From the Body, the Senses, the Site and the Community.* Chichester: Wiley, 2007.

Frey, J. H. *Survey Research by Telephone.* Thousand Oaks, CA: Sage, 1989.

Glushko, A. Participatory design in healthcare: Patients and doctors can bridge critical information gaps. *UX,* article no. 1028, May 31, 2013. http://uxmag.com/articles/participatory-design-in-healthcare.

Green, J. H. A collaborative process ties safety and efficiency to create Sacred Heart Medical Center's new design. *Healthcare Design,* June 30, 2008. www.healthcaredesignmagazine.com/article/collaborative-process-ties-safety-and-efficiency-create-sacred-heart-medical-centers-new-des.

Hall, J. Programming user needs. Unpublished paper, 1991.

Hardesty, T. Knowledge nurses need to participate on a design team. *Nursing Management* 19(3)49–57, March 1988.

Herssens J., and Heylighen, A. Haptic architecture becomes architectural hap. Paper presented in proceeding of Ergonomics for a Future: Annual Congress of the Nordic Ergonomic Society, Lisekil, January 2007. www.nordiskergonomi.org/nes2007/CD_NES.../A34_Herssens.pdf.

Heylighen, A., Devlieger, P., and Strickfaden, M. Design expertise as disability: And vice versa. Paper presented in proceedings of Communicating (by) Design, Brussels, April 2009. https://lirias.kuleuven.be/bitstream/123456789/206161/2/Heylighen09Design+Expertise+as+Disability.pdf.

Jensen, P. A. Inclusive briefing and user involvement: Case study of a media centre in Denmark. *Architectural Engineering and Design Management* 7(1):38–49, 2011. http://orbit.dtu.dk/en/publications/inclusive-briefing-and-user-involvement%28f73d66aa-98d5–42b0-a02a-28983433ea5b%29.html.

Johnson, B. H. Family focus. *Trustee* 52(3):12–15, March 1999.

Joseph, A., Bosch, S., and Frede, C. Researching the effectiveness of a participatory evidence-based design process. *Healthcare Design,* March 31, 2007. www.healthcaredesignmagazine.com/article/researching-effectiveness-participatory-evidence-based-design-process.

Kaplan, S., and Kaplan, R. *Cognition and Environment: Functioning in an Uncertain World.* New York: Praeger, 1983.

Kernohan D., Gray, J., Daish, J., and Joiner, D. *User Participation in Building Design and Management.* Oxford: Butterworth-Heinemann, 1992.

King, J., Marans, R. A., and Solomon, L. A. Pre-construction evaluation: A report on the full scale mock-up and evaluation of hospital rooms. Ann Arbor, MI: Architectural Research Laboratory, University of Michigan, 1982.

Kujala, S. User involvement: A review of the benefits and challenges. *Behaviour & Information Technology* 22(1):1–16, 2003. doi:10.1080/01449290021000055530. www.tandf.uk/journals.

Kujala, S., and Kauppinen, M. Identifying and selecting users for user-centered design. NordiCHI 2004. Proceedings of the third Nordic conference on Human-computer interaction. ACM New York, 297–303. doi:10.1145/1028014.1028060. www.academia.edu/366383/Identifying_and_Selecting_Users_for_User-Centered_Design.

Lawrence, R. J. Designers' dilemma: Participatory design methods. In P. Bart, A. Chen, and G. Francescato, editors. *Knowledge for Design: Proceedings of EDRA 13,* 261–71. Washington, DC: Environmental Design Research Association, 1982.

Lickhalter, M. How to be a good consumer (both buyer and manager) of programming services. Part I. *Journal of Health Administration Education* 6(4):741–49, 1988.

Lindamood, M. O. Getting your input into unit design. *Dimensions of Critical Care Nursing* 1(1):36–43, January–February 1982.

Madge, J. H. *The Tools of Social Science.* Garden City, NY: Doubleday, 1965.

Manasec, V., and Adams, J. Post-occupancy evaluation by hospitals. *Hospital Trustee* 11(5):5–7, September–October 1987.

Michelson, W. M., editor. *Behavioral Research Methods in Environmental Design.* Stroudsburg, PA: Dowden, Hutchinson, & Ross, 1975.

Moser, C. A., and Kalton, G. *Survey Methods in Social Investigation* (2nd ed.). Farnham, Surrey, UK: Ashgate, 1985.

Ogrodnik, T. M. The user of space programming and post-occupancy evaluation. *World Hospitals* 21(4):58–61, November 1985.

Pallasmaa, J. *The Eyes of the Skin.* Chichester, UK: Wiley, 2007.

Preiser, W. Learning from our buildings: A state-of-the-practice summary of post-occupancy evaluation. Federal Facilities Council Technical Report No. 145. Washington, DC: National Academies Press, 2002.

Reizenstein, J. E. Hospital design and human behavior: A review of the recent literature. In A. Baum and I. Singer, editors. *Advances in Environmental Psychology. Vol. 4, Environment and Health,* 137–39. Hillsdale, NJ: Erlbaum, 1982.

Reizenstein, J. E., and Grant, M. A. From hospital research to hospital design. Patient and Visitor Participation Project. Office of Hospital Planning, Research and Development, University of Michigan, Ann Arbor, 1982.

_____. Schematic design of the inpatient room. Unpublished research report No. 1. Patient and Visitor Participation Project, Office of Hospital Planning, Research and Development, University of Michigan, Ann Arbor, 1981.

Reizenstein, J. E., Simmons, D. A., Grant, M. A., and Dayanandan, A. *Hospital Design and Human Behavior: A Bibliography.* Architectural Series, A673. Monticello, IL: Vance Bibliographies, 1982.

Sanders, E. B.-N. Design research in 2006. *Design Research Quarterly 1,* September 1, 2006. www.maketools.com/articles-papers/DesignResearchin2006_Sanders_06.pdf.

Sanders, E. B.-N., and Stappers, P. J. Co-creation and the new landscapes of design. *CoDesign: International Journal of CoCreation in Design and the Arts* 4(1), March 2008. www.tandfonline.com/doi/full/10.1080/15710880701875068#.VEQid1fiJCo.

Sanders, E. B.-N., Brandt, E., and Binder, T. A framework for organizing the tools and techniques of participatory design. *PDC '10: Proceedings of the 11th Biennial Participatory Design Conference,* 195–98. New York, NY: AMC, 2010. doi:10.1145/1900441.1900476. www.maketools.com/articles-papers/PDC2010ExploratoryFrameworkFinal.pdf.

Sanoff, H. *Community Participation Methods in Design and Planning.* New York: Wiley, 2000.

_____. *Integrating Programming, Evaluation, and Participation in Design: A Theory Z Approach.* Farnham, Surrey, UK: Ashgate, 1992.

_____. *Methods of Architectural Programming.* New York: Dowden, Hutchinson, & Ross, 1977.

Schuler, D. Participatory design. 2014. www.publicsphereproject.org/node/235.

Sidhu, M., Berg, K., Endicott, C., Santulli, W., and Salem, D. The patient visits program: A strategy to highlight patient satisfaction and refocus organizational culture. *Journal on Quality Improvement* 28(11), November 2002.

Simonsen, J., and Robertson, T., editors. *Routledge International Handbook of Participatory Design.* New York: Routledge, 2013.

Sleeswijk Visser, F., Stappers, P. J., van der Lugt, R., and Sanders, E. B.-N. Contextmapping: Experiences from practice. *CoDesign: International Journal of CoCreation in Design and the Arts* 1(2), 2005. https://cmdconceptdevelopment.files.wordpress.com/2008/09/codesign2005sleeswijk.pdf.

Sommer, R. *Social Design: Creating Buildings with People in Mind.* Englewood Cliffs, NJ: Prentice-Hall, 1983.

Spohn, J. Imagining a better hospital room. *Healthcare Design* 7(9):59–70, November 2007.

Steen, M., Kuijt-Evers, L., and Klok, J. Early user involvement in research and design projects: A review of methods and practices. Paper for the 23rd EGOS Colloquium (European Group for Organizational Studies), July 5–7, 2007, Vienna. Theme 25: Dancing with users: How to organize innovation with consumers and users? www.academia.edu/2607698 /Early_user_involvement_in_research_and_design_projects_A_review_of_methods_and_practices.

Stern, A. L., MacRae, S., Gerteis, M., Harrison, T., Fowler, E., Edgman-Levitan, S., Walker, J., and Ruga, W. Understanding the consumer perspective to improve design quality. *Journal of Architecture and Planning Research* 20(1), Spring 2003. http://japr.homestead.com/files/STERN.pdf.

Stern, P. C. *Evaluating Social Science Research.* New York: Oxford University Press, 1979.

Walsworth-Bell, J. Think before you build. *Health Service Journal,* 596–97, May 1, 1986.

Webb, E. I., Campbell, D. T., Schwartz, R. D., and Sechrest, L. *Unobtrusive Measures.* Chicago: Rand-McNally, 1966.

Wohlwill, J. F., and Weisman, G. D. *The Physical Environment and Behavior: An Annotated Bibliography and Guide to the Literature.* New York: Plenum, 1981.

Zeisel, J. *Inquiry by Design: Environment/Behavior/Neuroscience in Architecture, Interiors, Landscape, and Planning.* New York: Norton, 2006.

Zeit, K. D. Patient-centered design: Next steps. *Healthcare Design,* January 14, 2013. www.healthcare -designmagazine.com/blogs/kristin-zeit/patient-centered-design-next-steps.

Zimring, C. *Guide to Conducting Healthcare Facility Visits.* The Center for Health Design, 1994. www .healthdesign.org/sites/default/files/Healthcare%20Facility%20Visits.PDF.

Zimring, C., Rashid, M. and Kampschroer, K. Facility Performance Evaluation (FPE). *Whole Building Design Guide,* 2014. http://www.wbdg.org/resources/fpe.php.

Zimring, C. M., and Reizenstein, J. E. A primer on post-occupancy evaluation. *American Institute of Architects Journal* 70(13):52–58, November 1981.

_____. Post-occupancy evaluation: an overview. *Environment and Behavior* 12(4):429–50, December 1980.

Sacred spaces, 403
   accessibility of, 377
   for all belief systems, 376
   design guidelines for, 377
   functional limitations and, 377
   furnishings for, 377
Safety
   bathrooms and issues of, 220, 247, 349
   commercial systems of, 48
   for older people, 334, 335–336, 358–359
   in outdoor space design, 293
   security and, 58
Sampling, with design research, 26
Satisfaction
   with ED waiting areas, 388, 389
   with food service areas, 374–375
Schematic design, 11
Seating. *See also* Benches; Chairs; Waiting
      area seating
   in ED waiting areas, 389
   in food service areas, 374, 376
   handrails and, 98, 110–111
   at Main Entrance, 46
Seating, for older patients and visitors, 361
   armrests with, 341, 342, 343
   with arthritis, 341
   biomechanics of rising with, 341, 343
   chair design for, 341
   clear space for, 342, 343
   firmness of, 342–343
   height of, 341, 342, 343
   important considerations for, 340
   with obesity, 343
   selection of, 343
   skin ulcers caused by, 342–343
Seating, in outdoor space design, 303–304
   benches for, 289–291
   capacity of, 290
   comfort of, 289–290
   in courtyards, 286, 287, 291, 292, 293
   design guidelines for, 289–291

evaluation of, 291–292
   layout and design of, 289
   orientation of, 289
   privacy of, 289
   variety of, 289–290
Section 504 of the Rehabilitation Act of 1973,
      316, 353
   contents of, 316
   discrimination prohibited by, 316
Security
   for parking, 49
   safety and, 58
   sense of, 122
Selection
   of artwork, 212
   of beds, 346
   of colors, 199
   of sign messages, 82–83
   of terminology, 84
   of user participation, in healthcare facility
      design, 434–435
Self-disclosure, in diagnostic and treatment
      areas
   environmental factors with, 158–159
Semi-private, visual privacy in, 192–193
Seniors, EDS for, 390–391, 409
Sense of community, with user participation,
      423
Sensitivity
   to lighting, 159
   to patient experience, 22
   to user needs, 31
Sensory overload, in ICUs, 233–235,
      258–259
Separate functional units, in EDs, 382
Serotonin, 199–200
Shops, 397–398, 412
Shower areas, in bathrooms, 223–224,
      255–256
Sidewalk design, 53
Sign language, 327

ED break rooms for, 384, 385

in ED waiting areas, 389

healthcare facility design relating to, 428

for hearing disabilities, 328, 329

outdoor spaces for, 278

STAI. *See* State-Trait Anxiety Inventory

Stairways

accidents on, 100

with blind or low-vision patients and visitors, 331

with older patients and visitors, 345–346

floor-to-floor travel on, 100–102, 112–113

guidelines for, 101

poor architectural design of, 346

treads on, 340

unplanned uses of, 102, 113

Stakeholders, in healthcare facility design, 424

State-Trait Anxiety Inventory (STAI), 135

Statistics

about hearing disabilities, 327

on users with disabilities, 312–313

Storage areas, 58. *See also* Places for belongings, in waiting areas

in acute care inpatient rooms, 204–207

bedside stands, 205, 251, 346

closets, 206

for clothing, 204

for EDs, 384, 385

overbed tables, 205, 250

for personal items, 204–205

for toiletries, 204

wardrobes, 205–206, 251

Stress. *See also* High-stress waiting areas

with disorientation, 73–74

facilitating recovery from, 275

of ICUs, 231

of patients and visitors, 9, 74

reduction of, 58, 274

sacred spaces for reprieve from, 376

wayfinding and, 75

Studies

about color, 196–199

about design research, 26, 32

about facility design, 7

about inpatient lounges, 227–228

about music, 164–165

about nature, 275, 296–298

about noise, 163, 238

about outside views, 213–215

about therapeutic music, 215–220

at University of Michigan Medical Center, 41, 78, 89, 93, 129, 184, 395

about waiting areas, 125

about waiting patients, 121

about YAH maps, 89–91

Sunlight, 199–200

Sunny vs sunless rooms, in ICUs, 241

Super-suite rooms, 191

Surgical procedures, therapeutic music during, 217–218

Symbolic meaning, of facility design, 10

Symbols and pictograms, with interior wayfinding, 84–85, 107

Tactile and thermal sensitivity changes, in older people, 333

Tactile signage, for blind or low-vision patients and visitors, 329–330

T-coil hearing-loop induction systems, 328

TDD/telephone relay services, 314

Technical considerations, of facility design, 5–6

Technologies

digital, 75

for hearing disabilities, 327–328

information, for EDs, 383

for interior wayfinding, 94, 109

VR, 168

Telephones, 314, 347, 363

Televisions
  in acute care inpatient rooms, 208–209, 251–252
  for older patients and visitors, 347
  positive distraction of, 208
  sharing of, 209
  types of, 208–209
  in waiting areas, 125–126, 142
Temporary disabilities, 311, 312
Terminology, 41, 82
  in diagnostic areas, 152
  for floor numbering, 79
  influence of, 83
  misunderstanding of, 83
  selection of, 84
  of YAH maps, 88
Texture, for older people, 338, 359
Therapeutic aspects, of facility design, 6–7
Therapeutic music
  for acute care inpatient rooms, 215–220, 253–254
  for anxiety and mood, 216
  choice of, 219
  culture and, 219
  for older people, 348
  guided imagery with, 217
  impact of, 219–220
  during medical procedures, 216
  for pain, 216–218
  physiological responses to, 218
  studies about, 215–220
  during surgical procedures, 217–218
  types of, 218–219
Therapy gym, for rehabilitation units, 392, 394
Threshold, of bathrooms, 221, 222
Timing, of user participation, in healthcare facility design, 433–434
Toilet areas, in bathrooms, 224–226, 256, 347, 364
Toiletries storage, 204

Towel racks, in bathrooms, 348, 364
Traditional care unit, with acute care inpatient rooms, 187
Training
  in design-relevant research, 32
  and experience, for research, 24
  in research methods, 31
Trauma area, in EDs, 385
Travel. *See* Floor to floor travel
Traveling, to healthcare facility, 37
  by bus, 38–39
  by car, 38
  by public transit, 38–39
  by taxi or van, 38
Treatment. *See* Diagnostic and treatment areas
Treatment rooms, for mobility disabilities, 324–326, 354
Trees, in outdoor space design, 285, 297
Triage, in front-end areas, of EDs, 384, 386, 387

Undressing and dressing, in diagnostic and treatment areas, 171
  accommodations for, 153–154
  dressing room design, 153, 154
  with functional limitations, 153
  hospital gowns, 152, 155, 159, 172
Unfamiliar environments, older people in, 344
Universal Design, 23–24, 320–321, 353
  automatic doors for, 318, 319
  barrier-free policies for, 318
  concept of, 318
  design for all, 318
  design principles for, 318, 319
  disability definition with, 318
  human-centered design as, 318
  inclusive design as, 318
  participation in, 317
  resources for, 322
  user/experts in, 319